Evidence-Informed Nursing with Older People

Edited by

Debbie Tolson, Joanne Booth and Irene Schofield

WILEY-BLACKWELL

A John Wiley & Sons, Ltd., Publication

This edition first published 2011
© 2011 by Blackwell Publishing Ltd

Blackwell Publishing was acquired by John Wiley & Sons in February 2007. Blackwell's publishing program has been merged with Wiley's global Scientific,Technical and Medical business to form Wiley-Blackwell.

Registered Office
John Wiley & Sons Ltd, The Atrium, Southern Gate, Chichester, West Sussex, PO19 8SQ, UK

Editorial Offices
9600 Garsington Road, Oxford, OX4 2DQ, UK
The Atrium, Southern Gate, Chichester, West Sussex, PO19 8SQ, UK
2121 State Avenue, Ames, Iowa 50014-8300, USA

For details of our global editorial offices, for customer services and for information about how to apply for permission to reuse the copyright material in this book please see our website at www.wiley.com/wiley-blackwell.

The right of the authors to be identified as the authors of this work has been asserted in accordance with the UK Copyright, Designs and Patents Act 1988.

Library of Congress Cataloging-in-Publication Data

Evidence informed nursing with older people/edited by Debbie Tolson, Joanne Booth, and Irene Schofield.
    p. ; cm.
  Includes bibliographical references and index.
    ISBN 978-1-4443-3113-4 (pbk. : alk. paper)   1. Geriatric nursing.   2. Evidence-based nursing.   I. Tolson, D. (Debbie)   II. Booth, Joanne.   III. Schofield, Irene.
[DNLM: 1. Evidence-Based Nursing–methods.   2. Nursing Care–methods.
3. Aged.   4. Nurse-Patient Relations. WY 152]
  RC954.E95 2011
  618.97′0231–dc22

                                                    2010041335

A catalogue record for this book is available from the British Library.

This book is published in the following electronic formats: ePDF 9781444340105; ePub 9781444340112

Set in 10/12.5pt Times by SPi Publisher Services, Pondicherry, India
Printed and bound in Malaysia by Vivar Printing Sdn Bhd

1   2011

Contents

Contributors

Yvonne Awenat, MPhil, BSc, RGN, ONC Hon
Research Fellow, School of Psychological Sciences, University of Manchester;
Trustee Board of Stockport & District MIND; Independent Nurse Consultant,
Manchester, England, UK

Janice Bianchi, MSc, BSc, RGN, RMN, Pg Cert, TLHE
Lecturer (Nursing), School of Health, Department of Adult Nursing, Glasgow
Caledonian University, Glasgow, Scotland, UK

Joanne Booth, PhD, BSc (Hons), BA, RN, RNT
Reader, School of Health, Department of Adult Nursing, Glasgow Caledonian
University, Glasgow, Scotland, UK

Jayne Brown, PhD, MMedSci, RNT, RGN
Senior Research Fellow, University of Nottingham, Sue Ryder Care Centre,
School of Nursing, Midwifery & Physiotherapy, Nottingham, England, UK

Kay Currie, BSc, PhD, MN, RN, RNT
Reader, School of Health, Department of Adult Nursing, Glasgow Caledonian
University, Glasgow, Scotland, UK

Tracy Day, Diploma in Hearing Therapy
Senior Audiologist/Hearing Therapist, Registered Clinical Physiologist,
NHS Grampian, Audiology Department, Aberdeen, Scotland, UK

Kathleen Duffy, PhD, MSc, BA, RGN, RNT
Senior Lecturer, School of Health, Department of Adult Nursing, Glasgow Caledonian
University, Glasgow, Scotland, UK

Katherine Froggatt, PhD, BSc (Hons)
Senior Lecturer, Division of Health Research, School of Health and Medicine,
Lancaster University, Lancaster, England, UK

Lyle Gray, PhD, BSc, MCOptom
Senior Lecturer & Postgraduate Tutor, School of Life Sciences, Department of Vision Sciences, Glasgow Caledonian University, Glasgow, Scotland, UK

Wolfgang Hasemann, RN, MNS
Clinical Nurse Specialist, University Hospital Basel, Department of Clinical Nursing Science, Basel, Switzerland

Jennie Jackson, BSc (Hons), PhD, RD, RNutr
Lecturer in Nutrition and Dietetics, School of Life Sciences, Glasgow Caledonian University, Glasgow, Scotland, UK

Derek Jones, BA (Hons), Dip COT, PhD
Senior Lecturer, School of Health, Department of Occupational Therapy, Physiotherapy & Social Work, Glasgow Caledonian University, Glasgow, Scotland, UK

Suzanne Kumlien, LMSc, BSc, PhD, RN, RNT
Senior Lecturer, Department of Neurobiology, Care Sciences and Society, Karolinska Institute, Huddinge, Sweden

Maggie Lawrence, PhD, MSc, MA (Hons), RGN
Research Fellow, School of Health, Department of Adult Nursing, Glasgow Caledonian University, Glasgow, Scotland, UK

Andrew Lowndes, MSc, BA, RNT, RCNT, RN
Practice Development Fellow, School of Health, Glasgow Caledonian University, Glasgow, Scotland, UK

Marie McAloon, RNT, RCNT, RN
Lecturer Practitioner (Gerontological Nursing), School of Health, Glasgow Caledonian University, NHS Greater Glasgow and Clyde, Glasgow, Scotland, UK

William McDonald, MSc, PgC, LTHE, BSc, RMN, FHEA
Lecturer, Mental Health Nursing, School of Health, Glasgow Caledonian University, Glasgow, Scotland, UK

Mike Nolan, BEd (Hons), MA, MSc, PhD, RMN, RGN
Professor of Gerontological Nursing, University of Sheffield, Sheffield, England, UK

Deborah Parker, RN, Grad Cert Gerontology (Bendigo), BA (FUSA), MSoc Sci (UniSA), PhD (FUSA)
Associate Professor, Director of the UQ/Blue Care Research and Practice Development Centre, Director of the Australian Centre for Evidence Based Community Care (ACEBCC), a Collaborating Centre of the Joanna Briggs Institute, School of Nursing & Midwifery, Toowong, Queensland, Australia

Susan Polding-Clyde, RGN, RSCN, DN, Dip Comm Care, BSc
Nurse Consultant, Care Commission, Paisley, Scotland, UK

Jacqui Reilly, PhD, BA (Hons), PgCE, LTHE, RN, RNT, LPE
Professor of Nursing, School of Health, Glasgow Caledonian University, Glasgow, Scotland, UK

Yvonne Robb, PhD, MSc, BSc (Hons), RGN, Dip Ned RNT
Lecturer, School of Health, Department of Adult Nursing, Glasgow Caledonian University, Glasgow, Scotland, UK

Irene Schofield, PhD, MSc (Gerontology), RNT, RGN
Research Fellow, School of Health, Department of Adult Nursing, Glasgow Caledonian University, Glasgow, Scotland, UK

Pat Schofield, RGN, PhD, PGDipEd, DipN
Director for Advanced Studies in Nursing (CASN), Centre for Academic Primary Care, University of Aberdeen, Aberdeen, Scotland, UK

Dawn Skelton, PhD, BSc (Hons)
Reader in Ageing and Health, HealthQWest, School of Health, Glasgow Caledonian University, Glasgow, Scotland, UK

John Timmons, MSc, BSc, RGN, PgCert TLHE
Clinical Education Manager, Smith and Nephew, UK

Debbie Tolson, PhD, MSc, BSc (Hons), RGN
Professor of Gerontological Nursing; Later Life Research Group Lead, Institute for Applied Health Research, School of Health, Glasgow Caledonian University; Director of the Scottish Centre for Evidence Based Care of Older People, a Collaborating Centre of the Joanna Briggs Institute, Glasgow, Scotland, UK

Anthony Tuckett, PhD, MA (Research), PGradDip (Phil), BNursing, RN
Senior Lecturer, University of Queensland, UQ/Blue Care Research & Practice Development Centre, Brisbane, Queensland, Australia

Yuli Zang, PhD, BMed, MMed, RN
Associate Professor, Associate Dean, Shandong University School of Nursing, Jinan, Shandong Province, China

Foreword

I feel both honoured and humbled to be asked to write the foreword for this excellent book. To support effective learning for all levels of nurses, we need up to date texts that achieve an accessible balance between theory, evidence and practice. Tolson, Booth and Schofield have assembled international experts to author chapters in *Evidence Informed Nursing with Older People* and I am delighted to see the range of examples of best practice they have selected and linked to the key health issues in later life. Problems such as sensory impairment, cognitive impairment, mobility impairment and incontinence, commonly known as the 'geriatric syndromes', don't affect every person over the age of 65, but all nurses need to recognise the red flags and ensure that they are addressed through evidence based person-centred practice. The essential knowledge on all of these clinical topics is comprehensively covered, with attention to cross-cutting issues such as relationships, communication and palliative care.

Evidence Informed Nursing with Older People is essential reading for all nurses, not just for specialists like me. With an ageing population, it is imperative that every nurse who works with adults is competent in caring for those who are old. The majority of hospital beds are already occupied by older people, the 'baby boomers' are entering retirement and the prospect of survival into very old age is more and more likely for those of us who are ageing behind them. It is not a question of choice, but of necessity, that nurses are equipped with the knowledge and skills to address the ensuing healthcare needs.

We are working in swiftly changing times in terms of the health economy, which inevitably impacts on the planning and provision of older people's services. Pragmatic choices have to be made, and this includes re-evaluating the role of the professional nurse and the future development of the workforce that will be needed. Textbooks age quickly, but in taking an approach that is mindful of the challenges in implementing evidence based practice, this one will, I am sure, age well itself.

It has been said in the past, many times, that 'geriatric nursing' has been associated with the 'Cinderella' label. Gerontological nurses have had a hard task to combat this, but through championship of older people's issues and with support of much enlightened policy and practice within health and social care, those of us who choose to work in care homes or health and ageing units no longer need fear the stigma or sneers from others that used to accompany that choice. It remains a fact, though, that promoting appropriate values about ageing is still as important a part of learning about gerontological nursing as is knowledge about the ageing process itself. This book gets the balance right, putting social gerontological issues into an appropriate professional health care context and unselfconsciously consolidating the position of professional gerontological nursing.

Lately, my concern has been more that in rooting out ageist attitudes and ensuring that older people are not discriminated against in healthcare, policy makers and healthcare providers risk underestimating the complex needs of frail older people, and the skills that are needed to address them. Advances in preventative treatment such as the use of anti-hypertensive medication have been hugely successful in supporting better health in older age, but health inequalities even within developed countries such as the UK mean that people are still surviving into very old age with multiple comorbidities and impairments. The need for skilled and informed healthcare provision for older people is not going away.

For me, the process of unravelling the complexities of the ageing process and interpreting it in health and social care has made gerontological nursing a fabulously rewarding and challenging speciality to choose. I've always looked out for texts that will help to support my personal learning and that of nurses I work with; rarely do books make the mark that this one has.

Fortunately, with a growing evidence base and the development of models such as the Caledonian Improvement Model, our personal and professional journeys can now be better supported than ever before. I savour the approach that this book provides and hope that other readers will do likewise.

Nicky Hayes
RGN, BA (Hons), MSc, PGCert (HE)
Nurse Consultant

Acknowledgements

In preparing this edited textbook we are indebted to the contributing authors and to individual older people, family carers and practitioners who provided insightful reflective contributions. We are grateful to Margaret McLay and Susan Cockburn from the School of Health administrative team at Glasgow Caledonian University who assisted with manuscript preparation and project management. Jane Wright, doctoral student, from the School of Health, assisted with literature searching and retrieval. We thank Professor Mike Nolan for his insightful advice and challenges which helped us to plan and structure the book.

Some of the figures and tables in this book are based on materials published elsewhere and have been reproduced or adapted and we thank the publishers and authors who generously permitted us to use their work.

Chapter 1

Principles of Gerontological Nursing

Debbie Tolson, Joanne Booth and Irene Schofield

Box 1.1 What matters to me: older person

'A good nurse to me is someone who knows what they are doing and can do it in a way that shows they care, care about me that is. They should speak to me with respect and not simplify information because I am eighty years old. I will ask when I don't understand.' (Ronald Newman, 81)

Introduction

Improvements in health and social care have contributed to demographic ageing around the world. This means that nurses who work with adults will increasingly be working with older people (people over retirement age, most often aged 60 years or more). The fastest growing group of the older population is the oldest old, i.e. those who are 80 years old or more. Globally in 2000, the oldest old numbered 70 million and their numbers are projected to increase to more than five times that over the next 50 years (Huber 2005). Adding years to life is a great achievement, particularly when this is accompanied by a good level of health and well being. For many people, however, longevity brings with it an array of challenges, some age related, others condition specific which impact on their lives and those close to them. Increased susceptibility to health problems and the cumulative effect of relatively minor problems coupled with a decreased recovery capacity explains the high demands for healthcare by this group. In addition to changes in states of physical and mental health, social determinants of health such as poverty and social isolation can compound an individual's problems. The susceptibility of older people to declining health and the global increase in numbers of people living into late old age make compelling reasons to mobilise nursing efforts and for us all to prioritise investment in the development of gerontological practices.

Evidence Informed Nursing with Older People, First Edition. Edited by Debbie Tolson, Joanne Booth and Irene Schofield.
© 2011 Blackwell Publishing Ltd. Published 2011 by Blackwell Publishing Ltd.

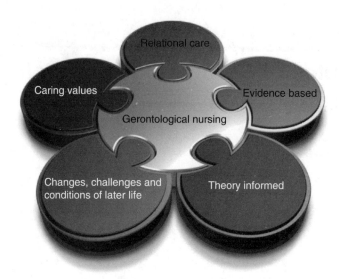

Figure 1.1   Essential connections for gerontological nursing practice.

Nurses are uniquely positioned to promote health in later life and to influence care outcomes and experiences for older people and their families. To do this effectively nurses need to draw on the best available evidence and adopt approaches to practice informed by health and medical sciences. Practice will also be influenced by conceptual and cultural understandings and reflect what is possible in the particular nursing situation. This book does not set out to be a definitive practice textbook *per se* – our intention is to explore the connections between practice, the value base of practice, emergent theory and the continually evolving evidence base which collectively informs how nurses can and do work with older people.

This foundational chapter will orientate readers to three fundamentally important and related issues which shape contemporary thinking about evidence informed nursing with older people:

(1) the meaning of gerontological nursing and its relationship to the evidence base;
(2) the importance of shaping evidence implementation through a culturally appropriate value base;
(3) the evidence informed management of common geriatric syndromes and health conditions.

Taking this unified view allows individual nurses to make essential connections to inform practice (Figure 1.1).

The introductory discussion is pivotal to understanding the contribution that nurses can and do make to the health and well being of older people. Importantly, we will introduce current debates and emergent ideas about the constituents of nursing practice at its best. The core premise is that nursing at its best occurs when practitioners make connections between the value base, evidence, underlying theory and gerontological practice know-how in the unique moment of care.

Meaning and scope of gerontological nursing

Over recent decades it is possible to trace debates in the literature as to whether nursing older people is a specialism or a component of general adult nursing. Kagan (2009) is critical of this preoccupation, contending that to progress we must focus on the promotion of gerontological principles when nursing people who for reasons of chronological age, illness, injury or genetic disposition manifest needs associated with later life. The Nursing and Midwifery Council of the UK now recognises that nursing older people is a specialism that requires highly skilled nurses who can respond to the complexity of health and social care needs of older people (Nursing and Midwifery Council 2009, p. 6). In addition to recognising the prerequisite skills that practitioners require to nurse older people, McCormack and Ford argued a decade ago that it is essential for nurses to be able to describe the contribution they make to older people's health and healthcare. If they fail to do so then it is likely that the trend, in some countries, to replace registered nurses with cheaper vocationally qualified support workers will continue (McCormack & Ford 1999).

We take the view that nurses who become expert in working with older people draw on knowledge from applied gerontology, geriatric medicine and generic nursing skills alongside knowledge of the older person, their family and life circumstances.

By describing nurses whose practice is guided by an explicit value base and informed by clinical and applied gerontological knowledge as 'gerontological' nurses, a distinction can be made between nurses with expertise, and those with a more general understanding of adult nursing. We believe this distinction is an important one to make as it signals the need for preparation specific to understanding clinical and psychosocial aspects coupled with an appreciation of the aspirations and felt needs of older people. We also concur with Kagan (2009) that all adult nurses should be equipped to apply gerontological principles within their practice.

Approaches to preparing nurses to work with older people vary and are influenced by views about underlying competencies and essential skills sets. Such views inevitably change with development of knowledge and theory and are reflective of national healthcare policies, priorities and service configurations. In the UK for example, recent health policies have promoted respectful and dignified care. These affective dimensions and the relationships within care are reflected in gerontological nursing competencies set out by the national agency for healthcare education in Scotland (NHS Education Scotland 2003). American and European alliances, whilst acknowledging the importance of these dimensions, highlight more clinically orientated perspectives including the differentiation of normal ageing from illness and disease processes, and assessment for syndromes and constellations of symptoms that may be manifestations of other underlying health problems (American Association of Colleges of Nursing 2004; Milisen *et al.* 2004). Such regional differences reflect local interpretations of nursing roles and functions in relation to older people rather than genuine differences in the underlying knowledge and skills sets which inform practice. In reality nurses need knowledge derived from clinical subjects and social sciences including the arts and humanities, so they can understand both what to do in a technical clinical sense and to convey their caring in ways that are safe and compassionate. There is an emerging consensus in the international literature that the scope of nursing older people embraces:

- health promoting aspects that enable people to optimise health, well-being and independence in later life;
- curative and rehabilitative dimensions that focus on functional or psychological recovery from illness or injury;
- facilitating self-care and enabling effective management of long-term conditions;
- providing care for those who become frail or with limited and/or declining self-care capacity;
- palliative and end-of-life care.

An important consideration for all countries is the attention afforded by pre-registration nursing courses in terms of preparing nurses to meet the varied and complex needs of an ageing population. Given the broad scope of gerontological nursing, working with older people offers ample opportunities for registered nurses to specialise in selective aspects of later life care. A challenge for the profession is to steer a transformative path to ensure a positive future for nursing older people and move away from negative legacies associated with ageist service mindsets and a general lack of investment in this area of healthcare (Hayes & Webster 2008).

We suggest that reframing thinking around the concept of gerontological practice contributes in several ways to the development of a positive mindset, which could facilitate progress (Kelly *et al.* 2005). Gerontological practice is a multi-professional and multi-agency endeavour, and although our discussions focus on nursing, it is with an appreciation that the clinical, theoretical, conceptual and ethical roots of much of our practice are shared and collaboratively developed with other health and social care disciplines.

The definition of this area of nursing presented in Box 1.2 reflects the previously listed scope of gerontological nursing. The definition was generated inductively through a social participatory programme of research undertaken over a 6-year period within Scotland (Kelly *et al.* 2005). The definition was formulated collaboratively with nurses from across Scotland working in a spectrum of specialist settings with older people, including acute hospital wards, rehabilitation units, long stay facilities, care homes, community and primary care (Tolson *et al.* 2006). Hence it has applicability across UK care environments and potentially beyond. An additional feature of the definition is that older people were also involved in its preparation. Critique and feedback on the original definition agreed in 2001 was invited from 11 gerontological nursing communities of practice over a period of 5 years (www.geronurse.com; Tolson *et al.* 2007, 2008) and it is noteworthy that the only requested amendment was made in 2004 when the concept of person-centred care was substituted with relationship-centred approaches. This suggests that the definition captures the contemporary meaning of gerontological nursing for practitioners and older people within Scotland and we also believe that it is in tune with international descriptions. Participants who collaborated in the development of this definition recognised that to realise their vision, a nurse would require in-depth, evidence informed gerontological nursing knowledge, skills and experience together with commitment to an explicit value base shared with members of their local multidisciplinary team. For some this definition represented an important stage in demonstrating professional identity, improving status and conveying their growing confidence in a new era of nursing with older people.

Box 1.2 Defining gerontological nursing

Gerontological nursing contributes to and often leads the interdisciplinary and multi-agency care of older people. It may be practised in a variety of settings although it is most likely to be developed within services dedicated to the care of older people.

It is a relationship-centred approach that promotes healthy ageing and the achievement of well-being in the older person and their family carers, enabling them to adapt to the older person's health and life changes and to face ongoing life challenges. See www.geronurse.com

Our definition (Box 1.2) highlights that gerontological nursing is relevant within any setting where older people receive healthcare and that it is not the exclusive domain of units dedicated to the care of older people. Importantly, the definition acknowledges the potential leading role played by gerontological nurses working as part of a multi-professional care team. Interestingly, most nurses who practise gerontological nursing do not use this term in their job title, preferring descriptions which are more meaningful to the public.

That said, an agreed definition and clarity about the principles of gerontological nursing are useful in that they enable nurses to describe their contribution or potential contribution to the healthcare of older people. Furthermore, it is an important step towards understanding the core gerontological knowledge and skills that underpin safe practice. This in turn should determine how we prepare practitioners to work with older people, either as a component of their general adult nursing role or as specialists with increased knowledge. Now that we have defined the area of practice and delineated the range of knowledge necessary to equip practitioners we can begin to examine the adequacy of our practice know-how, the underlying evidence base. Following this we can make theoretical connections to develop and advance practice. In this way we can demonstrate aspects of practice that are informed by evidence to be of demonstrable or perceived benefit to older people and reconsider aspects that are of questionable benefit. We will consider the issue of evidence, information use and appraisal within practice more closely in Chapter 2.

For now let it suffice to say that it is only by drawing on a credible inclusive evidence base that we can begin to understand how to optimise outcomes for older people and realise the potential of gerontological nursing. Griffiths (2008) suggests that by focusing on outcome indicators with older people, nurses have an opportunity to move beyond traditional approaches of identifying the problems and needs of older people. Rather, Griffiths (ibid.) argues that we should begin by identifying the desired outcomes of healthcare with the person and from this position recognise the nursing contribution to their care, plan and deliver appropriate nursing interventions. Heath and Phair (2009a) also advocate outcomes frameworks, which focus on older people's abilities, aspirations, health and well-being. To do so, they argue, values activities such as listening and being compassionate which research has shown are important to older people (Way *et al.* 2008). Furthermore, given that our definition of gerontological nursing (Box 1.2) recognises the importance of family carers it would be inconsistent to ignore them in our consideration of care outcomes.

If we accept the above arguments, we need ways to orientate our thinking towards person and family carer experiences, their expectations of care in addition to responding to the individual's presenting clinical symptoms and life changes.

Additionally, it would be inappropriate to restrict the nursing view of outcomes for the management of clinical symptoms to narrow measures based upon treatment efficacy alone; this has been the tendency of evidence based medicine (Jutel 2008). A more relevant approach for nursing is to take a broader view to accommodate the practical benefits experienced by patients and their close family members. Schulz *et al.*'s (2002) review of intervention studies specific to the caregivers of people with dementia provides a useful basis for a more relevant and inclusive description of clinical significance. They identify four core concepts that are clinically significant: symptomatology, quality of life, social significance and social validity. Intuitively these constructs have relevance to both the family carer and older people and to conditions other than dementia, including the spectrum of geriatric conditions and syndromes. Table 1.1 provides an overview of clinical significance based on the analysis of Schulz *et al.* (2002) using as exemplars two common geriatric conditions (urinary incontinence and hearing loss) to demonstrate the nursing contribution and outcomes within healthcare.

We will return to clinical conditions and features in the latter part of this chapter, but first we will turn our attention to the values underpinning practice and connections between these and the evidence base.

Linking evidence with beliefs about caring

Evidence based practice has in many ways become the mantra of contemporary healthcare policy and practice (Rycroft-Malone 2006). However, debates continue within nursing as to what constitutes meaningful evidence. Jutel (2008) is highly critical of the narrow scientific preoccupation of evidence based medicine and advocates that nurses should engage in information appraisal that goes beyond traditional evidence based tools which are subservient to evidence hierarchies.

We agree with this stance and acknowledge the view that evidence is contextually bound and socially constructed (Dopson *et al.* 2002). Philosophically, this means that the way nurses understand and relate to evidence is a function not only of the evidence itself but the interplay of how nurses think about practice and their beliefs about the constituents of good care. This may or may not embrace contemporaneous research. In a postal survey of registered nurses' understanding and interpretation of evidence based practice, Rolfe *et al.* (2008) found that nurses cited three influences on their practice: their own past experiences (69%), patient preferences (63%) and local evidence based guidelines (49%). This suggests that the way nurses make decisions and judgements in practice is a function of much more than their awareness of what may be recommended within care guidance. We have confirmed, within the Scottish Gerontological Nursing Practice Project, that when evidence is presented in ways that explicitly align with nurses' underlying beliefs about practice and caring, then they are more likely to adopt and sustain evidence based change (Tolson *et al.* 2008).

Many authors contend that caring is the core essence of nursing, describing it in terms of conveying a sense of concern, a desire to protect and ameliorate suffering in others.

Table 1.1 Exemplifying the nursing contribution using Schulz's framework for clinical significance.

Clinical significance core concepts	Focus	Geriatric condition 1: urinary incontinence (UI)		Geriatric condition 2: hearing loss	
		Nursing contribution	Outcome	Nursing contribution	Outcome
Symptomotology	Physical and mental health symptoms	Comprehensive assessment and determination of type of UI	Type of UI identified: targeted intervention applied	Screening using voice testing	Person gains insight into level of hearing impairment crucial to adaptation
		Agreeing continence-promoting intervention with older person	Bladder rehabilitation not palliative containment	Determination of need for a hearing referral for audiological assessment	Rehabilitation options known
		Support for self-management of urinary symptoms Evaluate effects	Reduced urinary incontinence or cure	Development of self-care skills for hearing aid	Timely referral Optimal hearing aid benefit
Quality of life	Perceptions of life quality which includes relationships with others	Measures of symptom distress and impact on quality of life	Reduced experience of symptom distress, reduced social isolation and improved quality of life	Measures of hearing-related hassles and family relationships	Reduction in hearing hassles Improved relationship with communication partners
Social significance	Includes service utilisation and broader impacts on society, such as delaying institutionalisation	Appropriate use of specialist continence, urodynamic and urology services	Enables coping Delays need for institutionalisation Appropriate use of continence equipment	Appropriate referral to specialist audiological services	Inappropriate consultations avoided Reduction in level of hearing aid rejection
Social validity		Support to appropriately manage urinary incontinence to prevent curtailment of life-enhancing activities	Improved self-esteem and participation	Informed and sensitive response to age-related hearing loss Augmentation of specialist audiological rehabilitation	Improved self-esteem Enhanced communication opportunities Improved levels of participation

Other authors, however, concede that caring is an elusive concept that defies definition, being a culturally and contextually bounded experience. Cronqvist *et al.* (2004) describe caring as a relational concept that involves caring about someone. For Cronqvist *et al.* the qualities that characterise caring include compassion, conscience and commitment, competence, sharing and mutual respect. Specific to expert gerontological nursing, McCormack and Ford (1999) propose five caring attributes: holistic knowledge and practice, saliency, knowing the patient, moral agency and skilled know-how. In an analytical exploration of the four core concepts of person-centred nursing in relation to nursing older people, McCormack (2004) describes:

- *being in relation* as concerned with relationships with people;
- *being in a social world* as highlighting the essential sociability of a person;
- *being in place* as the context in which personhood is articulated; and
- *being with self* is about being recognised, respected and trusted and its impact on our sense of who we are.

On a theoretical level it becomes clear that relationships are central to caring, and that to create a sense of care involves reciprocity founded on trust and demonstrable respect for the individual. This highlights the centrality of attitudinal dimensions and communication in nursing older people. In thinking about how to promote quality in our communications with people, Fredriksson and Eriksson (2003) advocate that we focus on what they describe as the caring conversation. This they explain is rooted in an appreciation that conversation occurs at a number of levels extending from being with (the ontological perspective), to a means of gaining knowledge (epistemological perspective), as a process which focuses on communication technique (methodological) and as an ethical encounter intended to do the person good. Recognition of the ethical dimensions of the caring conversation we believe to be pivotal to the relationships that nurses and others can form with older people and their family carers. This is reflected in the evidence surrounding perceptions of truth telling which we explore in Chapter 4.

Rights based care

International rights movements have highlighted the principles of fairness, respect, equality, dignity and autonomy. For many readers these principles will resonate with their own core values. The United Nations adopted five principles for the care of older persons in 1991 concerning independence, participation, care, self-fulfilment and dignity (United Nations 1999). These principles, reflecting the rights of older people are considered to be globally relevant and form the basis of an international action plan agreed in Madrid in 2002 (United Nations 2002). Some of the rights are related to essential elements for survival such as access to food and water, whilst others extend to opportunities for social engagement and participation in community life. The intention is that countries will embrace these five dimensions and create appropriate policies and mechanisms to ensure that these rights are observed.

In terms of healthcare policy imperatives a number of important UK developments reflect principle based care rooted in a system of older people's rights. The Department of Health in England produced a National Service Framework for Older People which introduced a set of national standards for the care of older people in England and Wales (Department of Health 2001). A major ambition of the National Service Framework was to root out age discrimination in health services and promote person-centred care. However, Nolan *et al.* (2004) have suggested that whilst this development was a major step forward some tensions have emerged from the narrow focus on the individual, which excludes the many supportive relationships within care. The importance of relationship-centred care, with a focus on the individual, will be further explored in Chapter 3.

A different stance to promoting principle based care of older people has been adopted in Australia. Rather than mandating standards of care, as in the English system, the Australian health ministry established an overarching framework for health services to use in their management of older people services (AHMAC 2004). Australian providers were duly expected to review their underlying principles and practices to ensure that they:

- adopted principles and practices that enable older people to access appropriate forms of care, support and treatment;
- optimise older people's health outcomes and functional independence;
- take the older person's wishes into account where possible;
- provide a supportive environment during decline and end of life (AHMAC 2004).

The importance of the involvement of family and significant others in care is enshrined within the Australian aged care standards of practice (Haesler *et al.* 2006). In regions of New Zealand, where this scheme has been partially adopted, the Treaty of Waitangi provides a framework to address cultural and inequality issues for older Maori people (Waikato District Health Board 2009).

An interesting feature of the Australian scheme is the emphasis placed on the evidence base. Principle 1 states that health treatment and care delivered to older people will be based on strong evidence (AHMAC 2004, p. 6). What is not explained in the document is the meaning or form of the evidence that might be considered strong.

As we move beyond rights based service frameworks to explore the value base espoused by specific disciplines such as nursing, the core concepts of human rights remain implicit. In many countries this can in part be attributed to legislative frameworks such as the European Convention on Human Rights and professional codes of practice (Nursing and Midwifery Council 2009).

The value base for gerontological nursing

In many care environments, unit philosophies and value statements explaining the caring culture to staff and clients are displayed in public areas or distributed in written material. The intention of such statements is to demonstrate organisational commitment to shared values designed to promote good quality care. However, such overt displays of group ethics are no guarantee that individual practitioners believe or act in accordance with the declared value base. This situation was reflected in early findings from the Scottish Gerontological Nursing Practice Project as will be explained in Chapter 2. An initial step in building a sense of cohesion among participants of the newly formed community of practice was to invite the group of 36 nurses working in different care environments to scrutinise the care philosophies in their own workplace (Tolson *et al.* 2005). In the majority of cases the origins of the workplace value statements were unknown and only a minority of the nurses could illustrate the influence that these values had on current practice. Nonetheless, the community of practice members were adamant that alignment of their personal values and that of their team would be a key determinant as to whether they would be willing to implement best practice care guidance (Tolson *et al.* 2005). It thus became a key activity for the community of practice to locate or develop an explicit set of values that resonated with their own and their team's values. These values would then be used as a lens through which to filter the care guidance (best practice statements) which the group were concurrently constructing (Tolson *et al.* 2006; Booth *et al.* 2007).

As with the definition shown in Box 1.2 refinement of these values is an ongoing process. Kelly *et al.* (2005) noted that the list of 10 values may appear an oversimplification of the philosophical foundations of practice. However, the project participants saw simplicity of expression as the key to the future utility of the values. The brief value statements were subsequently used as a filter through which to present the written care guidance and in doing so made an explicit connection between the nurses' shared beliefs and the evidence base (Booth *et al.* 2007). This strategy avoided a common pitfall in care guidance preparation, that of failing to reflect practitioners' beliefs.

McCormack (2004) describes the notion of authentic consciousness whereby principles for action or care embody the beliefs of both nurse and patient. As Dewing (2004) elaborates, it is the act of making values transparent which provides the basis upon which the negotiated relationship between the nurse and older person can develop. In the dynamic of a caring relationship then, an explicit value base enables the practitioner to view the evidence in new light. This is an essential beginning for trust and for working in partnership with older people and their families (Tolson *et al.* 2007).

The values set out in Box 1.3 were developed collaboratively by nurses involving older people, and the inductive approach used in the Scottish Gerontological Nursing Practice Project ensured that practitioners could express their values in familiar language. Kelly *et al.* (2005) acknowledge that although developed by and for nurses, these values have a generic quality and are arguably meaningful for the multi-professional gerontogical practice team. Explication of the multi-professional practice value base is an important step to promoting consistent approaches to care. The achievement of conceptual and attitudinal clarity is critical to the delivery of optimal care and enrichment of the practice environment. However, as can be seen in the definitions of expert practice already reviewed, affective and moral considerations form only part of the totality of attributes required by gerontological nurses. Other key attributes are clinical and therapeutic aspects.

Key clinical features in later life care

It is timely to revisit and reinforce the importance of some key features of clinical geriatric care. The term 'geriatric' is used here in its true sense, as pertaining to the healthcare needs of older people. Although it is often used in a derogatory manner, it must be acknowledged that it is a term which is used in leading contemporary medical research

Box 1.3 Practice values agreed within the Scottish Gerontological Nursing Study

Commitment to relationship-centred care

Recognition that the older person is best understood in the context of their relationships with others and that while the focus of care is the individual, they are part of a network of complex relationships that may impact on the person's care processes and which should be acknowledged for the most successful care to be achieved. Promoting continuity of care that values the older person's unique past, present and future individuality and respects the person's role and contribution to family and wider society.

Commitment to negotiating care decisions

Recognising that the older person has the right to make informed choices, with assistance from family members if they wish. The older person's choices and priorities are respected and may include an element of risk.

Promoting dignity and respect

Promoting dignity and respect for the older person in all aspects of care, regardless of setting, including consideration for the person's privacy and confidentiality.

Maximising potential

Recognising that caring events are also therapeutic opportunities and developing attitudes, knowledge and skills to empower the older person to live a life that reflects their individuality and enables them to achieve their potential.

Commitment to an enabling environment

Promoting a positive work culture together with a supportive physical and organisational environment in order to create an enabling living or care environment that conveys a sense of hope and achievement for the older person.

Establishing equity of access

Striving to secure on behalf of all older people the same access to services as other age groups and challenging evidence of age discrimination.

Commitment to developing innovative practice

Adopting strategies to promote evidence based gerontological nursing, acknowledging the value of multiple forms of evidence including practice expertise. Recognising the importance of choosing to specialise in gerontological nursing as a prerequisite to successful advancements in practice.

Consistency of vision

Developing a shared care philosophy that clearly enunciates the value base of gerontological nursing and the standards of care older people and their families can expect.

Commitment to team working

Working as part of a team who recognise, seek out and respect each other's contribution and commitment to the care of the older person. Directing the collective effort towards attaining goals negotiated with the older person and their family according to their needs and wishes.

The value of reciprocity

Recognising the value of mutual respect between all parties involved in the giving and receiving of care and the dynamic nature of the interactions in which benefits for all are appreciated.

papers and associated literature. Knowledge contributed by different disciplines forms part of the overall knowledge base relating to older people's health and well-being. Nurses working in older people's specialist teams must therefore necessarily have a comprehensive knowledge of the presentation of changes in health status in later life, of contemporary holistic responses to such changes, and an appreciation of the contribution of colleagues from other disciplines. We would argue that nurses who work with older people in any setting require a working knowledge of such health changes in order to contribute to safe and effective care for older people. The key clinical features include the altered presentation of disease; multiple pathology; the concept of frailty; 'geriatric syndromes' (Anderson 1985; Inouye *et al.* 2007), also referred to as 'geriatric conditions' (Cigolle *et al.* 2007); and the 'domino effect' whereby a single event can trigger a knock-on series of events that lead to rapid deterioration or death of an older person (Isaacs 1981). These key features (Box 1.4) will form the basis of selected chapters, or they will be considered in each chapter, and their significance is now outlined.

The presentation of changed health status itself can be different in older people. Signs of illness are often atypical or 'altered' and this is mainly due to age-related changes in physiology. For example, pain may not always be a reliable indicator of myocardial infarction and fractured femur, and temperature may not be elevated in infection. Instead an older person in pain or with an infection may present with cognitive impairment, as in the development of delirium. The atypical presentation of a change in health status is often complicated by the presence of multiple pathology. Even when conditions are minor, they can have a cumulative effect on the older person's overall condition to the extent that the individual rapidly loses functional and cognitive capacity. For each separate medical condition the older person may require medication and the resulting polypharmacy may lead to toxic drug reactions and interactions, which in turn culminates in the loss of functional and cognitive capacity.

Geriatric syndromes (Inouye *et al.* 2007) and geriatric clinical conditions are commonly seen in older people, especially those who are frail, and where changes in health status do not fit into discrete disease categories. Common, serious and debilitating conditions such as delirium, falls, pain, urinary incontinence, low body mass index, hearing impairment, and immobility, where people describe themselves or are described by others as 'going off their legs', are examples of geriatric syndromes. The syndromes are indicative of a change in health status but frequently do not represent the specific disease condition or conditions which are causing that change. Furthermore, the organ systems affected, such as the

Box 1.4   Key clinical features in later life care

- Altered disease presentation
- Multiple pathology
- Polypharmacy
- Frailty
- Geriatric conditions and syndromes
- Domino or cumulative effect

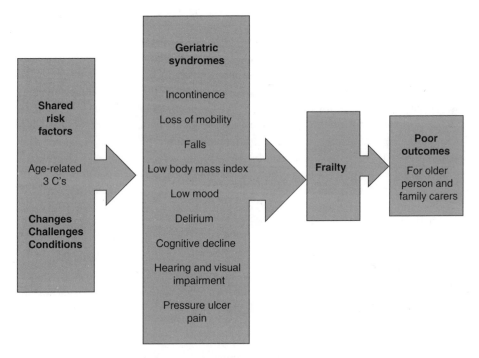

Figure 1.2   Geriatric syndromes and link to poor care outcomes. (Adapted from Inouye *et al.* 2007 with permission.)

bladder in urinary tract infection, may be distinct and distant from the system involved in its presentation (the brain in delirium). When geriatric syndromes occur together, precipitated by multiple underlying conditions, the interrelationships are increased in complexity. Figure 1.2 shows the link between the shared risk factors which give rise to geriatric conditions and the link with frailty and, if unmanaged, poor outcomes of care.

Geriatric syndromes will play an ever more prominent role with the increasing numbers of very old people. Despite this, within the UK and USA, the policy focus is on the management of single disease long-term conditions such as diseases of the heart and lungs and diabetes. However, a large US prevalence study of geriatric conditions and their effect on health and disability in older people living in their own homes found that some geriatric conditions were as common as chronic diseases, and strongly associated with disability (Cigolle *et al.* 2007). Whilst we would not argue against nurses playing a role in the care trajectories of long-term conditions, a failure to address the key features of geriatric care will result in inadequate and substandard care for potentially preventable disability for older people.

Frailty is currently a much debated concept and understandings of frailty vary. According to Campbell and Buckner (1997) it is a syndrome associated with underlying physiological and metabolic changes to the extent that minor alterations in a person's health status can cause increased disability or death. Another approach is an understanding of frailty as a collective of risk factors which might result in an increased state of vulnerability or even death (Ravaglia *et al.* 2008). Topinkova (2008) describes frailty as a 'geriatric condition' which belongs to the larger family of 'geriatric syndromes'. She cites a consensus of geriatricians working in Europe, Canada and America to the effect that frailty is a state of increased vulnerability to stressors, resulting from a decrease in physiological reserves and a degree of failure in multiple organ systems. Fried *et al.* (2004) describes frailty as a clinical syndrome characterised by multiple pathologies of weight loss, fatigue or weakness, low levels of physical activity, slow movement, abnormalities of balance and gait and with the added possibility of cognitive impairment. Frail individuals are particularly vulnerable to hospitalisation and medical procedures, sustaining falls and developing delirium, the latter resulting from age-associated changes in neuromuscular functioning and activity of endocrine and immune systems. It has been suggested that frailty can be reversed, by treating underlying conditions, under-nutrition and weakness. A recent definition of frailty from the nursing literature is provided by Heath and Phair (2009b):

> *a weakened state of being in which a person's reserve capacity is reduced to an extent where health, functioning and wellbeing are compromised. In the Precursor Stage a range of indicators can identify people who are vulnerable to frailty. Advanced frailty threatens life. Complications of frailty occur when the care delivered fails to compensate for the impact of frailty...*

This definition is important for our book as prevention or compensatory care in relation to common clinical conditions will be addressed in the case study chapters.

Heath and Phair (2009b) suggest that ill health characterised by the 'domino effect' affects older people who are described as being 'frail', such as those people who already have impaired cognition, impaired physical function and mobility. A single event such as a fall in a frail individual can result in a cascade of events, such as immobility, pressure ulcers, dehydration, urinary tract infection, delirium, and prolonged or lasting cognitive impairment. It may sometimes be burdensome and futile to search for an underlying condition, and it may be most appropriate to focus care on the presenting syndrome or to begin end-of-life care (National Confidential Enquiry into Patient Outcome and Death, 2009). Chapters 5–13 explore aspects of evidence informed nursing care based on the key features of clinical geriatric care, within a framework that is relationship centred and appropriate to the context in which it is delivered.

Summary

Our discussion has offered an explication of the nursing contribution to the healthcare of older people and their family carers. We have advocated investment in the promotion of gerontological nursing principles and the development of expert gerontological nursing practice as a legitimate way to meet the needs of the growing number of people around the world. Importantly, we have set out the essential connections that nurses need to make between theory, practice values and evidence in response to the policy imperative to deliver evidence informed care. This key messages contained within this introductory chapter are highlighted in the box below. Furthermore, by making these connections nurses will be better placed to respond to the reasonable request of older people as illustrated in our opening quote (Box 1.1) to work with older people in appropriate age-sensitive ways. Interestingly, in reviewing literature on health professionals' views and engagement with quality improvement, Davies *et al.* (2007) conclude that nurses think differently about what constitutes best care to other professional groups. In particular Davies notes that nurses have a tendency to place greater emphasis on achieving patient satisfaction, meeting both psychosocial and physical care and on the relationships that they form with the person. In doing this, we suggest, nurses show that they intuitively begin to make connections between the evidence, clinical knowledge and more conceptual understandings about ethical dimensions and relational aspects within the dynamics of care delivery. Our task in the chapters which follow is to explicate this in relation to nursing with older people.

Key messages

By making connections between theory, evidence, values, relational care and knowledge of the three C's (age-related changes, life challenges and conditions), nurses are equipped to deliver safe and effective nursing with older people.

References

AHMAC (Australian Health Ministers' Advisory Council) (2004) *Age-friendly Principles and Practices. Managing Older People in the Health Service Environment*. Victorian Government Department of Human Services, Melbourne, Australia. Available at www.health.vic.gov.au/acute-agedcare

American Association of Colleges of Nursing (2004) *Nurse Practitioner and Clinical Nurse Specialist Competencies for Older Adult Care*. Hartford Geriatric Nursing Initiative. Available at www.aacn.nche.edu/Education/dpf/APNCompetenceis.pdf (accessed 25 August 2009).

Anderson F (1985) An historical overview of geriatric medicine: definition and aims. In: Pathy MSJ (ed.) *Principles and Practice of Geriatric Medicine*. John Wiley & Sons, Oxford.

Booth J, Tolson D, Hotchkiss R, Schofield I (2007) Using action research to construct national evidence-based nursing care guidance for gerontological nursing. *Journal of Clinical Nursing* **16**, 945–953.

Campbell AJ, Buckner DM (1997) Unstable disability and the fluctuations of frailty. *Age and Ageing* **26**, 315–318.

Cigolle CT, Langa K, Kabeto MU, Tian Z, Blau CS (2007) Geriatric conditions and disability: The Health and Retirement Study. *Annals of Internal Medicine* **147**, 156–164.

Cronqvist A, Theorell T, Burns T, Lutzen P (2004) Caring about–caring for: moral obligations and work responsibilities in intensive care nursing. *Nursing Ethics* **11**, 63–76.

Davies H, Powel A, Rushmer R (2007) *Healthcare Professionals' Views on Clinician Engagement in Quality Improvement: A Literature Review*. The Healthcare Foundation, London.

Department of Health (2001) *National Service Framework for Older People*. Department of Health, London. Available at www.doh.gov.uk/nfs/olderpeople.htm

Dewing J (2004) Concerns relating to the application of frameworks to promote person centredness in nursing with older people. *International Journal of Older People Nursing* **13**, 39–44.

Dopson S, Fitzgerald L, Ferlie E, Gabbay J, Locock L (2002) No magic targets! Changing clinical practice to become more evidence based. *Health Care Management Review* **27**, 35–47.

Fredriksson L, Eriksson K (2003) The ethics of the caring conversation. *Nursing Ethics* **10**, 138–148.

Fried LP, Ferrucci L, Darer J, Williamson JD, Anderson G (2004) Untangling the concepts of disability, frailty and comorbidity: implications for improved targeting and care. *Journals of Gerontology A. Biological Sciences and Medical Sciences* **59**, 255–263.

Griffiths P (2008) Metrics for nursing. *Nursing Management* **15**, 10–11.

Haesler E, Bauer M, Nay R (2006) Factors associated with constructive staff–family relationships in the care of older adults in the institutional setting. *International Journal of Evidence Based Healthcare* **4**, 288–336.

Hayes N, Webster J (2008) Give old people a seat at the modernisation table. *Health Service Journal* 5 June.

Heath H, Phair L (2009a) Shifting the focus: outcomes of care for older people. *International Journal of Nursing Older People* **4**, 142–153.

Heath H, Phair L (2009b) The concept of frailty and its significance in the consequences of care or neglect for older people: an analysis. *International Journal of Older People Nursing* **4**, 120–131.

Huber B (2005) Implementing the Madrid Plan of Action on Ageing. United Nations Department of Economic and Social Affairs, Mexico.www.un.org/esa/population/meetings/EGMPopAge/EGMPopAge_21_RHuber.pdf

Inouye S, Studenski S, Tinetti ME, Kuchel GA (2007) Geriatric syndromes: clinical, research, and policy implications of a core geriatric concept. *Journal of the American Geriatrics Society* **55**, 780–791.

Isaacs B (1981) Is geriatrics a specialty? In: Arie T (ed.) *Health Care of the Elderly*. Croom Helm, London.

Jutel A (2008) Beyond evidence-based nursing: tools for practice. *Journal of Nursing Management* **16**, 417–421.

Kagan SH (2009) Guest Editorial: Boundaries and barriers: redefining older people nursing in the 21st century. *International Journal of Nursing Older People* **4**, 240–241.

Kelly T, Tolson D, Schofield I, Booth J (2005) Describing gerontological nursing: an academic exercise or prerequisite for progress? *International Journal of Nursing Older People* **14**, 1–11.

McCormack B (2004) Person-centredness in gerontological nursing: an overview of the literature. *International Journal of Nursing Older People* **13**, 31–38.

McCormack B, Ford P (1999) The contribution of expert gerontological nursing. *Nursing Standard* **13**, 42–45.

Milisen K, De Geest DE, Schuurmans M *et al.* (2004) Meeting the challenges for gerontological nursing in Europe: the European Nursing Academy for Care of Older Persons (ENACO). *Journal of Nutrition, Health and Aging* **8**, 197–199.

NHS Education for Scotland (2003) *Continuing Professional Development Portfolio. A Route to Enhanced Competence in Caring for Older People*. NES, Edinburgh.

National Confidential Enquiry into Patient Outcome and Death (2009) *Deaths in Acute Hospitals: Caring to the End?* NCEPOD, London.

Nolan MR, Davies S, Brown J, Keady J, Nolan J (2004) Beyond person centred care: a new vision for gerontological nursing. *International Journal of Nursing Older People* **13**, 45–53.

Nursing and Midwifery Council (2009) *Guidance for the Care of Older People*. NMC, London.

Ravaglia G, Forti P, Lucicesare A, Pisacane N, Rietti E, Patterson C (2008) Development of an easy prognostic score for frailty outcomes in the aged. *Age and Ageing* **37**, 161–166.

Rolfe G, Sergott J, Jordan S (2008) Tensions and contradictions in nurses' perspectives of evidence-based practice. *Journal of Nursing Management* **16**, 440–451.

Rycroft-Malone J (2006) The politics of the evidence based practice movements: legacies and current challenges. *Journal of Research in Nursing* **11**, 95–108.

Schulz R, O'Brien A, Czaja S *et al.* (2002) Dementia caregiver intervention research: in search of clinical significance. *The Gerontologist* **42**, 589–602.

Tolson D, McAloon M, Schofield I, Hotchkiss R (2005) Progressing evidence based practice: an effective nursing model? *Journal of Advanced Nursing* **50**, 1–10.

Tolson D, Schofield I, Booth J, Kelly TB, James L (2006) Constructing a new approach to developing evidence based practice with nurses and older people. *World Views on Evidence Based Nursing* **3**, 62–72.

Tolson D, Schofield I, Booth J, Kelly T (2007) Partnerships in best practice. In: Nolan M, Hanson E, Grant G, Keady J (eds) *User Participation in Health and Social Care Research: Voices and Evaluation*. Open University Press, Berkshire, pp. 33–49.

Tolson D, Booth J, Lowndes A (2008) Achieving evidence based practice: impact of the Caledonian Development Model. *Journal of Nursing Management* **16**, 682–691.

Topinkova E (2008) Aging, disability and frailty. *Annals of Nutrition and Metabolism* **52** (Suppl. 1) 6–11.

United Nations (1999) International Year of Older Persons (IYOP) in Asia and the Pacific. Social Development Division, United Nations ESCAP, 16 December 1991. 74th plenary meeting: Implementation of the International Plan of Action on Ageing and Related Activities. Available at www.unescap.org/ageing/res/res46-91.html

United Nations (2002) Madrid International Plan of Action on Ageing. Report of the Second World Assembly on Ageing, Madrid, 8–12 April 2002. United Nations, New York. Available at www.un.org/esa/socdev/ageing/madrid_intlplanaction.html

Waikato District Health Board (2009) *Principles of Best Practice in Older Persons Care: Towards Integrated Services Delivery*. WDHB Hamilton, New Zealand.

Way R, Lynch T, Bridges J (2008) Learning from older people who use urgent care services. *Emergency Nurse* **16**, 20–22.

Chapter 2

Applying the Evidence to Practice

Joanne Booth, Debbie Tolson, Irene Schofield
and Maggie Lawrence

Introduction

The purpose and role of evidence in healthcare is to inform practitioner decision-making, enable effective judgements to be made and best practice to be delivered. Applying evidence within practice is an essential component of safe and effective nursing care. However, when we talk about evidence informed practice in relation to nursing older people, what is meant by the term 'evidence' is not always clear. For some practitioners this is about compliance with evidence based clinical guidance but this can be problematic when they are not convinced by the strength or breadth of the evidence used to inform recommendations for practice. A further challenge is to find a way to implement evidence informed care that aligns with what nurses and older people believe to be important based on their own values, preferences and experiences. Despite the rapid development of the evidence based practice movement and apparent global acceptance of its validity to inform the best clinical decisions, there are many unresolved tensions and continued debates. These include different views about the nature of evidence and the practical challenges of equipping practitioners to access and apply the evidence where they work. Finding methods to translate evidence into nursing practice in ways that improve care experiences and contribute to better outcomes for older people has been the preoccupation of implementation scientists and practice development leaders around the world.

This chapter focuses on one improvement model, which was collaboratively constructed with health practitioners, older people and family carers, healthcare providers and policy makers to promote best nursing practice within Scotland. The Caledonian Improvement Model is grounded in user experiences, adopts an inclusive view of evidence and uses a community of practice framework to pool expertise and know-how in the quest to achieve sustainable evidence informed improvements in practice (Tolson *et al*. 2006). A brief overview of the theoretical influences supporting the various components of the model will be provided and the genesis and research base of the model will be explained, followed by its description. Discussion of evidence sources, critical appraisal and methods for summarising evidence will be integrated within this discussion, which begins by exploring the link between evidence and the decisions that nurses make in their everyday practice.

Evidence Informed Nursing with Older People, First Edition. Edited by Debbie Tolson, Joanne Booth and Irene Schofield.
© 2011 Blackwell Publishing Ltd. Published 2011 by Blackwell Publishing Ltd.

Understanding decision-making

All nurses will make decisions during the course of their care. Making accurate and appropriate clinical decisions to effectively nurse older people requires thorough and accurate data gathering processes, the possession of a sound theoretical knowledge base and the ability to utilise and integrate the two in forming judgements from which the decision is made (Thompson & Dowding 2002). It is an assumption of evidence based practice that knowing the options for best intervention automatically leads to the older person receiving this. However, we know that clinical decision-making is more complex than indicated by this linear relationship and that the numerous other factors that shape judgements are equally, or more influential, than the cold hard facts. While many benefits accrue from the effective and appropriate use of evidence, some argue that adhering to evidence based guidelines may result in a recipe approach to healthcare decision-making and reduce the need for clinical experience and judgement. Fears have been expressed that this results in the erosion of professional expertise and a stifling of creative approaches to caring and health improvement (Rashotte & Carnevale 2004). However, the suggestion that nurses' experience and judgement is marginalised is not borne out in practice, where paradoxically the evidence suggests that the sources of greatest influence on healthcare decision-making are the clinical experiences of the practitioner, their interactions with patients and local opinion leaders (McCaughan 2002; Gabbay & Le May 2004; Rolfe *et al.* 2008). Thus, it is rarely the case that decision-making processes directly reflect the systematic, phased, evidence informed approaches presented in guidelines and policy documents. As Redelmeier *et al.* (2001, p. 358) point out, clinical judgement is

> the exercise of reasoning under uncertainty when caring for patients... A process including missing data, conflicting information, limited time and long-term trade-offs.

This description seems to better reflect the 'messy' reality of nursing older people and takes account of the competing demands, which each decision-maker must deal with on a regular basis (Schofield 2008). If an evidence informed approach is to be successful, ways to deal with this complexity and uncertainty must be found.

There is increasing recognition of different approaches to decision-making based on the nature of the decision task (see cognitive continuum theory, Hamm 1988). The more complex a decision task, the less likely nurses will use analytical decision processes, instead preferring the use of intuitive forms of information processing (Dowding *et al.* 2009); these may rely largely on tacit knowledge. Whilst uncovering tacit knowledge is a useful adjunct to decision-making in complex situations, the specific types of decisions nurses commonly make have not been subject to close examination, the reason being that research in this area has tended to focus on the *processes* of decision-making. Although there is no current evidence underpinning the types of decisions made by nurses working specifically with older people, a six-category decision-making taxonomy has been identified for acute care nurses, whose work predominantly includes those in the older age ranges (McCaughan 2002). This is shown in Table 2.1.

Table 2.1   Types of decisions made by acute care nurses.

Decision type	Description
Intervention/effectiveness	Involves choosing between interventions
Targeting	Subcategory of intervention whereby the nurse chooses which patient will benefit most from the intervention
Timing	Subcategory of intervention whereby the best time to deliver the intervention is selected
Communication	Focuses on choices about ways of delivering to and receiving information from patients, families and colleagues
Service organisation, delivery and management	Concerns the configuration or processes of service delivery
Experiential, understanding or hermeneutic	Relates to the interpretation of cues in the process of care

The decision type most commonly observed relates to choice of intervention, including who should receive it and at what point. This reflects the reality of nursing where care delivery forms the bulk of the nurses' clinical practice and contrasts with medicine, where there is greater emphasis on diagnosis, management, epidemiological and non-clinical decisions as well as decisions about type of treatment (Ely *et al.* 1999). Given that nurses make different types of clinical decisions from medical practitioners, it is perhaps more understandable that they both require and respond to different types of evidence to support their decision-making. Furthermore, this explains the poor applicability and credibility of many clinical guidelines for nursing care and their lack of acceptance by many practitioners (Day *et al.* 2009).

It is not only the types of decisions but the nature of the decision-making process that influences the quality of care delivery. In the main nurses practise shared decision-making, drawing on collective knowledge and experiences when they feel their own to be inadequate for a particular decision (McCaughan 2002; Dowding *et al.* 2009; Rycroft-Malone *et al.* 2009). This collaboration with colleagues occurs frequently, both for making a decision and for feedback on whether it is the right thing to do. Only rarely do nurses make lone decisions, suggesting that the sharing of concerns, dilemmas and challenges, together with the options and solutions that have worked for others, is part of the nursing culture. This presents an opportunity to enhance an evidence informed approach to care using collaborative methods underpinned by social learning theory, as in the communities of practice advocated by Wenger *et al.* (2002).

A consideration for many nurses, particularly those working in hospitals or care homes is the competing demands and priorities in caring for a group of older people. Prioritising and decision-making in a communal setting such as an acute care ward brings different challenges to the clinical encounters in single-patient episodic situations most familiar to community nurses for example. In complex group situations nurses are often required to 'juggle' their activities in order to meet diverse and fluctuating needs. In addition, needs and decisions may change quickly and nurses are frequently required to respond with decisions in the 'moment of care' (Case study 2.1).

Case study 2.1

You are a staff nurse in a small independent care home and you have 14 older people in your care. Among this group are the following.

- Mrs Jackson, who is physically fit and enjoys walking outside in all weathers. She has vascular dementia, with moderately impaired memory, reasoning, orientation and communicative functions. She requires to be accompanied when walking outside the care home. She has vision and hearing loss and has fallen on three occasions in the past year.
- Miss Johnson, who has multiple physical and communicative disabilities following her third stroke. She is dependent on staff for her care needs. She has severe urinary urgency and frequency but remains continent when her toileting needs are met in time.
- Mr Bruce, who has end-stage COPD and who has developed a chest infection the previous day. He is confined to bed and is receiving continuous oxygen therapy. The decision has been made that he will not be transferred to an acute hospital and that he will receive palliative care in the care home. The local hospice outreach team will contribute to his care. He requires regular monitoring as he has now developed delirium and needs to be given fluids and food. He also needs mouth care, and attention to his physical comfort needs. Both Mr Bruce and his wife need psychological support.
- Mrs McLeod, who has severe Parkinson's disease, and rheumatoid arthritis. She is recovering from recent surgery to repair a fractured neck of femur. She requires regular oral analgesia to control pain as a result of the surgery. In addition she requires 3-hourly administration of her Parkinson's medication.

You are on duty with three care assistants. It is lunchtime and you have five other residents who need assistance to eat and drink. Mrs McLeod is due her medication at 12.30 and she will 'freeze' when she tries to walk if this is not given on time. Miss Johnson is indicating she needs to go to the toilet for which she needs two members of staff and a hoist. Mrs Jackson is pacing up and down in front of the door and showing signs of agitation. You know that this situation can sometimes escalate into verbal and physical aggression. Mr Bruce's wife is distressed by her husband's discomfort and is asking you to come and spend time with him.

Reflective points
- What care will you prioritise?
- Explain your reasoning and decision-making. What evidence informs your decisions?
- How do you balance the competing demands for care?

Successfully managing this situation requires great knowledge and skill. It is challenging in the extreme yet is not unusual and many readers will recognise similarities with their own practice experiences.

The case study illustrates the many factors that influence decision-making and the challenges of applying evidence at the point of caring for older people. Adhering to clinical guidance on falls prevention (National Institute for Clinical Excellence 2004; Australian Commission on Safety and Quality in Health Care 2009), continence promotion (International Continence Society 2009) and delirium (National Institute for Clinical Excellence 2010) will involve most of the staffing complement for extended periods of time, regardless of the needs of the other residents. In such cases, as supported by cognitive continuum theory, the necessity for multiple rapid judgements and decisions in the face of limited evidence and other information cues supports the reliance on more intuitive modes of cognition and approaches to decision-making. This is where the individual nurse's core belief system and values are important, as a clinical and moral guide, which impact directly on the activities prioritised and ultimately the care decisions made. It is imperative to the delivery of best practice that these are uncovered and recognised for their influence on care provision (see Chapter 1 for discussion of gerontological nursing values system).

Of course decisions about care are not only made by nurses and other *healthcare* practitioners. Contemporary practice has active involvement and partnerships with older people as an imperative central to the delivery of best practice in health and social care (Davies & Nolan 2003; Andrews *et al.* 2004; Kelly *et al.* 2006; Department of Health 2008; Nursing and Midwifery Council 2009). There is increasing recognition of the benefits that accrue for older people, their families and nurses when decisions about care are shared, although the methods to successfully achieve this continue to evolve. However, decision-making by older people is known to differ from that of younger adults. Thought deliberation, including speed of information processing and working memory, deteriorate with normal ageing (Peters *et al.* 2007), and this may lead to an impression of reduced capacity to make informed decisions. In contrast there is an increase in attention towards the emotional content of information provided and a tendency to focus on the positive rather than the negative. This potentially influences the ways the older person interprets the information provided and suggests the possibility of a limited consideration of risks and consequences of proposed health or care strategies. The full implications of these complex differences have yet to be understood. Nevertheless, it is important that they are recognised and taken into account by nurses when older people are making important personal healthcare decisions.

It is known that for all age groups, beliefs and values shape their interpretation of information. However, altered decision-making processes in older age may explain the influence that individual beliefs may exert on decisions about healthcare risk (Michaels *et al.* 2008). Indeed it is likely that the greater wealth of life experience that accompanies old age may serve to embed personal values and deepen beliefs. In recognition of this it is our view that delivery of best nursing practice is not possible unless the diverse preferences of older people and their family carers are considered fully in decision-making processes. In an ethically conscious society individual rights and responsibilities conform to principles of informed consent. However, in order to contribute to decision-making a dynamic process of information exchange must take place so that those responsible for the decision are fully informed about the different options, and the benefits and risks, before making their choice. Furthermore, our commitment to a relationship-centred care philosophy (Nolan *et al.* 2006), as detailed in Chapter 3, supports the need to involve those within the older person's family, if this is what the older person wants.

Thus we argue that consideration of the practitioner and older person's values are essential components in the delivery of evidence informed practice and that there should be mechanisms in place to ensure values are considered in the decision-making process. This aspect has been neglected in the evidence implementation models proposed previously. The Caledonian Improvement Model recognises diverse evidence presented as meaningful, accessible guidance. Furthermore, in order to reflect best practice, such guidance must be interpreted through the lens of older people's and practitioner values, in their particular delivery context. These elements connect to enable the delivery of best nursing practice with older people. Having explored the individual elements to be considered in constructing a model for practice improvement, we will now describe the model itself.

Background influences on the Caledonian Improvement Model

In 2001 the Scottish Strategy for Nursing and Midwifery, Caring for Scotland, called for the promotion of best practices in caring for older people and those with long-term conditions (Scottish Executive 2001). This strategic imperative was the catalyst for a 6-year programme of research that led to the development of the Caledonian Improvement Model.

The primary research question addressed was 'How can best practice in the nursing care of older people be promoted across Scotland?' As in many other countries, nurses in Scotland work with older people in a range of care settings which reflect the scope of gerontological nursing described in Chapter 1. Provision ranges from state-provided health and social care services to services such as care homes provided by commercial companies. The project ambition was to find an approach that would influence and improve care across provider and sector boundaries. The underlying assumption was that older people have a right to nursing care informed by the best available evidence irrespective of the care setting.

As the project was concerned with improvement on a large scale and capital resources were, and remain, limited, a cost-effective and efficient approach was sought that would create the conditions to:

- translate knowledge into evidence informed nursing practice;
- lead to sustainable change within care environments;
- change professional behaviour and improve practices;
- achieve demonstrable benefits for older people.

Theoretical influences on planning, what was to become known as the Scottish Gerontological Nursing Demonstration Project, were rooted in achieving the four conditions listed above. Conceptual and theoretical influences include theories of organisational and behavioural change, learning theories, practice development models and implementation science. The range of influences reflects the complexity of addressing the deceptively simple research question. Indeed there was no 'off the shelf' solution and although many potentially useful and increasingly popular approaches were described in the literature, their demonstrable impact on care outcomes was negligible and at that time theoretical underpinnings unclear.

Thus the project design included consideration of emerging descriptions of practice development within the nursing literature, which highlighted the important interplay and interdependence of evidence, context and facilitation in activities designed to develop practice (Kitson *et al.* 1998). Facilitation is known to take many forms when the desired outcome is to change professional behaviour and practice in ways that are sustainable. A number of approaches were therefore explored, including use of new technologies to support the processes.

Accumulating evidence indicated that education *per se* was a necessary but insufficient condition for behaviour change leading to the improvement of practice (Robertson & Jochelson 2006). As Michie *et al.* (2005) argue, there are three additional important psychological constructs that must be addressed for the individual practitioner and discipline:

(1) beliefs about evidence based practice
(2) professional role and identity
(3) beliefs about consequences.

Thus strategies to encourage nurses to adopt new evidence informed ways of working with older people must resonate with their beliefs and be relevant to their practice role and professional identity. Nurses must also believe that the new way is beneficial to older people and feasible where they work.

In any development activity the role of learning is a crucial part in the process. As the Scottish project was focused on registered nurses, we sought a learning framework appropriate to the experienced practitioner. Mindful of demands on practitioner time we recognised that our design would need to be flexible, accommodate working patterns and create opportunities for brief episodes of learning, which could transform thinking. We opted for a blended approach mixing a range of learning and reflective strategies designed for individual and group learning, with a mix of classroom-based and internet-enabled learning experiences. Elmore (2003) provides a useful overview integrating learning and change theories, which highlight the strength of work-based and problem-based approaches to support professional learning. Henri and Pudelko (2003) present compelling arguments for work-based learning using group approaches, concluding that communities of practice offer the greatest potential for bridging between individual and group learning, and learning in order to transform practice.

A community of practice is a group of people who share a concern or passion for something they do, and learn how to do it better as they interact regularly (Wenger 1998). Knowledge is shared and created through social relationships – thus learning is situated, taking place in the setting where it will be applied, rather than seen as a distinct activity that takes place in isolation from practice. Wenger *et al.* (2002) argue that there are three distinguishing dimensions of communities of practice in comparison to other types of group:

• they have a purpose, or joint enterprise, that brings the members together;
• the members possess relevant knowledge and bond with fellow members to form a social group;
• the members build their capability in practice by developing shared resources using the accumulated knowledge of the community.

With these characteristics the community of practice was a suitable framework around which to construct the practice improvement model.

Sustainability as an essential determinant of success was a major consideration for the Scottish project team. In the context of developing practice, sustainability is about the capacity of people (practitioners) and organisations (e.g. care home, hospital) to learn and change (as summarised in Box 2.1).

Box 2.1 Sustainable practice change

- Capacity of the individual and team to learn and change the way they think about practice and what they do in practice.
- Capacity of the organisation to learn and embed change in service provision.

In relation to our project this was seen as the capacity of nurses to deliver evidence informed practice and the capacity of the care provider to embed new approaches within its systems of organisation, care policies and care culture. New ways of working become sustainable through individual and collective responsibilities and actions. This view is supported by normalisation process theory, which purports that sustainable change only occurs when the new intervention, or way of doing things, becomes routine or taken for granted (May & Finch 2009). Grimshaw *et al.* (2004) agree that change is more likely to be embedded in practice if organisational and national-level strategies support individuals at the level of practice. This emphasises the importance of high-level political drivers.

Given the above theoretical considerations, we recognised that the most appropriate way forward was to form a collaborative alliance of stakeholders and adopt social participatory research methods. To this end an alliance was formed to steer the project comprising researchers, educators, practice developers, service providers, practitioners and older people.

Project design

We adopted an enhancement approach to action research which encourages practitioners to use theory and values to advance their practice (Holter & Schwartz-Barcott 1993). Each cycle of action drew on the principles of realistic evaluation to determine what was working well and to plan how to continually strengthen the impact of approaches that seemed to work (Pawson & Tilley 1997).

From 2001 to 2006, five action cycles were completed which sought to develop:

- an internet-based practice development college with an agreed development agenda;
- mechanisms to promote the involvement of older people;
- the development of shared principles underpinning the evidence based nursing care of older people;
- a methodology to construct legitimate, credible and achievable care guidance for nursing (best practice statements);
- a practice development model with demonstrable impact (the Caledonian Improvement Model).

A range of research methods were used to collect process and outcome evaluation data (Tolson *et al.* 2006). These are shown in Box 2.2.

Box 2.2   Evaluative research methods used

- Individual and group interviews
- Case studies
- Analysis of virtual college archive and user statistics
- Action plan evaluation
- Baseline and outcome practice audits
- Knowledge surveys
- SWOT analyses
- Work satisfaction questionnaires
- Perceptions of workplace change surveys
- Assessment of caring attributes
- Computer skills surveys need

The Caledonian Improvement Model

The model is grounded in research undertaken with 11 communities of practice. Much of the evidence gathering and experiences of practitioners who took part will be detailed in the book's case study chapters. They illustrate in practice how the Caledonian Improvement Model is a vehicle for achieving evidence informed practice (Figure 2.1). The communities of practitioners work together to champion best practice both locally and nationally. Momentum to improve practice is generated by the combination of practitioner knowledge and a need to answer specific questions about practice using knowledge from a range of evidence. Practice improvements and learning in the demonstration sites provide encouragement and templates for success for the members of the community of practice. Successful development of best practice stimulates continued efforts to improve. The model blends elements associated with both the technical and emancipatory approaches to practice improvement described in the literature and user involvement is integral to it. Figure 2.1 offers a diagrammatic representation showing the link between the integration of the different forms of evidence and practitioner knowledge, the learning that takes place in the community of practice and application of the knowledge to achieve evidence based practice. The linked turning of the arrows creates the momentum to enable practitioners to progress towards evidence informed practice. Lack of progress in one part of the system delays overall progress or stops it. Thus clinical practice stagnates when practitioners lack a spirit of inquiry and continue to rely on old routines.

Operationally, the model includes three core elements that provide the dimensions and mechanisms to support communities of practice in their quest for practice improvement:

(1) infrastructure and communication mechanisms
(2) knowledge conversion processes
(3) learning and development processes.

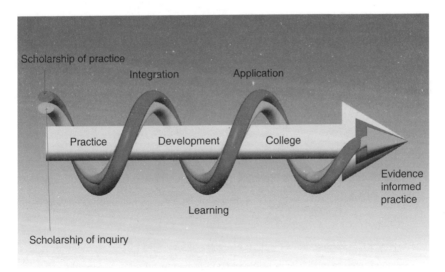

Figure 2.1 Caledonian Improvement Model. (Reproduced from Tolson *et al.* 2006 with permission from John Wiley & Sons.)

Box 2.3   Gerontological community of practice

A group of practitioners, educators and older people who pool expertise and share learning in order to develop practice. The community of practice achieves:

- shared values through an explicit and agreed care philosophy;
- a shared understanding of best practice as an inclusive evidence based description aligned to shared values;
- shared implementation solutions and resources/toolkits;
- improved care experiences and outcomes for older people.

We begin our explanation of the model by sharing our understanding of communities of practice. We defined a community of practice in the demonstration project as shown in Box 2.3.

An internet-based 'virtual' college provided the collaborative workplace and communication systems to connect individual members of each community (Figure 2.2). A definition of gerontological nursing and a value base developed by the community helped the members to bond with each other. A novel guideline development methodology for practitioners (Booth *et al.* 2007) and a method for older people to develop their own companion resources (Kelly *et al.* 2006) were developed to enable evidence to be effectively presented. A transformational learning journey equipped practitioners and teams for implementation of the specific best practice guidance. The practitioners' enhanced capacity to improve practice resulted in an enhanced confidence and development of their leadership skills (Tolson *et al.* 2008).

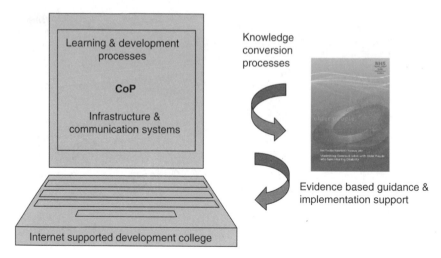

Figure 2.2   Overview of core components of Caledonian Improvement Model.

Infrastructure and communication mechanisms

The design of the internet-based practice development college was influenced by the community of practice members. The prototype college used freely available software and was based on a building metaphor with easily identifiable 'rooms' for community members to work in (Buggy *et al*. 2004). This initial system became unstable due to increasing demands and the college was transferred onto a managed learning environment platform called Blackboard (Lowndes *et al*. 2007). The college was password protected and members entered via the public website www.geronurse.com. The virtual college provides a safe place for members to collaborate, learn, report progress, discuss development challenges and share implementation solutions. It is accessible at any time, which is of benefit to rostered nurses, and user statistics have shown activity throughout the 24-hour period, with peak activity between 9 and 11 p.m. (Tolson *et al*. 2008). The virtual college enables communication between geographically dispersed community members for whom attending face-to-face meetings is challenging. Its many facilities include real-time or synchronous meetings in addition to threaded discussions or asynchronous communication, and learning activities. The community members can contribute to these at any point. All learning materials developed are archived for access by college members at any time (Lowndes *et al*. 2007).

Knowledge conversion processes

The evidence used to inform practice is socially negotiated in that it must conform to an accepted definition of what constitutes knowledge (Nutley *et al*. 2003). It is the prevailing dominant paradigm that dictates the nature of the evidence generally recognised to have merit (Pearson *et al*. 2007). Currently within healthcare this means the use of objective scientific research evidence to drive clinical decision-making. However, nurses in the project considered this narrow approach limiting to their practice and unsuited to the different types of clinical decisions they made (McCaughan 2002). Thus there was support to include forms of knowledge such as clinical experience, patient and carer experiences and local contextual information (Rycroft-Malone *et al.* 2004) and evidence from research designs other than the clinical trials favoured by other guideline developers.

In addition, evidence was seen as being interpreted by each individual, including older recipients of nursing, in light of their values, priorities and the practice context. Thus evidence that was considered to inform nursing care of older people encompassed the sources shown in Box 2.4.

Box 2.4   Sources of evidence that inform nursing with older people

Scientific research evidence
Knowledge that is derived from biomedical and social scientific research, both quantitative and qualitative in approach. Inclusive approach including clinical trials, other experimental designs and meta-analysis as well as mixed methods' studies, qualitative interviews, observational designs and others.

Clinical experience
Includes both explicit knowledge, which is knowledge that can be stated, and tacit knowledge, which is known to the individual but cannot be easily articulated or transferred and is often context specific. Both forms of knowledge are fundamental to professional practice but explicit knowledge is sometimes considered more valuable. Yet an inclusive evidence base is built by also understanding contributions made by tacit knowledge to decision-making. The model seeks to uncover its methods and details, in effect making the unspoken explicit.

Values and beliefs
Deeply held convictions that mould behaviour and shape attitudes and perspectives yet are rarely explicitly examined. Individual, organisational and cultural in nature, they represent powerful influences on practice.

Older people and their carers
Previous experiences underpin health-related beliefs and values that direct healthcare preferences and decision-making and are an important evidence source in caring for older people.

Local context and environment
Recognition of the association between practice culture, context and outcomes of care and the active contribution of context to knowledge translation process (Dopson 2007). Evidence must be adapted to the particular contextual conditions in which it is being implemented or utilised.

Policy documents
Evidence from government committee reports, national audits and other forms of non-research evidence such as published and unpublished care guidance and protocols that shape the direction and priorities for healthcare of older people.

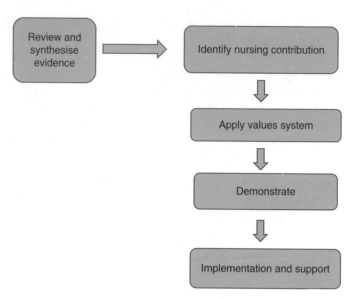

Figure 2.3   Guideline development methodology. (Reproduced from Booth *et al.* 2007 with permission from John Wiley & Sons.)

The methodology developed to prepare the evidence informed guidance (best practice statements) for nurses working with older people was framed around a critical review and synthesis of the range of evidence sources in Box 2.4 (Booth *et al.* 2007). The critical appraisal of the evidence is a cornerstone of evidence informed practice and is the process undertaken to systematically evaluate evidence. It is a technique that is designed to answer specific practice questions through a process of extracting relevant information to succinctly summarise the extent of what is known about a particular area. There is no single universally accepted approach to critical appraisal, but there are a number of useful resources and tools to support the development of appraisal skills. It will be no surprise to find that most of these resources focus on the systematic evaluation of specific research designs only, in line with the hierarchical models previously mentioned, for example Critical Appraisal Skills Programme (CASP) (www.phru.nhs.uk/Pages/PHD/resources.htm, accessed 20 January 2010), where effectiveness and the randomized controlled trial are most highly valued.

The consensus of the communities of practice who collaborated in the Scottish project was that nursing issues and the questions that nurses may have for the delivery of best practice are rarely addressed in published guidelines (Booth *et al.* 2007), a view endorsed by others (Miller & Kearney 2004; Rycroft-Malone *et al.* 2004; Rowat *et al.* 2009). The gerontological nursing project guideline methodology, as shown in Figure 2.3, sought to redress this deficit in two ways: firstly, through combining a robust appraisal and synthesis of diverse forms of evidence and, secondly, by extracting the nursing contribution and making judgements about the quality of the evidence and its relevance to practice. The agreed values system was applied to the resulting draft guidance which was then pilot tested in demonstration sites to determine achievability in the real world of practice (Booth *et al.* 2007). The key challenges to implementation uncovered by the demonstration sites are noted in the resultant guidance for others to benefit from.

To date five best practice statements have been produced using this method (Nursing and Midwifery Practice Development Unit 2002; NHS Quality Improvement Scotland 2004, 2005a–c). The development of each statement was led by a community of practice supported by a clinical expert advisor. Each community of practice included links to teams of nurses in demonstration sites. The demonstration sites included hospital wards, day hospitals, care homes and community settings. The published guidance provided an evidence based rationale for provision of best practice in a particular area of nursing, indicating the strength and source of underlying evidence supporting the practice. In addition how practice areas could demonstrate compliance was noted. For example, this might be about the routine use of validated screening instruments, evidence of collecting relevant patient data and responsive care planning that captures individual preferences.

Learning and development processes

The community of practice exists specifically to enable members to pool practice-based knowledge and enrich professional practice. In this respect communities of practice provide the conditions through which learning can occur where learning is brought about through social interaction and is situated in the practitioners' work context. This produces knowledge that is a blend of culture, context and activity which is embedded in practice (Lave & Wenger 1991; Brown & Duguid 2001; Breu & Hemingway 2002). Learning in a community of practice takes place through active processes of participant sharing, which leads to the creation of practice knowledge.

As members of a community of practice working in a virtual college, each practitioner undergoes a transformational learning journey (Figure 2.4). Engagement with the different activities within the virtual college is associated with a variety of positive effects on the road to achieving improved care. Nurses become active members of a community of practice and are facilitated to explore and reconcile their value base, and through this process articulate their understanding of the principles of gerontological nursing (see Chapter 1). The effects of this process are described as empowering and result in enhanced confidence levels and the development of a positive identity as gerontological nurses within the community (Kelly *et al.* 2005a; Tolson *et al.* 2005). In turn this improved identity energises the nurses, enabling them to focus on their local priorities and set practice improvement goals. The nurses' active participation in the preparation of the best practice statements fosters a sense of ownership and helps them to tailor and implement the care guidance within their work context. A range of personal development outcomes are inherent within this model.

Members of each community share the journey, focusing on 'seeing possibilities for improvement' and finding solutions to local implementation challenges. Online facilitation was used to support practitioner-centred learning. It did not simply focus on developing virtual college content for all to access but also recognised the value of practitioner interaction. The experience of the practitioners in itself became a vast learning and practical resource. Exchange of experiences and solutions were seen as empowering and validatory of development work, in addition to eliciting practice know-how to make tacit knowledge explicit, thus enabling others to access it. Online facilitation sessions were

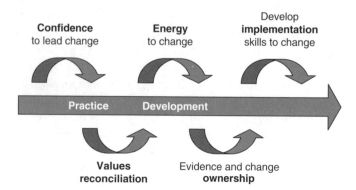

Figure 2.4   The practitioner's journey. (Adapted from Tolson *et al.* 2006; © Glasgow Caledonian University.)

aimed at enabling participants to identify strategies to resolve real challenges in developing areas of practice.

On average it takes nurses 18 months to complete their first practice development journey and demonstrate better care locally. This involves them in cascading learning through their teams and implementing revised local policies and practices in line with the best practice statements. Subsequent efforts to improve practice locally are swifter and less reliant on virtual college based facilitation. Accessible implementation resources and periodic external facilitation appears to speed up local achievement of subsequent best practices. Importantly, the way that each community evolves gives it inbuilt capacity to integrate new members (Kelly *et al.* 2005b). This is essential given workforce issues facing healthcare teams' intent on improving care as to so do requires sustained effort and continuity.

Impact of Caledonian Improvement Model

A study to determine the impact of the Caledonian Model on practice outcomes was completed in 2008. The previous action cycles had provided evidence of positive effects for participants and older people but had relied on self-report methods of evaluation, including unverified benchmarking activities, and stories about change experiences from individual perspectives or caring dyads (Booth *et al.* 2005; Kelly *et al.* 2005b; Tolson *et al.* 2005). While providing a range of evidence suggestive of benefit, further more objective evidence of effect was required. Three communities of practice were formed by 24 nurses from 18 different practice sites. Each community was formed by nurses, working in one of three contrasting care environments: NHS day hospitals, NHS long-term care wards and independent care homes. Their purpose was to select and implement a best practice statement. Evidence of impact at the ward/unit level and at the level of individual patients was examined using baseline and 6-monthly outcome patient and facilities audits (Booth *et al.* 2005). The impact on the nurses was explored using the Revised Nursing Work Index (Aiken & Patrician 2000) and focus group interviews. The results, as verified by an independent auditor, showed that 80% of the patient-related audit criteria

Table 2.2 Audit changes at 6-month outcome evaluation.

Community of practice	Patient	Facilities
Wards (5) Depression BPS	+86%	+32%
Day hospital (7) Activity BPS	+82%	+41%
Care homes (6) Nutrition BPS	+73%	+33%

and 35% of the facilities audit criteria were achieved. Table 2.2 indicates the improvements made in each of the three care environments.

Externally verified data

For the participating nurses the Revised Nursing Work Index indicated that they experienced greater autonomy in their roles ($P = 0.019$) and increased organisational support ($P = 0.037$). The focus groups revealed a deepening organisational support for the initiative over time, illuminating work-based learning challenges and overall enthusiasm for the approach. The conclusion of the study was that the Caledonian Improvement Model was an effective approach to developing evidence informed nursing practice and improving care standards, and that it constituted value for money in time and budgetary restricted health services.

Nevertheless, although the results look impressive in terms of the pace of guideline implementation, sustainability may not be claimed until changes are seen in facility level policies and procedures and as is shown this was less easily influenced. Furthermore, it must also be acknowledged that three national agencies – NHS Education Scotland (NES), NHS Quality Improvement Scotland (QIS) and Scottish Government Health Department – were funding the work, which may have given greater impetus for success.

Summary

One criticism of evidence based practice has been the lack of well-described models, informed and shaped by relevant theory. Evidence informed practice is recognised as the way forward for health and care services for older people, although there is a relative dearth of effective, realistic and achievable methods to enable nurses to achieve this ambition. Demonstrating that nursing older people is a therapeutic amalgam of relevant evidence, an agreed values system and the preferences of older people all tailored to the local care context is the aim of nurses who work with older people. The Caledonian Improvement Model provides a mechanism to enable the connections between these components of best practice to be achieved (see Key messages). The communities of practice framework facilitates the pooling of knowledge and sharing of practical solutions to care challenges, expediting time and resource efficient practice improvement while simultaneously developing the confidence and creativity of the nurses to foster commitment, motivation and capability to engage in continual improvement activities.

In contrast to other approaches this is an improvement model that develops a sense of ownership among those who engage with it, as its success is largely reliant on the collective and sustained contributions of the community members. It has been shown to be effective in a range of care contexts and is flexible and affordable, accommodating the needs of nurses working across the spectrum of health and care contexts with older people.

Key messages

- Evidence informed decision-making is best practice.
- To enable evidence informed decision-making and delivery of best practice, evidence must:
  - o be described and presented in a format applicable to nurses
  - o reflect older people's and nurses' values
  - o be demonstrable in a range of practice contexts.
- The Caledonian Improvement Model includes all these elements and impacts positively on nursing practice with older people.

References

Aiken L, Patrician P (2000) Measuring organizational traits of hospitals: the revised Nursing Work Index. *Nursing Research* **49**, 146–153.

Andrews J, Manthorpe J, Watson R (2004) Involving older people in intermediate care. *Journal of Advanced Nursing* **46**, 303–310.

Australian Commission on Safety and Quality in Health Care (2009) *Preventing Falls and Harm From Falls in Older People: Best Practice Guidelines for Australian Hospitals, Residential Aged Care Facilities and Community Care.* www.safetyandquality.gov.au/internet/safety/publishing. nsf/Content/FallsGuidelines (accessed 14 February 2010).

Booth J, Leadbetter A, Francis M, Tolson D (2005) Implementing a best practice statement in nutrition for frail older people. *Nursing Older People* **16**, 26–28.

Booth J, Tolson D, Hotchkiss R, Schofield I (2007) Using action research to construct national evidence-based nursing care guidance for gerontological nursing. *Journal of Clinical Nursing* **16**, 945–953.

Breu K, Hemingway C (2002) Collaborative processes and knowledge creation in Communities of Practice. *Creativity and Innovation Management* **11**, 147–153.

Brown J, Duguid P (2001) Knowledge and organization: a social practice perspective. *Organization Science* **12**, 198–213.

Buggy T, Andrew N, Tolson D, McGhee M (2004) Evolution of a virtual Practice Development College for nurses. *ITIN. Journal of the British Computer Society Nursing Specialist Group* **16**, 4–11.

Davies S, Nolan M (2003) Learning from experience. *Quality in Ageing: Policy, Practice and Research* **4**, 2–5.

Day J, Higgins I, Koch T (2009) The process of practice redesign in delirium care for hospitalised older people: a participatory action research study. *International Journal of Nursing Studies* **46**, 13–22.

Department of Health (2008) *Darzi Report: High Quality Care for All: Next Stage Review, Final Report*. The Stationery Office, London.

Dopson S (2007) A view from organizational studies. *Nursing Research* **56** (4S), S72–S77.

Dowding D, Spilsbury K, Thompson C, Brownlow R, Pattenden J (2009) The decision making of heart failure specialist nurses in clinical practice. *Journal of Clinical Nursing* **18**, 1313–1324.

Elmore R (2003) A plea for strong practice. *Educational Leadership* **61**, 6–10.

Ely J, Osheroff J, Ebell M *et al.* (1999) Analysis of questions asked by family doctors regarding patient care. *British Medical Journal* **319**, 358–361.

Gabbay J, Le May A (2004) Evidence based guidelines or collectively constructed mindlines? Ethnographic study of knowledge management in primary care. *British Medical Journal* **329**, 1013–1018.

Grimshaw J, Thomas R, MacLennan G *et al.* (2004) Effectiveness and efficiency of guideline dissemination and implementation strategies. *Health Technology Assessment* **8** (6).

Hamm RM (1988) Clinical intuition and clinical analysis: expertise and the cognitive continuum. In: Dowie J, Elstein AS (eds) *Professional Judgment: A Reader in Clinical Decision Making.* Cambridge University Press, Cambridge, pp. 78–105.

Henri F, Pudelko B (2003) Understanding and analysing activity and learning in virtual communities. *Journal of Computer Assisted Learning* **19**, 474–487.

Holter IM, Schwartz-Barcott D (1993) Action research: what is it? How has it been used and how can it be used in nursing? *Journal of Advanced Nursing* **18**, 298–304.

International Continence Society (2009) *Fourth International Consultation on Incontinence* Health Publications Ltd, Paris.

Kelly T, Tolson D, Schofield I, Booth J (2005a) Describing gerontological nursing: an academic exercise or prerequisite for progress? *International Journal of Older People Nursing* **14**, 1–11.

Kelly T, Lowndes A, Tolson D (2005b) Advancing stages of group development: the case of virtual nursing community of practice groups. *Groupwork* **15**, 17–38.

Kelly T, Tolson D, Schofield I, Booth J (2006) The use of online groups to involve older people in influencing care guidance. *Groupwork* **16**, 69–94.

Kitson A, Harvey G, McCormack B (1998) Enabling the implementation of evidence-based practice: a conceptual framework. *Quality in Health Care* **7**, 149–158.

Lave J, Wenger E (1991) *Situated Learning: Legitimate Peripheral Participation.* Cambridge University Press, Cambridge.

Lowndes A, Smith J, Tolson D, Buggy T (2007) Evolution of a virtual practice development college for nurses (stage 2). *ITIN. Journal of the British Computer Society Nursing Specialist Group* **18**, 8–13.

McCaughan D (2002) What decisions do nurses make? In: Thompson C, Dowding D (eds) *Clinical Decision-making and Judgement in Nursing.* Churchill Livingstone, Edinburgh, chapter 6.

May C, Finch T (2009) Implementation, embedding, and integration: an outline of Normalization Process Theory. *Sociology* **43**, 535–554.

Michaels C, McEwan M, McArthur D (2008) Saying 'no' to professional recommendations: client values, beliefs, and evidence-based practice. *Journal of the American Academy of Nurse Practitioners* **20**, 585–589.

Michie S, Johnston M, Abraham C, Lawton R, Parker D, Walker A (2005) Making psychological theory useful for implementing evidence based practice : a consensus approach. *Quality Safety in Health Care* **14**, 26–33.

Miller M, Kearney N (2004) Guidelines for clinical practice: development, dissemination and implementation. *International Journal of Nursing Studies* **41**, 813–821.

NHS Quality Improvement Scotland (2004) *Best Practice Statement: Working with Older People Towards Prevention and Early Detection Of Depression*. NHSQIS, Edinburgh.

NHS Quality Improvement Scotland (2005a) *Best Practice Statement: Working with Older People Towards Promoting Movement and Physical Activity*. NHSQIS, Edinburgh.

NHS Quality Improvement Scotland (2005b) *Best Practice Statement: Working with Dependent Older People to Achieve Good Oral Health*. NHSQIS, Edinburgh.

NHS Quality Improvement Scotland (2005c) *Best Practice Statement: Maximising Communication with Older People Who Have Hearing Disability*. NHSQIS, Edinburgh.

National Institute for Clinical Excellence (2004) The assessment and prevention of falls in older people. Royal College of Nursing, London.

National Institute for Clinical Excellence (2010) *Delirium: prevention, diagnosis and management*. NICE, London.

Nolan M, Davies S, Brown J (2006) Transitions in care homes: towards relationship-centred care using the 'Senses Framework'. *Quality in Ageing* **7**, 5–15.

Nursing and Midwifery Council (2009) Guidance for the care of older people. Available at www.nmc-uk.org/aDisplayDocument.aspx?DocumentID=5593 (accessed 16 February 2009).

Nursing and Midwifery Practice Development Unit (2002) *Nutrition for Physically Frail Older People. Best Practice Statement*. NMPDU, Edinburgh.

Nutley S, Walter I, Davies HTO (2003) From knowing to doing: a framework for understanding the evidence-into-practice agenda. *Evaluation* **9**, 125–148.

Pawson R, Tilley N (1997) *Realistic Evaluation*. Sage Publications, London.

Pearson A, Wiechula R, Court A, Lockwood C (2007) A re-consideration of what constitutes 'evidence' in the healthcare professions. *Nursing Science Quarterly* **20**, 85–88.

Peters E, Hess T, Vastfjall D, Auman C (2007) Adult age differences in dual information processes. *Perspectives on Psychological Science* **2**, 1–23.

Rashotte J, Carnevale F (2004) Medical and nursing clinical decision making: a comparative epistemological analysis. *Nursing Philosophy* **5**, 160–174.

Redelmeier DA, Ferris L, Tu V, Hux J, Schull M (2001) Problems for clinical judgement: introducing cognitive psychology as one more basic science. *Canadian Medical Association Journal* **164**, 358–360.

Robertson R, Jochelson K (2006) *Interventions that Change Clinician Behaviour: Mapping the Literature*. Unpublished review commissioned by National Institute for Health and Clinical Excellence, London.

Rolfe G, Segrott J, Jordan S (2008) Tensions and contradictions in nurses: perspectives of evidence-based practice. *Journal of Nursing Management* **16**, 440–451.

Rowat A, Lawrence M, Horsburgh D, Legg L, Smith LN (2009) Stroke research questions: a nursing perspective. *British Journal of Nursing* **18**, 100–5.

Rycroft-Malone J, Seers K, Titchen A, Harvey G, Kitson A, McCormack B (2004) What counts as evidence in evidence-based practice. *Journal of Advanced Nursing* **47**, 81–90.

Rycroft-Malone J, Fontenla M, Seers K, Bick D (2009) Protocol-based care: the standardisation of decision-making? *Journal of Clinical Nursing* **18**, 1490–1500.

Schofield I (2008) *A critical discourse analysis of how nurses understand and care for older patients with delirium in hospital*. PhD thesis. Glasgow Caledonian University, Glasgow.

Scottish Executive Health Department (2001) *Caring for Scotland: The Strategy for Nursing and Midwifery in Scotland*. The Stationery Office, Edinburgh.

Thompson C, Dowding D (eds) (2002) *Clinical Decision-making and Judgement in Nursing.* Churchill Livingstone, Edinburgh.

Tolson D, McAloon M, Schofield I, Hotchkiss R (2005) Progressing evidence based practice: an effective nursing model? *Journal of Advanced Nursing* **50**, 1–10.

Tolson D, Schofield I, Booth J, Kelly T, James L (2006) Constructing a new approach to developing evidence based practice. *World Views Evidence Based Practice* **3**, 62–72.

Tolson D, Booth J, Lowndes A (2008) Achieving evidence-based nursing practice: impact of the Caledonian Model. *Journal of Nursing Management* **16**, 682–691.

Wenger E (1998) *Communities of Practice: Learning, Meaning and Identity.* Cambridge University Press, Cambridge.

Wenger E, McDermott R, Snyder W (2002) *Cultivating Communities of Practice.* Harvard Business School Press, Boston.

Chapter 3

Understanding Relationships within Care

Jayne Brown, Yvonne Robb, Andrew Lowndes, Kathleen Duffy, Debbie Tolson and Mike Nolan

Our world does not consist of separate things but of the relationships we co-create.
Bradbury & Reason (2003)

Introduction

Practitioners working with older people, and nurses in particular, have often struggled to clearly articulate the goals of their care. Early pioneers of gerontological nursing, such as Doreen Norton (Norton *et al*. 1962), argued that nursing older people represented 'true nursing' and that it was an area of practice in which the profession should excel. However, following a major study of nurses working with older people some 20 years later, Wells (1980) considered that 'nurses do not know why they do what they do'. In other words, they lacked a model for delivering care, and an approach to their care that provided a sense of purpose and direction for their activities. Whilst at the time the same might have been true of nursing in general, stating clearly the goals of their care was a particular challenge for gerontological nurses, especially those working in non-acute settings.

Older people, and particularly frail older people, as much of this book will demonstrate, often experience age-related changes and have conditions that cannot be cured. As such many of their needs do not fit easily into a healthcare system that focuses primarily on acute illness, where the primary goal is cure and the restoration of function. Of course these are the goals of choice, when they are achievable, but for many older people they are not appropriate. Consequently, frail older people have often been portrayed as creating 'problems' for the system, being called 'bed blockers' when they cannot be discharged rapidly once the acute illness is over, or 'frequent flyers' when they require repeated admissions because they have been discharged too quickly before their often complex needs have been adequately addressed. Furthermore despite being highly skilled, work with older people is often seen as 'low tech' and has never been accorded particularly high status or value. Such tensions are long-standing and can be traced back to the emergence of our present-day healthcare system in the mid-19th century when the

Evidence Informed Nursing with Older People, First Edition. Edited by Debbie Tolson, Joanne Booth and Irene Schofield.
© 2011 Blackwell Publishing Ltd. Published 2011 by Blackwell Publishing Ltd.

acute curative medical model became the dominant philosophy (see Wilkin & Hughes 1987 for an excellent account). This largely remains the case today.

Consequently, such issues remain highly relevant, with major concerns about the quality of care older people receive in acute care settings being voiced both by nursing organisations (Royal College of Nursing 2008; Nursing and Midwifery Council 2009) and older people's organisations (Age Concern 2006; Help the Aged 2008). Indeed, as technology continues to provide ever more sophisticated 'cures' for once untreatable conditions, those older people who are not responsive to such interventions, and the nurses who care for them, are once more at risk of being marginalised by the healthcare system and society in general.

The aim of this chapter is to present an approach to care, 'relationship-centred care', and a way of applying it to practice, the 'Senses Framework', that seeks to create equal partnerships between practitioners, older people and their families so that the needs of each group is valued and seen as important. We begin with a brief consideration of the broader policy background before outlining the challenges in implementing such policy in the day-to-day reality of care delivery. We then explore some of the current policy goals such as promoting dignity in care, as well as the difficulties that practitioners experience in realising such aims.

Subsequently, the emergence of the Senses Framework is discussed, and the rest of the chapter turns attention to a major new development in the use of Senses in the form of the Profiles of Learning Achievements in Care Environments (PLACE) toolkit. This development is important in terms of driving cultural reforms within care healthcare settings in tune with the principles and values of gerontological nursing as described within Chapter 1.

Policy: turning principles into practice, rhetoric into reality

Policies, and the legislation and the practice guidance that flow from them, are the Government's way of stating the overall goals and direction of their activity. Policy addresses numerous areas and takes many forms, but in the present context we are primarily concerned with those health and social care policies that impact on the experiences of older people and their family carers. Even if we confine attention to these areas, the issues involved are complex and extend beyond this chapter, and indeed this book as a whole. However, policy across the board poses similar challenges, the main one being how to translate often abstract ideas into something that can be applied in the real world.

It has long been recognised that policies deal in the language of 'general' principles (Henwood 1992) and that they focus on the needs of the population as a whole rather than those of specific individuals (Kendig & Brooke 1999). Practice, on the other hand, is much more about the 'preferences, resources and situations' of individuals (Kendig & Brooke 1999). In order to appeal to the public imagination (and some would say thereby win votes), governments tend to use 'buzzwords' (Gilloran *et al.* 1994) that promote their ideas as being inherently good (Williamson 1992). However, just because we all use these words does not mean that we define and understand them in the same way (Kellaher & Peace 1990). As Brechin (1998) argues, many of the words we use in both policy and practice are 'simple in their expression but highly complex to translate into behaviour'; in other words, they are 'easy to say, but far more difficult to do'. You can probably think of many such words but 'dignity' is a very topical one. Everyone would agree that providing older people with 'dignified' care is essential; in other words we see it as being an 'inherently' good goal (Williamson 1992). Similarly as 'dignity' is a word that we all use (Kellaher & Peace 1990), it might be assumed that it means the same thing to all of us. However, recent extensive reviews of the literature (Coventry 2006; Gallagher *et al.* 2008; Cass *et al.* 2009) have failed to find a common or shared meaning for dignity, and it is now widely recognised as being a highly complex idea; in other words, it is easy to say but far harder to achieve (Brechin 1998).

The major difficulty in translating policy into practice is that policies promote 'aspirational' visions without indicating how such aspirations can be achieved (Goodrich & Cornwell 2008). This is especially true of policy for frail older people and their family carers. To make matters worse policy is not always 'joined up'. For example, policy for older people and policy for family carers is often developed in isolation without considering the shared needs of both groups. To compound difficulties even policies for the same section of the population may not be developed in a similar fashion. For example, health and social care policies are not necessarily cohesive. Nevertheless, certain key ideas (buzzwords) have underpinned policy over the last 20 years or so. Of particular interest here are the notions of independence, autonomy, participation and partnerships.

Dalley (2000) argues that independence and autonomy have become the 'watchwords' of social policy (including healthcare) for successive governments, and that this is part of the emergence of a 'new language' of social policy based on ideas such as empowerment and participation (Bernard & Phillips 2000). These ideas reflect wider principles in the literature. Minkler (1996), for example, believes that 'empowerment' has been a unifying concept in the critical gerontology movement that aims to ensure equal status and rights for all older people, irrespective of their physical or mental frailty. Empowerment, she argues, should result in 'power with' or 'power to' older people rather than 'power over' older people. Such ideas lie at the heart of recent reforms to the NHS in the UK (Hodgson & Canvin 2005), with users and carers now being expected to play a much more active role, not only in determining individual treatment options, but also wider policy goals. The Labour Government's vision of creating a 'New NHS' (Department of Health 1997) was underpinned by the belief that services should be led by the aspirations of users and carers rather than by those of service providers. This was meant to herald a new approach to how the quality of care is determined, which in the past was seen to have paid too much attention to 'counting numbers, measuring activity, logging what could be logged' (Department of Health 1998), and consequently tended to ignore the needs of patients and carers. Since then the idea of patients and carers becoming active 'partners' in their care has been widely accepted and underpins the most recent Government initiatives, such as the Darzi review of the NHS (Department of Health 2008), and has also been incorporated into the standards of care for nurses working with older people (Nursing and Midwifery Council 2009).

The idea of people, especially those with long-term conditions, being partners in their care is not new and has long been promoted within the academic literature (see, for example, Corbin & Strauss 1991; Rolland 1994) based on the belief that such individuals know more about what it is like to live with a long-term condition than do the so-called expert practitioners. This has led to developments such as the expert patient programme in the NHS (Department of Health 2001). Similar principles have also been applied to family carers who, it is suggested, should be viewed as 'co-experts' in the care of frail older people in need of support (Nolan *et al.* 1996).

Therefore, whilst the principle of working in partnership is well accepted, there is still the challenge of making such ideas work in practice. For this to happen there needs to be far greater recognition of the differing forms of knowledge and expertise that are needed to provide a complete understanding of the complex needs of older people and their carers. For example, current ideas about what constitutes evidence for healthcare practice too often place 'research' evidence, produced by experts using certain, usually experimental, approaches, at the top of the hierarchy. Such 'evidence' is seen as being superior to other ways of 'knowing' the world which are based on personal experience or intuition; a fuller discussion of such issues can be found in Chapter 2 and in Nolan *et al.* (2007).

However, there is now growing recognition of the need to draw upon both the 'abstract' knowledge of practitioners and the 'personal' knowledge of users (Barnes 1999), in order to generate insights that help to bring together the psychological and experiential aspects of illness with the physical consequences (Evans 1999). A fuller understanding of the complex needs of people with long-term conditions will only be achieved when we utilise the 'outsider' expertise of practitioners and the 'insider' expertise of older people and their family carers. Achieving this raises questions about the current importance attached to ideas such as independence and autonomy.

Towards relationship-centred care

Policies promoting partnerships, participation and empowerment, and the acknowledgement of differing forms of knowledge and expertise are essential to the provision of high-quality care and support for older people and their families and this suggests that the promotion of autonomy and independence may not be appropriate goals. Indeed, there is considerable debate and disagreement in this area. For some people only the absolute empowerment of users and carers is an appropriate goal, whereas others argue that partnerships have to be based on the recognition that each person brings something of value and that every contribution is equally important (see Nolan *et al.* 2007 for a fuller discussion). Our belief is that the latter of these two positions is the correct one and that if older people and their families, especially those who are very frail, are to participate fully, then nurses may have to assist them to do so. Liaschenko (1997), for example, argues that nurses need to bring together several types of knowledge.

- *Case knowledge*, i.e. knowledge about a particular condition, for example stroke.
- *Patient knowledge*, i.e. about an individual's circumstances such as their home environment, the availability of family support and so on.
- *Person knowledge*, i.e. about an individual's life history, biography and particular needs, preferences and aspirations.

Similarly Griffin (1997) suggests that nurses need to draw upon several types of knowledge to ensure the best possible care.

- *Structural knowledge*: about the way that health and social care systems work.
- *Communicative knowledge*: about the type of language used between people. This not only refers to a patient's 'native' language, but also the use of technical jargon and so on.
- *Cultural knowledge*: about the wider belief systems of differing groups.
- *Social knowledge*: of a given individual and their background.

The way that practitioners 'blend' these differing types of knowledge largely determines how complete an understanding is achieved (Harvath *et al.* 1994). However, if such 'blending' is to become part of skilled practice, then such 'work' needs to be seen as important. There is now widespread concern, both amongst nursing groups and older people's organisations, that currently the emphasis is largely given to the 'acquisition of technical skills' that are needed to 'fix' conditions, to the detriment of the interpersonal and relational aspects of care (Goodrich & Cornwell 2008; Help the Aged 2008; Royal College of Nursing 2008; Nursing and Midwifery Council 2009). Over a decade ago Davies (1998) argued that one of the greatest intellectual challenges for the future was to create a new alliance between competence (in a technical sense) and caring (in a relational sense). For this to occur, Brechin (1998a,b) contended that caring requires practitioners to achieve the appropriate balance between dependence, independence and interdependence.

Several people have argued that the emphasis now placed on independence and autonomy potentially creates an image of the 'super-aged', which many frail older people cannot hope to achieve (Feldman 1999), and that what is needed is a better understanding of 'ordinary' ageing (Coleman 1997) if we are to promote realistic goals for the majority of older people. This will require a greater recognition of the interdependence that underpins relationships within healthcare settings (Nolan *et al.* 2004) if advances in technological treatments is not to be at the expense of care at a fundamentally human level (Youngson 2007, 2008).

Encouragingly, there is now growing recognition of the importance of attending to the 'social' processes that shape the healthcare experience (Goodrich & Cornwell 2008), and of the need to prevent the 'clinical and technical' dimensions of care eclipsing the 'human and organisational' (Bate *et al.* 2008). However, whilst there is an emerging consensus in this area, the challenge remains of how to ensure that such ideals are translated into practice. For this to happen we have to move beyond the language of general principles (Henwood 1992) and to present potentially complex ideas in a way that is 'ordinary, accessible, jargon free and commonly understood' (Goodrich & Cornwell 2008). It is here that we believe the Senses Framework has much to offer.

The Senses Framework

The Senses Framework was originally suggested in 1997 (Nolan 1997) and has been developed over a number of years (Davies *et al.* 1999; Nolan *et al.* 2001, 2006; Brown 2006; Brown *et al.* 2007, 2008). Its initial purpose was to provide some therapeutic direction for staff working in long-term care settings, especially care homes. Such environments have never been highly regarded and staff who work there have not been accorded the status they deserve.

Because of the curative orientation of modern day healthcare, and the dominance of the medical model, frail older people who cannot be cured or rehabilitated have tended to be provided with little other than 'aimless residual care' (Evers 1991) or 'good geriatric care' (Reed & Bond 1991), where the main aim is to keep people fed and clean. However, Nolan (1997) argued that work with such people was in fact highly complex and required specialist skills, much as Norton had argued over 40 years ago (Norton *et al*. 1962). He suggested that staff working in care homes should create an environment in which older people experience six senses:

- sense of security
- sense of belonging
- sense of continuity
- sense of purpose
- sense of achievement
- sense of significance.

However, he also believed that if staff were to create these Senses for others, then they had to experience the Senses for themselves. As the framework was developed, it was clear that the Senses also applied to staff and older people in acute care settings, and that family carers needed to experience the Senses as well (see Davies *et al*. 1999; Nolan *et al*. 2001). Following several detailed studies the Senses were defined as shown in Table 3.1.

Further work also demonstrated that if student nurses were to enjoy work with older people, and to select this area as a future career option, then they also needed to experience the Senses themselves (Nolan *et al*. 2002; Brown 2006; Brown *et al*. 2007, 2008). A care environment in which all groups experience the Senses has been termed an 'enriched' environment (Nolan *et al*. 2002) and is one in which the best care is likely to be delivered, and staff are more likely to experience high levels of job satisfaction and morale. This is captured in the matrix shown in Table 3.2.

As the matrix suggests, the Senses Framework is underpinned by ideas of 'interdependence' rather than independence and highlights the importance of relationships within and between people. It was therefore argued that concepts such as person-centred care, which focus mainly on the needs of the patient, do not fully capture such interactions and that relationship-centred care was a better model to adopt (see Nolan *et al*. 2004). The term 'relationship-centred care' was originally used by a major task force in the USA (Tresolini and the Pew-Fetzer Taskforce 1994) who were searching for a model of care delivery that better reflected the needs of people with long-term conditions. The Taskforce argued that the current system placed too much emphasis on acute illness and cure, whereas the major health challenges of the future are posed by individuals with ongoing needs. A similar set of beliefs underpin the Senses Framework and, whilst the two ideas were developed entirely independently, they share many of the same principles.

Recently, Youngson (2007, 2008) has made an essentially similar set of arguments in promoting compassion as the key to better health services. He argues that there is a need for a move away from a health service based on 'fixing' things, where the goal is to

Table 3.1   The six Senses in the context of caring relationships.

A sense of security	
For older people	Attention to essential physiological and psychological needs, to feel safe and free from threat, harm, pain and discomfort. To receive competent and sensitive care
For staff	To feel free from physical threat, rebuke or censure. To have secure conditions of employment. To have the emotional demands of work recognised and to work within a supportive but challenging culture
For family carers	To feel confident in knowledge and ability to provide good care (to do caring well; Schumacher *et al.* 1998) without detriment to personal well-being. To have adequate support networks and timely help when required. To be able to relinquish care when appropriate
A sense of continuity	
For older people	Recognition and value of personal biography. Skilful use of knowledge of the past to help contextualise present and future. Seamless consistent care delivered within an established relationship by known people
For staff	Positive experience of work with older people from an early stage of career, exposure to good role models and environments of care. Expectations and standards of care communicated clearly and consistently
For family carers	To maintain shared pleasures/pursuits with the care recipient. To be able to provide competent standards of care, whether delivered by self or others, to ensure that personal standards of care are maintained by others, to maintain involvement in care across care environments as desired/appropriate
A sense of belonging	
For older people	Opportunities to maintain and/or form meaningful and reciprocal relationships, to feel part of a community or group as desired
For staff	To feel part of a team with a recognised and valued contribution, to belong to a peer group, a community of gerontological practitioners
For family carers	To be able to maintain/improve valued relationships, to be able to confide in trusted individuals to feel that you're not 'in this alone'
A sense of purpose	
For older people	Opportunities to engage in purposeful activity facilitating the constructive passage of time, to be able to identify and pursue goals and challenges, to exercise discretionary choice
For staff	To have a sense of therapeutic direction, a clear set of goals to which to aspire
For family carers	To maintain the dignity and integrity, well-being and 'personhood' of the care recipient, to pursue (re)constructive/reciprocal care (Nolan *et al.* 1996)
A sense of achievement	
For older people	Opportunities to meet meaningful and valued goals, to feel satisfied with one's efforts, to make a recognised and valued contribution, to make progress towards therapeutic goals as appropriate
For staff	To be able to provide good care, to feel satisfied with one's efforts, to contribute towards therapeutic goals as appropriate, to use skills and ability to the full
For family carers	To feel that you have provided the best possible care, to know you've 'done your best', to meet challenges successfully, to develop new skills and abilities
A sense of significance	
For older people	To feel recognised and valued as a person of worth, that one's actions and existence are of importance, that you 'matter'
For staff	To feel that gerontological practice is valued and important, that your work and efforts 'matter'
For family carers	To feel that one's caring efforts are valued and appreciated, to experience an enhanced sense of self

Source: adapted from Davies *et al.* (1999), Nolan (1997) and Nolan *et al.* (2001).

Table 3.2   Creating an 'enriched' care environment.

Senses \ Stakeholder	Older person	Staff	Family carers	Students
Security				
Belonging				
Continuity				
Purpose				
Achievement				
Significance				

Table 3.3   Factors promoting high-quality care for older people: people, place and processes.

Royal College of Nursing (2008)	Nursing and Midwifery Council (2009)
Place: the physical environment and culture of the organisation	**Place**: Is care managed and resourced effectively? Does the environment encourage an element of calculated risk?
People: attitudes and behaviours of others	**People:** Are they competent, assertive, reliable, empathic, compassionate?
Processes: nature and conduct of care activities	**Processes**: Is there open communication and partnerships between patients, colleagues and families?

provide a service, to one where the main aim is to be *of service* in order to create a 'healing' environment. Conceptualising what such an environment looks like is the next challenge, but we would assert that an 'enriched environment' as reflected by the Senses, captures the interdependency that Youngson promotes.

Interestingly, both the Royal College of Nursing (2008) and the Nursing and Midwifery Council (2009) have recently suggested similar models of care comprising three elements, which are again based on ideas of interdependence, as illustrated in Table 3.3. It is therefore the interactions that occur between the *place* in which care is delivered, the *people* involved and the *processes* that they employ that shape the nature and quality of the care experience. If true partnerships are to be created then nurses need a way of ensuring that all parties learn from each other. It is here that the Profile of Learning Achievements in Care Environments (PLACE) has a potentially important role to play.

Research case: the PLACE (Profile of Learning Achievements in Care Environments) project

W.B. Yeats (1865–1939), the dramatist and poet, is credited with saying that 'education is not the filling of a pail but the lighting of a fire'. In a few words Yeats captures the need to inspire a learner's passion for a subject, whilst also suggesting that it is not the quantity but the quality of the learning experience that is paramount. This widely used quote can be applied to any situation in which learning takes place, and within environments where older people are cared for it captures the importance of igniting a learner's passion for the specialty, whether the learners are students, care workers, qualified staff or indeed older people and their family carers.

The learning needs of staff in healthcare environments are commonly assessed during performance appraisal, and have often been met by them undertaking courses away from the workplace. However, there is an increasing move towards work-based learning for staff of all grades, and a need to further understand how they perceive their learning needs to be met within individual care settings. Moreover, staff are not the only group that have learning needs within the care environment, and greater attention should also be given to the needs of older people and family carers, especially with regard to the most effective ways of giving and receiving of information. However, poor communications in healthcare is one of the most frequently voiced concerns of older people and family carers and the ways in which learning needs are met for this group within specific care environments could help to facilitate more effective communications.

The research with student nurses that we referred to earlier (Nolan *et al.* 2002; Brown 2006; Brown *et al.* 2007, 2008) not only demonstrated that the students enjoyed working with older people in care environments where the Senses were created, but also identified straightforward and practical ways in which ward staff might create such an 'enriched environment'. For example, a sense of belonging was created for students who were expected on placement and they received a welcome letter prior to their arrival. Traditionally, institutions of higher education have audited student placements to ensure that they provide the range of learning resources and experiences to meet students' learning needs and student satisfaction questionnaires have been used to monitor their perceptions and experiences of placements. However, it was evident from our research over a number of years that healthcare professionals, older patients and family carers relied on one another to fulfil their individual learning needs. So, for example, a student nurse may work with a care assistant learning to provide essential care or ask an older person if they can describe their care as part of their course; a family carer may learn about stoma care from a nurse, and placement staff may learn from a student who shares an article with them. Our research also demonstrated that the Senses, and subsequently an enriched environment of care and learning, could only be created for students when such an environment was also created for staff, older patients and family carers. What was less clear was how managers could gauge if the learning needs of staff, older patients, family carers, and students were being met. With this in mind the aim of the PLACE project was to develop a toolkit that would tap into the nature of an 'enriched' learning environment from multiple perspectives. The toolkit was intended to capture areas of success and achievement in creating an enriched learning environment as well as highlighting areas in need of improvement in a wide range of care settings.

Developing toolkits: achieving the Senses

As it was felt that the learning needs of each group (older people, family carers, nurses, care assistants and student nurses), would be related but different it was decided that the toolkit should contain five questionnaires, one for each group. As we have discussed earlier the concept of empowerment and the idea of patients and carers becoming active partners now lie at the heart of government health policy; and these concepts were also central to this work. This study was designed to give an opportunity for all voices to be heard and therefore all groups including older people and their family carers were actively involved as equal partners in developing the PLACE toolkit. In order to do this we used a research approach that engaged all stakeholder groups in generating the relevant questionnaires: the Event Frequency Approach (Faulkner *et al.* 2006) (for a more detailed discussion of the way in which this approach was used in the PLACE project see Brown *et al.* 2009).

We held focus groups and individual interviews with family carers ($N = 30$), older people ($N = 30$), nurses ($N = 30$) and care assistants ($N = 30$) about their teaching and learning needs and the factors which acted as barriers and facilitators to that learning in medical, surgical, continuing care, inpatient, outpatient and community settings We then extracted the statements which directly related to the teaching and learning needs of each group from those interviews. We had already undertaken extensive interviews with students (Brown 2006; Nolan *et al.* 2006) and were able to use these to extract statements relating to students learning needs. The statements from all of the interviews reflected the Senses and were grouped accordingly. This gave us five lists of statements, all over 100 items long, generated by each group of learners, from which to develop the questionnaires. Obviously, questionnaires of over 100 items are not practical and so we had to find a way of discovering which of the statements were the most important. We did this by asking groups of 30 older people, family carers, qualified nurses, care assistant and student nurses to rank the statements in order of importance. This enabled us develop much shorter questionnaires that represented the most important statements for each group.

What we found

The relationships and interdependency between the groups was evident in the interviews and it was clear that participants were unable to consider their own learning and information needs without considering those of others. Nurses and care assistants clearly thought that what they did to facilitate learning for others was as important as the factors needed to support their own learning. For example, the item in the care assistant questionnaire 'Training is offered to me in a way that is comfortable to me' clearly addresses the needs of the care assistant as learner. However, the item 'I have a role in helping students understand what we are doing' addresses the learning of others. Whilst the items in the student nurse questionnaire focused mostly on their own learning needs, the importance of good relationships with staff, patients and family carers was highlighted. For example in the item 'I get to go on my break with members of the team', students are indicating their wish to feel part of the team; and the item 'Older patients and family carers recognise the contribution of students' shows how much they value the views of older people and family carers. Similarly, while family carers are keen to have their need for information met, they also wish to provide information to staff to facilitate caregiving (e.g. 'Staff involve me in decision-making about my relative's care'), and older people also thought it important to provide staff with information (e.g. 'Staff asked me about my home circumstances').

Table 3.4 The Senses in the context of place, people and processes.

	Place: physical environment and culture of the organisation, resources, effective management, encourage calculated risk	*People*: attitudes and behaviours. People being competent, assertive, reliable, empathetic and compassionate	*Processes*: nature and conduct of care. Communication and partnerships between patients, staff and families
Older people	It was clear who was in charge	Staff relieved my concerns about being here	I was encouraged to interact with other patients
Family carers	I feel that the environment is conducive to good care	My attempts to make things easier for staff are recognised	The routine of care is flexible enough to meet the wishes of my relative
Nurses	I have access to a resource room	I get the opportunity to use and develop a variety of skills	I feel supported in dealing with grieving families
Care assistants	I get to spend quality time with patients	I feel able to motivate and encourage patients when I am giving care	Staff tell me when I have done a good job
Student nurses	If I challenge practice I will still be supported by placement staff	I know where I stand with a mentor, the boundaries are clear	The link tutor from the university comes regularly to talk issues through with me

The interviews conducted as part of the PLACE project have shown that the creation of the Senses for a given individual is important in promoting learning in a care environment with every Sense being represented in each questionnaire. We also learnt more about the Senses Framework itself in the completion of this research. Firstly, it was evident that how the Senses are created in a learning environment was influenced by the interactions of the three elements of place, person and process described earlier (Royal College of Nursing 2008; Nursing and Midwifery Council 2009). In Table 3.4, examples of statements from each group are mapped onto these three elements.

It also become evident that the creation of the Senses is contextual; that is to say, what creates a Sense for one group of people in a given situation varies from what creates that Sense for the same group in another context or for a different group in the same context. Once again this is influenced by the care being given (process), the person giving the care (people) and where the care occurs (place). This can be best illustrated if we look at a single Sense and what creates that Sense for each group (examples of what creates a sense of continuity are outlined in Table 3.5). From this we can see that the factors that create a sense of continuity are very different for each group. However, all the statements reflect feelings about bringing together the past, present and future and connecting significant places like home or university with the experience of the care environment, and connecting significant people and organisations to members of the groups, such as university tutors with students, family members with patients, linking placements with universities

Table 3.5   Factors creating a sense of continuity for different groups.

Older people	I was given relevant information prior to discharge
	Staff asked me about my home circumstances
Family carers	Staff discuss the options available for the future care of my relative with me
	Staff members are able to discuss my relative's care with me
	I see the same staff members on a regular basis
Nurses	Relationships with other care agencies are strong
	I feel able to make time to provide family carers with information about their relative's condition
	I feel able to apply material from courses to clinical practice
Care assistants	I get to know the patient as a person by learning about their life
	I try to find out about patients likes and dislikes
Student nurses	My mentor and the senior nurse on the placement have a good working relationship with the university link tutor
	Placement staff have recent experience of education and value learning

Table 3.6   The relative importance of the Senses for differing groups.

	Security	Belonging	Continuity	Purpose	Achievement	Significance
Older people	44%	11%	11%	6%	6%	22%
Family carers	30%	13%	13%	3%	7%	33%
Nurses	17%	7%	10%	37%	10%	17%
Care assistants	6%	12%	3%	45%	9%	24%
Student nurses	25%	25%	8%	17%	8%	17%

and care provider organisations with one another. In this way a sense of continuity high-lights the interdependency not only of individuals within the care environment but also to people's wider social networks and draws attention to the way in which relationships between organisations impact.

We have indicated that all the Senses were relevant to creating an enriched learning environment for each group. However, it was evident that some of the Senses were of greater importance to some groups than to others, and in developing the questionnaires we were careful to ensure that the balance amongst the Senses in each questionnaire accurately reflected the balance in the interview data. So, for example, 44% of the statements extracted from the interviews with older people concerned a sense of security, and so we ensured that this was reflected in the relevant questionnaire. Table 3.6 shows the percentage of each questionnaire related to each Sense by group.

Interestingly, for those people who are relatively brief visitors and are largely 'passing through' a care environment (i.e. older people, family carers and students), a sense of security figures prominently, and is the most important sense for older people and students.

This has intuitive appeal as such groups are likely to feel the most vulnerable. Students also accord a sense of belonging great value and this again captures their need quickly to feel 'part of things' within an established team. Tellingly, for carers it is a sense of significance that matters most and this reflects the wider literature, which indicates that family carers' needs are often overlooked by staff in all care environments (see Hanson *et al.* 2006). On the other hand, for more permanent staff it is a sense of purpose that is most important and again this is indicative of the work we cited earlier highlighting the challenges that gerontological nurses face in stating clearly what they do and why. A sense of achievement figured rather less prominently but a sense of significance mattered to all groups. Therefore whilst the Senses were never intended to be hierarchical, prior work with students showed that some Senses were more important at differing points in time, for example a sense of security and belonging were very important to students at the start of their training but tailed off as they became more confident during training, only to emerge to the fore again upon qualification (Brown 2006; Brown *et al.* 2007, 2008). The current work would suggest that changes in the importance of the senses applies to all groups, further reinforcing their contextual nature.

Summary

We have based this chapter on the belief that when working with frail older people the best care is most likely to be experienced by all groups when an 'enriched' environment of care is created. In such an environment partnerships are valued and people recognise interdependency as one of the core values. This is a rather different approach to that promoted by models of person-centred care and current policy initiatives that are underpinned by notions of independence and autonomy (Department of Health 2009). We do not suggest this change in emphasis lightly and it is underpinned by 15 years of research that has actively involved older people, family carers and staff, nor is it simply a matter of using different words to say the same thing. The Senses are about changing the way that we think about working with older people and their carers and the PLACE project is the latest product of such thinking. We have yet to further develop and test the PLACE toolkit in practice but, as with other approaches that are based on the Senses – for example the Combined Assessment of Residential Environments (CARE) profiles (Faulkner *et al.* 2006) – PLACE potentially provides practitioners with a way of turning what might be 'aspirational' goals into a workable reality. Our experience tells us that the Senses speak to all the relevant groups in a language that is commonly understood but, as we have demonstrated, what creates the Senses is likely to vary by both group and care settings, as reflected in the interactions between place, people and processes. We view this as a strength rather than a weakness as it expands the application of the Senses to a wide range of care settings and potentially to client groups other than frail older people and their carers. We do not present a relationship-centred model of working as an alternative to a curative model; indeed we see the latter as essential when cure is achievable. However, the experience of acute care can be enhanced for everyone if the Senses are applied and in other contexts we believe that the Senses can provide the underpinning rationale for the care given.

Although we have been working with the Senses for some time now, the journey is only just beginning and we invite you to join us as together we develop such ideas further. Here are some things to think about.

Key messages

- Independence, autonomy and empowerment have become the watchwords of health and social policy. Government policy relates to abstract ideas and the challenge is turning that into action that can be applied in the real world.
- Relationships between people offer a way of working in partnership that is accessible and readily understood.
- An enriched environment of care (where partnerships are valued and people recognise interdependency as a core value) is created when the Senses are experienced by all groups.
- The Profiles of Learning Achievements in Care Environments (PLACE) project used the Senses Framework to develop a toolkit to capture the areas of success, and areas for improvement in creating an enriched learning environment from the perspective of a range of learners in equal partnership (older people, family carers, nurses, care assistants and student nurses).
- The PLACE toolkit offers a practical way of bringing the abstract concepts of empowerment and partnership working to the issues of teaching/learning, information giving and receiving in the care environment.

References

Age Concern (2006) Q is for Quality: The Voices of Older People on the Need for Better Quality Care and Support. Available at www.ageconcern.org.uk/AgeConcern/policy-QisforQualityreport. asp (accessed 8 January 2009).

Barnes M (1999) Public expectations: *From Paternalism to Partnership, Changing Relationships in Health and Health Services*. Policy Futures for UK Health, No. 10. Nuffield Trust, London.

Bate P, Mendel P, Robert G (2008) *Organizing for Quality: The Improvement Journeys of Leading Hospitals in Europe and the United States. Briefing Paper*. The Nuffield Trust, London.

Bernard M, Phillips J (2000) The challenge of ageing in tomorrow's Britain. *Ageing and Society* **20**, 33–54.

Bradbury H, Reason P (2003) Issues and choice points for improving the quality of action research. In: Minkler M, Wallerstein N (eds) *Community-Based Participatory Research for Health*. Jossey-Bass, San Francisco, CA.

Brechin A (1998a) Introduction. In: Brechin A, Walmsley J, Katz J, Peace S (eds) *Care Matters: Concepts, Practice and Research in Health and Social Care*. Sage, London, pp. 1–12.

Brechin A (1998b) What makes for good care? In: Brechin A, Walmsley J, Katz J, Peace S (eds) *Care Matters: Concepts, Practice and Research in Health and Social Care*. Sage, London, pp. 170–187.

Brown J (2006) *Student nurses' experience of learning to care for older people in enriched environments: a constructivist inquiry*. PhD Thesis, University of Sheffield.

Brown J, Nolan M, Davies S (2007) Bringing caring and competence into focus in gerontological nursing: a longitudinal, multi-method study. *International Journal of Nursing Studies* **45**, 654–667.

Brown J, Nolan M, Davies S, Nolan J, Keady J (2008) Transforming students' views of geronto-logical nursing: realising the potential of 'enriched' environments of learning and care. A multi-method longitudinal study. *International Journal of Nursing Studies* **45**, 1214–1232.

Brown J, Robb Y, Duffy K, Lowndes A (2009) Enhancing learning in care settings: the Profile of Learning Achievements in Care Environments (PLACE) project. *Quality in Ageing* **10**, 24–33.

Cass E, Robbins D, Richardson A (2009) Dignity in Care. Available at www.scie.org.uk/publications/guides/guide15/files/guide15.pdf.

Coleman P (1997) The last scene of all. *Generations Review* **7**, 2–5.

Corbin JM, Strauss A (1991) A nursing model of chronic illness management based upon the Trajectory Framework. *Scholarly Inquiry for Nursing Practice* **5**, 155–174.

Coventry ML (2006) Care with dignity: a concept analysis. *Journal of Gerontological Nursing* **32**, 42–48.

Dalley G (2000) Defining difference: health and social care for older people. In: Warnes A, Warren L, Nolan M (eds) *Care Services for Later Life: Transformations and Critiques*. Jessica Kingsley, London.

Davies C (1998) Caregiving, carework and professional care. In: Brechin A, Walmsley J, Katz J, Peace S (eds) *Care Matters: Concepts, Practice and Research in Health and Social Care*. Sage, London, pp. 126–138.

Davies S, Nolan M, Brown J, Wilson F (1999) *Dignity on the Ward: Promoting Excellence in Care*. Help the Aged, London.

Department of Health (1997) *The New NHS, Modern Dependable*. The Stationery Office, London.

Department of Health (1998) *A First Class Service: Quality in the New NHS*. Department of Health, London.

Department of Health (2001) *National Service Framework for Older People*. The Stationery Office, London.

Department of Health (2008) *Darzi Report: High Quality Care for All: Next Stage Review, Final Report*. The Stationery Office, London.

Department of Health (2009) *Shaping the Future of Care Together*. Department of Health, London.

Evans M (1999) *Ethics: Reconciling Conflicting Values in Health Policy*. Policy futures for UK Health, No. 9. Nuffield Trust, London.

Evers HK (1991) Care of the elderly sick in the UK. In: Redfern SJ (ed.) *Nursing Elderly People*. Churchill Livingstone, Edinburgh.

Faulkner M, Davies S, Nolan MR (2006) Development of the combined assessment of residential environments (CARE) profiles. *Journal of Advanced Nursing* **55**, 664–677.

Feldman S (1999) Please don't call me 'dear': older women's narratives of health. *Nursing Inquiry* **6**, 269–276.

Gallagher A, Li S, Wainwright P, Rees Jones I, Lee D (2008) Dignity in the care of older people: a review of the theoretical and empirical literature. *BMC Nursing* **7**, 11.

Gilloran A, McGlew T, McKee K, Robertson A, Wight D (1994) Measuring the quality of care in psychogeriatric wards. *Journal of Advanced Nursing* **18**, 269–275.

Goodrich J, Cornwell J (2008) *Seeing the Person in the Patient: The Point of Care Review*. The King's Fund, London.

Griffin F, Ndidi U (1997) Discovering knowledge in practice settings. In: Thorne SE, Hayes VE (eds) *Nursing Praxis: Knowledge and Action*. Sage, Thousand Oaks, CA, pp. 39–53.

Hanson E, Nolan J, Magnusson L (2006) *COAT: The Carers Outcome Agreement Tool. A New Approach to Working with Family Carers*. Getting Research into Practice (GRiP) Report No 1, University of Sheffield.

Harvath TA, Archbold PG, Stewart BJ (1994) Establishing partnerships with family caregivers: local and cosmopolitan knowledge. *Journal of Gerontological Nursing* **20**, 29–35.

Help the Aged (2008) *On Our Own Terms: The Challenge of Assessing Dignity in Care*. Help the Aged, London. Available at http://policy.helptheaged.org.uk.

Henwood M (1992) *Through a Glass Darkly: Community Care and Elderly People*. King's Fund Institute, London.

Hodgson P, Canvin K (2005) Translating health policy into research practice. In: Lowes L, Hulatt I (eds) *Involving Service Users in Health and Social Care Research*. Routledge, London.

Kellaher L, Peace S (1990) From respondent to consumer resident: shifts in approaches to quality assurance: the last decade. Paper given at BSG Annual Conference, University of Durham.

Kendig H, Brooke C (1999) Social perspectives on community nursing. In: Nay R, Garrat S (eds) *Nursing Older People: Issues and Innovations*. Maclennan and Petty, Sydney, pp. 40–63.

Liaschenko J (1997) Knowing the patient. In: Thorne SE, Hays VE (eds) *Nursing Praxis: Knowledge and Action*. Sage, Thousand Oaks, CA.

Minkler M (1996) Critical perspectives on ageing: new challenges for gerontology. *Ageing and Society* **16**, 467–487.

Nolan MR (1997) Health and social care: what the future holds for nursing. Keynote address at Third Royal College of Nursing Older Person European Conference and Exhibition, Harrogate.

Nolan M, Grant G, Keady J (1996) *Understanding Family Care: A Multidimensional Model of Caring and Coping*. Open University Press, Buckingham.

Nolan MR, Davies S, Grant G (2001) *Working with Older People and their Families: Key Issues in Policy and Practice*. Open University Press, Buckingham.

Nolan MR, Davies S, Brown J, Keady J, Nolan J (2002) *Longitudinal Study of the Effectiveness of Educational Preparation to Meet the Needs of Older People and Carers: The AGEIN Project*. English National Board, London.

Nolan MR, Davies S, Brown J, Keady J, Nolan J (2004) Beyond 'person-centred' care: a new vision for gerontological nursing. *International Journal of Older People Nursing* **13**, 45–53.

Nolan MR, Brown J, Davies S, Nolan J, Keady J (2006) *The Senses Framework: Improving Care for Older People Through a Relationship-centred Approach*. Getting Research into Practice (GRIP) Series No. 2, University of Sheffield.

Nolan MR, Hanson E, Grant G, Keady J (2007) *User Participation in Health and Social Care Research: Voices, Values and Evaluation*. Open University Press, Buckingham.

Norton D, McLaren R, Exton-Smith AN (1962) *An Investigation of Geriatric Nursing Problems in Hospital*. National Corporation for the Care of Old People, reprinted in 1976 by Churchill Livingstone, London.

Nursing and Midwifery Council (2009) Guidance for the care of older people. Available at www.nmc-uk.org/aDisplayDocument.aspx?DocumentID=5593 (accessed 8 January 2009).

Reed J, Bond S (1991) Nurses assessment of elderly patients in hospital. *International Journal of Nursing Studies* **28**, 55–64.

Rolland JS (1994) *Families, Illness and Disability: An Integrative Treatment Model*. Basic Books, New York.

Royal College of Nursing (2008) *Defending Dignity: Challenges and Opportunities for Nursing*. Royal College of Nursing, London.

Schumacher KL, Stewart BJ, Archbold PG, Dodd MJ, Dibble SL (1998) Family caregiving skill: development of the concept. *Image: Journal of Nursing Scholarship* **30**, 63–70.

Tresolini CP and the Pew–Fetzer Task Force (1994) *Health Professions Education and Relation-ships-Centred Care: A Report of the Pew–Fetzer Task Force on Advancing Psychosocial Education*. Pew Health Professions Commission, San Francisco.

Wells TS (1980) *Problems in Geriatric Nursing*. Churchill Livingston, Edinburgh.

Wilkin D, Hughes B (1987) Residential care of elderly people: the consumers' views. *Ageing and Society* **7**, 399–425.

Williamson C (1992) *Whose Standards? Consumer and Professional Standards in Health Care*. Open University Press, Buckingham.

Youngson R (2007) People-Centred Health Care. International Symposium on People-Centred Health Care: Reorientating Health Systems in the 21st Century. The Tokyo International Forum, 25 November.

Youngson R (2008) *Compassion in Healthcare: The Missing Dimension of Healthcare Reform?* The NHS Confederation. Available at www.debatepapers.org.uk (accessed 21 May 2009).

Chapter 4

Truth-Telling and the Evidence

Anthony Tuckett and Debbie Tolson

Introduction

In the preceding chapters we have explored the connections between the evidence base and gerontological nursing practice and promoted relational approaches. Our attention now turns to one of the key determinants of the trust that can develop between nurses and older people: truth-telling within care. Much of the evidence we use in this chapter comes from studies completed within Australian care homes. Generally, we take telling the truth as indicative of a person's integrity and moral standing: an honest person is someone we can trust to tell us the facts. Similarly, the way the older person perceives how the nurse speaks with them and what they say is inextricably linked to the concept of truth-telling.

An interest in telling the truth, and the practical complexities of lying and deception, begin for all of us in early childhood. It therefore follows that the evidence base for truth-telling is our shared experience and knowledge. Philosophers, ethicists, researchers and commentators across a range of disciplines and across time have concerned themselves with examining truth-telling, lying and deception in a number of contexts.

In this chapter, three core tenets are recommended as guides for truth-telling in practice.

(1) Do not confuse telling the truth with the abstract concept of seeking to understand the 'truth'. Intention is integral to the former whereas the latter is a nebulous concept.
(2) Do not assume what an older person wants to know, nor assume what is important for them. Ask them.
(3) Do not make assumptions about truth-telling based on race, nationality or language and always ask the person how informed he or she wishes to be.

Communication in the relationship

Communication is the basis of our relationships with people and it is recognised that nurse communication behaviours exert a powerful influence on the views older people form about them and on the development of trust. Citing Wilmot's five-point model

Evidence Informed Nursing with Older People, First Edition. Edited by Debbie Tolson, Joanne Booth and Irene Schofield.
© 2011 Blackwell Publishing Ltd. Published 2011 by Blackwell Publishing Ltd.

(Wilmot 1995), Tuckett (2005) describes relationships and communication as symbiotic in that each gives form and adds to the development of the other. It follows that the relationships which develop between the older person and the nurse are influenced by their shared communications and their individual perception of the relationship they have with each another. Tuckett (2005) goes on to to explore the link between the context of care and the organisational culture in terms of defining and shaping developing relationships. This means that relationships are contextualised by the care setting and that communication behaviours of the nurse are in part a function of the caring culture. With the exception of brief isolated contacts, as might occur during emergency triage, it is important to remember that 'relationships are not static, linear processes' but are continually renegotiated and influenced through power dimensions and degrees of intimacy or closeness (Euswas & Chick 1999). In Nussbaum's (1990, 1991) explorations of interactions between older people and nursing aides, both identified friendship as an important determinant within the caring relationship. Interestingly, the staff group were more concerned with achieving efficiency and control than developing a close bond.

Information sharing or not sharing is one way in which people can exert control over others. Several authors suggest that in the care environment the management of information or failure to inform people about their healthcare is an issue primarily about control (Tuckett 2005). Parathian and Taylor (1993) acknowledge that even though some patients want more information from nursing staff, socialisation processes that govern information disclosure may inhibit them from asking. Furthermore, their research suggests that nurses have a tendency not to invite patients to ask questions, which may be linked with perceived divisions of labour and responsibilities within healthcare. Kendall (1995) agrees with this analysis and highlights the tension this creates between the desire to be honest with people and a reluctance to disclose information perceived to belong to medicine. Such imposed censorship of information due to issues of professional identity creates a dilemma that undermines relational aspects of care.

Information disclosure is one aspect of communication central to the development of trust; another important dimension is the *how* of communication. It is not uncommon for studies within hospitals and care homes to report that staff direct admission enquiries and information giving to accompanying or visiting relatives rather than the older person (Nussbaum 1993). Patronising talk and oversimplification of the message is another strategy that deliberately or unintentionally restricts opportunity for meaningful conversation which may be interpreted as an act of disempowerment and control (Hummert & Morgan 2001). A failure to remediate sensory impairments, such as hearing loss (see Chapter 9), also serves to restrict communication opportunity and might also be interpreted in a similar vein and be seen as a non-caring act.

Codes of conduct

Codes of ethics for nurses in Australia (Australian Nursing and Midwifery Council 2008) and the UK (Nursing and Midwifery Council 2008) concur. That is, both codes variously guide the nurse to facilitate the person or family in their care to follow the path of self-determination or self-governance. In so doing, the nurse is guided to promote the person's autonomy. Consequently as guides, these codes both embrace truthfulness in the care encounter.

The Nursing and Midwifery Council (NMC) code of ethics for nurses and midwives, when advocating trust in the therapeutic relationship, specifically directs the nurse or midwife to be 'open and honest' which in turn means 'to treat peoples as individuals and respect their dignity'. Clearly enunciated, the code further states that the nurse or midwife 'must share with people, in a way they can understand, the information they *want* or need to know about their health' (our emphasis) (Nursing and Midwifery Council 2008). Just as the NMC code guides nurses towards open disclosure, so too does the Australian Nursing and Midwifery Council (ANMC) code.

The ANMC code comprises eight value statements. Not exhaustively analysed here, a number of these specifically guide the nurse to value:

- respect and 'recognise [the person's] capacity for active and informed participation in their own healthcare';
- the diversity of people and 'responding to their culture…[means responding] effectively to the cultural and communication needs of people in their care';
- 'processes for open disclosure [of adverse events] to persons affected during the course of their care'.

Honesty and information sharing

While information sharing is inextricably linked to perceptions of honesty within healthcare, Tuckett (2005) argues that nurses afford less value to both than patients do. Tuckett's literature review draws on a range of qualitative and quantitative studies to evidence his assertion. In this review it becomes clear that the evidence base is reliant on relatively small-scale pieces of research, and the findings which may appear contradictory need to be considered in relation to the specific characteristics of the people who participated in the various studies. In other words, caution is needed in making generalisations from isolated studies as the findings may be peculiar to the particular groups studied rather than applicable to the wider population of older people. As we now illustrate, despite this caution it is possible to take some key messages from research to guide nursing practice. In 1980 Casselith *et al.*, based on findings of a small study, contended that older people sought less detailed information, preferred less involvement in treatment decisions and 'wanted minimal or only good information'. This can be challenged by the seminal survey completed by Erde *et al.* (1988) which involved 224 general medical outpatients, the majority of whom wanted to be told a diagnosis of Alzheimer's disease. A later survey involving 156 older people living in the community also revealed a strong preference among respondents for being told if they had a diagnosis of either Alzheimer's disease or cancer (Holroyd *et al.* 1996). Interestingly, one-third of the sample stated that they did not want their spouse to be told if it were them (the husband or wife) who had been diagnosed with dementia. This creates a potential caring dilemma, in that a relative may ask the nurse not to disclose information to the person, but the person may desire this information and in many countries has a right to personal medical information about themselves.

A study by Maestri-Banks and Goseny (1997) reported that if asked not to disclose diagnostic information to an older person by relatives, that 56% of the sample nurses from older people's units would respect the wishes of the family.

More recently, Jenkins *et al.* (2001) surveyed over 3000 people living in the UK, 13% of whom were over the age of 70 years. They reported that older people preferred to leave the disclosure of a bad diagnosis such as cancer to the doctor and would like additional information and involvement in making decisions about their care. Ajaj *et al.* (2001) concur with this, reporting that 88% of their sample of 270 people aged between 65 and 94 years would like to be told about their health.

A study comparing older care home residents' perceptions of the most important caring behaviours with those of nurses, completed by Smith and Sullivan (1997), revealed some interesting differences between the two groups. A striking finding was that older people rated 'staff being honest with them' as one of the most important behaviours but this caring attribute did not appear in the top ten behaviours thought to be important by nurses. However, both nurses and older people highlighted the importance of listening to each other and using straightforward language. Tuckett *et al.* (2009) investigated the relative importance of caring behaviours among care home residents and nurses by asking them to rank items from a series of scales. In this study both residents and nurses rated 'explains and facilitates' as the least important subscale, and yet this subscale included items about being honest with the resident and telling them about their condition or illness and treatment prospects. From this Tuckett *et al.* (2009) reasonably concluded that is inappropriate to assume that all older people desire the same level of information and it is important for nurses to clarify an individual's preferences.

An evidence base of older people's perspectives on such an approach is illuminating. Tuckett (2007) revealed the care home as a place of suspicious awareness and mutual pretence. What does this mean? In the research findings, both the care providers and the older persons in residential aged-care spoke about family demanding of the care providers 'Don't tell Mum'. That is, both understood that family ask that information not be disclosed about the health of a relative/resident. Paradoxically, the care providers revealed that they knew residents often know anyway what is going on and the residents revealed their observing 'quiet conversations' and first hand experiencing family demanding 'Don't tell Mum'. Hence, the resident can be both suspicious about what is known and try to verify same and/or the resident and care provider pretend not to know what really is (mutual pretence) (Glaser & Strauss 1965).

Best interest and harm prevention

Explorations of how nurses and other health professionals behave in relation to sharing bad news with people provides fascinating insights into the assumptions that we so easily make in our practice. An extreme view is that we can be complicit in a paternalistic lie and withhold information under the guise of therapeutic privilege (Drickamer & Lachs 1992; Hebert 1994). A more reasonable view is that a reluctance to share bad news is perhaps understandable as it conflicts with our duty of benevolence and non-maleficence (Sidgwick 1966). Deception is thus justified as a way to protect (Pfiffner 1999) and avoid causing a patient unnecessary distress (Rosner *et al.* 2000).

Furthermore, in the absence of strong evidence nurses might reasonably rationalise that older people do not want to hear bad news (Reeder 1988; Sprigler 1996). Interestingly Bok's seminal work completed in the 1970s dismissed interpreting truth as harmful and not in the best interests of another's well-being as a rare phenomenon, unsubstantiated through evidence (Bok 1973). More recently, Wright *et al.* (2002) added to the growing literature endorsing Bok's position. As Tuckett (2005) concludes, if asked many patients want to know the truth and the evidence of the benefits of truth-telling on older people's quality of life in care homes (Barkay & Tabak 2002) and the positive impacts on well-being (Irurita 1999; Tuckett 2004) outweigh perceived risks (Gillian *et al.* 2000). In our earlier consideration of the scope of gerontological nursing, in our opening chapter, the goals of independence and personal autonomy were central to our practice model. Miettinen *et al.* (2001) contends that failure to be truthful to a person diminishes their opportunity to be autonomous and we would add that it would also undermine the quest for quality within gerontological nursing. Parathian and Taylor (1993) portray truth-telling in relation to equality and maintenance of competent adulthood. If we accept this view, we might also argue that truth-telling is integral to considerations of health inequalities in later life.

Cultural influences

In a review of international literature on truth-telling, Tuckett (2004) concluded that truth-telling practices and preferences emerge as a cultural artefact. In countries such as China a terminal illness is not generally discussed with the person, disclosure being the prerogative of the family (Ross *et al.* 2001). Blackhall *et al.* (1995) in their study of people aged 65 years and older found that Mexican-Americans and Korean-Americans were less likely than European-Americans and African-Americans to believe that older people with a serious life-limiting illness should be told the diagnosis and truth about their prognosis. Studies of physician interaction in Tuckett's (2004) review consistently show the influence of ethnicity on a person's beliefs about truthful diagnostic and prognostic honesty. For nurses, it is important to understand cultural influences on an older person and family carers' perceptions of truth-telling. It is equally also important to appreciate the changing views that occur across generations over time. As explained in Chapter 1, the international rights movements contends that older people have as much right to self-determination and dignity as their younger counterparts (United Nations 1991). This implies that failure to directly share the complete truth as it is known and understood with an older person, no matter how well intentioned, might currently be interpreted as a violation of their human rights.

A review of literature (Mystakikdou *et al.* 2004) to examine the cultural influences on the attitudes of healthcare professionals working with cancer patients and families towards truth-telling practices revealed that doctors in the USA, northern Europe and Anglo-Saxon countries tell the truth to both patients and their spouse. These authors contrast this with doctors from southern and eastern Europe, Africa, France, Iran, Panama, Japan, Singapore and Saudi Arabia who conceal the truth, adding however that there is an emerging trend in these nations towards disclosure. According to their review, nurses in the Netherlands, Spain and Greece are reluctant to reveal a cancer diagnosis to cancer patients. The familial influence in countries like Spain, Italy, Greece, Saudi Arabia, Egypt, Singapore, China and Japan means the family sanctions truth-telling to the patient, and disclosure of the cancer diagnosis is revealed to the family first (Mystakikdou *et al.* 2004). Specifically in Japan, the Professional Ethics Guidelines for Physicians provide guidance for doctors in the context of informed consent. The guidelines provide advice for both pathways: that is, on the one hand, advising to inform the patient and, on the other, not to inform the patient but to tell only the family (Akabayashi *et al.* 2006).

The consensus is that the majority of persons of western European background want to know their diagnosis and prognosis of serious illness. However, an established writer in this area provides the take-home wisdom: do not make assumptions based on race, nationality or language and, furthermore, ask the patient how informed he or she wishes to be (Surbone 2004). Two more recent studies support the 'do not make assumptions' about truth-telling view: firstly, research amongst oncology outpatients in Singapore demonstrated generally similar preferences with regard to communication of 'unfavourable news' as compared with patients in Western countries (Chiu *et al.* 2004); and, secondly, in a study to describe the disclosure preferences about serious illness of Korean-Americans, the conclusion was drawn that healthcare professionals need to determine the disclosure preferences about serious illness of older Korean-Americans and avoid stereotypical assumptions that do not apply to many in this population (Berkman & Eunjeong 2009).

Evidence informed understanding of truth-telling

Our analysis of truth-telling has so far shown that it is a complex area of practice that is contextualised by the care environment, rooted in our personal and professional beliefs, and influenced by ethical codes, communicative style and cultural interpretations. Our truth-telling behaviours are shaped by many subtle influences, the assumptions we make about others and professional socialisation processes that are difficult to disentangle and sometimes justify. The case study which follows provides insight into the complexity of studying truth-telling in nursing practice and draws on Tuckett's (2006) study of truth-telling from the perspective of the Australian registered nurse in the care home.

A research case

An overview of the study design is presented in Box 4.1. (The previously published text has been reproduced with permission of eContent Management.) An extract of narrative data is presented to exemplify what we can learn through such in-depth analytical work. In the extracts below we see how the clinical manager and registered nurse distinguish between truth and non-truth.

> *I guess the thing about truth-telling is that of the opposite that you're not telling the truth. It's telling lies. But there is truth-telling and there is sort of omitting pieces that you sort of feel again to be harmful or damaging or upsetting so it's more ... you're easing and omitting. And it sort of comes back to I guess to that truth-telling concept that it is what we don't say almost, that becomes kind of truth-telling or otherwise. You are not telling a lie, you're just not telling them all the pieces.* [Clinical manager]

Box 4.1   Research design overview

Primary purpose

To understand what care providers and residents in residential aged-care (nursing homes) think and feel about truth-telling in practice.

Objectives

- To understand what care providers and aged residents think and feel with regard to truth-telling in practice, and how they act on these.
- Reveal the conditions in which these understandings and actions occur.
- Examine the consequences of these beliefs, feelings and actions.

Conceptual framework

Social constructionism (Berger & Luckmann 1966; Crotty 1998) and symbolic interactionism (Mead 1934; Blumer 1969).

Type of research

Qualitative.

Methods

Group discussion, journaling, in-depth interview, field-notes.

Analysis

Thematic analysis informed by grounded theory (Strauss & Corbin 1998).

Research setting

Five residential aged-care facilities (nursing homes) in Queensland, Australia.

Participants

15 registered nurses, 23 personal care assistants, 19 residents.

Source: Tuckett (2006).

The registered nurses in the same group discussion gave support to this view, explaining that this meant 'you are not giving a whole story' and not giving 'all the truths'. A clear distinction is made in this nursing home context between truth-telling as telling a full-truth, and truth-telling as communicating a partial, edited or tempered truth. It is the latter understanding of truth which is operationalised and justified for benevolent reasons. The telling of an edited or 'minimised truth' was considered a 'reasonable' practice by another registered nurse at a follow-up interview.

> *Yes, I think that is reasonable. We're not going to say 'Look…Mum is dying. She's not going to be here forever', but 'She's deteriorating slowly…she's frail' etc. Yes, there is the gradual easing of people into the idea so they're not totally shocked when Mum…*

does die… We're not… hitting them over the head with it. I don't know that we omit enough that people will not get a true picture.

This registered nurse concurs, suggests 'easing and omitting' aims to prevent the burden associated with telling the truth. She also understands this titrated information, whilst not necessarily false, does not present all that is known. Agreeing with this understanding, another registered nurse (at nursing home B) added her own rationale for truth-telling as an edited or 'minimised truth'.

Like possibly they [we] leave out some information for a daughter who might be sensitive but tell the son everything. You still tell the truth but, or is it lying by deception? But sometimes when you know people well, not all they want to hear but what they can't cope with or what would be unnecessary and possibly cruel to tell them some things.

This registered nurse is ambivalent about her practice, questioning whether it may be 'lying by deception' to omit parts of the truth. Premised on the nurses' judgements about sensitivity to information, others admitted that parts of the 'whole picture' (disclosure) are often not revealed. A registered nurse manager suggested:

Yeah… So I guess they can't come back and say 'Well you didn't tell me the truth'. Well it's pretty well like 'Well I didn't tell on that bit'. I just didn't broach the subject because for one reason or another I felt that I shouldn't or I couldn't or it was perhaps unnecessary for them to know because it was a distress.

Here we find the claim that 'minimised' disclosure is not quite the same as an outright false utterance. A registered nurse (at nursing home E) articulated a similar understanding during the nurses' group discussion, suggesting they understand and operate from 'the basis of the truth' but agreeing with her colleague that in practice 'it is about what is not said, about omitting, that truth-telling is understood'. A registered nurse and nurse manger (in the D group) expressed a similar view, stating that 'failing to mention all of the truth' is in fact 'truth-telling by layers'. Truth-telling in practice, then, can be understood as stratal.

Forming a relationship with the resident's relative facilitates the registered nurses' 'judging' or 'gauging' of what should be told and how it should be told. As Carol explains:

You would be able to feel how much that relatives need to know, how much they could cope with at any given time and what they would comprehend.

In addition, Doris, a registered nurse (a team leader from nursing home D), is asked at interview about information being omitted. The researcher seeks to test his understanding by stating 'You omit to disclose to family an event or resident behaviour "gauged", "judged", to cause family upset and over which the family has no control. This event or behaviour will not impact on the resident's care plan'. The nurse responded:

I agree with that…it's sort of on a need to know basis…if it's an event that isn't really going to alter anything as far as the way we care for the resident…then the relatives don't need to know. Then yes, I think we would omit it.

Within the same follow-up interview, Doris explains what is meant by a 'need to know'. She draws a distinction between 'conditions and changes' which impact on the overall care (a need to know) and disclosure about a resident being 'noisy and difficult' (does not need to know):

The basic sort of things about [their relative's] condition and changes to the care, type of care we're giving them. That's something they [the relatives] need to know. That they have developed a chest infection…they are becoming more frail…that they aren't communicating as much…

The person is deteriorating physically, we'll tell them that…they're not eating so well…not drinking so well…becoming less mobile…

It may upset them. They don't have any control over it, but it will alter the care plan. It's part of their need to know…

Different things like they [the relatives] will get the picture without having to know. They're [the resident] being noisy and difficult…

Furthermore, the registered nurse commented that if the resident's relatives do not need to know:

…we wouldn't say…She's [the resident] been screaming the place down all day, they can't do anything about it, they can't change it…We won't tell them [the relative] that they [the resident] are faecal smearing…there's just some things, I guess they're taboo that you just don't talk about it…it is upsetting.

Registered nurses in the nursing home differentiate between telling a relative what they determine a relative 'needs to know' and what they determine the relative does not 'need to know'. Adhering to the instrumental or task function of truth-telling, it cannot be ignored that openness about *changes to care* is judged to be beneficial to all. This strategy, which depends on their everyday authority, maintains control in the workplace. Clearly, undisclosed but observable alterations to a resident's care would otherwise attract a relative's questioning. On the other hand, silence protects a resident's relative from knowing about behaviours perceived by the registered nurse to be 'upsetting' and embarrassing. These registered nurses do not take into account the possibility of harm occurring as a result of the accidental and unplanned discovery of an undisclosed truth, nor are they guided in their work by the view that disclosure and good communication might assist relatives or residents to cope.

Some nurses express the view that 'keep(ing) back…things' and not telling the 'full story' is used as a means to minimise the emotional distress experienced by the nurses themselves, and that it is not always the best approach.

What this research exemplar reveals is that in everyday practice nurses must negotiate truth-telling with older people. The decisions that nurses make and their truth-telling behaviours, although well intended, are not necessarily always the most helpful for the

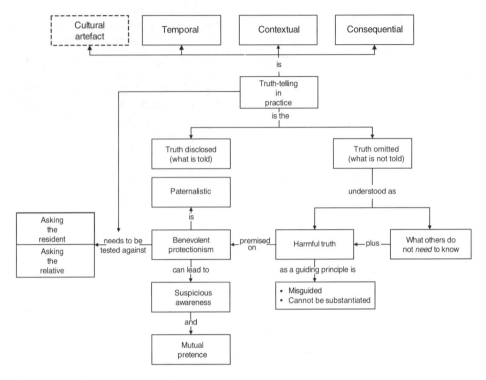

Figure 4.1   Truth-telling in practice: an evidence base.

person, their relatives or themselves. The evidence base in this area is not easy to interpret and the challenge is compounded by the complexity of the ethical and philosophical under-pinnings. Furthermore, people often have strong views about truth-telling, polarising it as either beneficial or harmful, and these views can exert a strong influence over their rela-tionships with others and particularly older people within caregiving situations. This research exemplar highlights the importance for registered nurses to be thoughtful and informed about an individual's capacities to cope with the truth and to do this within the context of relationship-centred caregiving. Being informed involves asking the person directly about their preferences for information and truth rather than reliance in what oth-ers might believe they want to be told.

Summary

This chapter has dealt with the practical realities of telling the truth in the clinical encoun-ter, specifically with the older person in residential aged-care. We have set out to provide the evidence base (Figure 4.1) in a way that is both thought provoking and guiding. In effect, what is offered here is the translation of evidence into practice that justifies the three core tenets recommended as guides for truth-telling in practice at the beginning of this chapter.

Key messages

- Communication is central to relationship-centred care.
- In telling the truth (sharing information honestly) intention is important.
- Truth-telling actually contributes to physical and psychological well-being.
- Nurses' truth-telling practices in residential aged-care risk manifesting suspicious awareness and mutual pretence.
- Good and safe nursing care means discussion with, listening to and providing the person with individualised relevant information.
- Not every person wants to know all that there is, nor wants to be actively involved in decision-making: respect the rights of those who do not wish to know.
- The Australian Nursing and Midwifery Code of Ethics for Nurses and the UK Nursing and Midwifery Council Code: Standards of Conduct, Performance and Ethics for Nurses and Midwives both guide nurses and midwives towards acting openly and honestly.
- In the aged-care setting the recommendation is not to assume what a resident wants to know, nor assume what is important for them but rather ask the resident.
- Do not make assumptions based on race, nationality or language and always ask the person how informed he or she wishes to be.

References

Ajaj A, Singh MP, Abdulla AJ (2001) Should elderly patients be told they have cancer? Questionnaire survey of older people. *British Medical Journal* **323**, 1160.

Akabayashi A, Taylor Slingsby B (2006) Informed consent revisited: Japan and the US. *American Journal of Bioethics* **6**, 9–14.

Australian Nursing and Midwifery Council (2008) *Code of Ethics for Nurses in Australia*. ANMC, Canberra, Australia.

Barkay A, Tabak N (2002) Elderly residents' participation and autonomy within the geriatric ward in a public institution. *International Journal of Nursing Studies* **8**, 198–209.

Berger P, Luckmann T (1966) *The Social Construction of Reality: A Treatise in the Sociology of Knowledge*. Penguin, London.

Berkman C, Eunjeong K (2009) Preferences for disclosure of information about serious illness among older Korean American immigrants in New York City. *Journal of Palliative Medicine* **12**, 351–357.

Blackhall L, Murphy S, Frank G, Michel V, Azen S (1995) Ethnicity and attitudes toward patient autonomy. *Journal of the American Medical Association* **274**, 820–825.

Blumer H (1969) *Symbolic Interactionism: Perspective and Method*. Prentice Hall, Englewood Cliffs, NJ.

Bok S (1973) *Lying: Moral Choices in the Public and Private Life*. Quartet Books, New York.

Cassileth B, Zupkis R, Sutton-Smith K, March V (1980) Information and participation preferences among cancer patients. *Annals of Internal Medicine* **92**, 832–836.

Chiu LQ, Lee WS, Gao F, Parker P, Ng GY, Toh CK (2004) Cancer patients' preferences for communication of unfavourable news: an Asian perspective. *Support Care Cancer* **14**, 818–824.

Crotty D (1998) *The Foundations of Social Research: Meanings and Perspectives in the Research Process*. Allen & Unwin, St Leonards, NSW, Australia.

Drickamer M, Lachs M (1992) Should patients with Alzheimer's disease be told the truth? *New England Journal of Medicine* **326**, 947–951.

Erde E, Nadal E, Scholl T (1988) On truth-telling and the diagnosis of Alzheimer's disease. *Journal of Family Practice* **26**, 401–406.

Euswas P, Chick N (1999) On caring and being cared for. In: Madjar I, Watson J (eds) *Nursing and the Experience of Illness: Phenomenology in Practice*. Allen & Unwin, St Leonards, NSW, Australia, pp. 171–188.

Gillian J, Webber J, Riley M (2000) Is it wrong to lie to patients, even if it seems to be in their best interests? *Nursing Times* **96**, 30.

Glaser B, Strauss A (1965) *Awareness of Dying*. Aldine Publishing Company, Chicago.

Hebert P (1994) Truth-telling in clinical practice. *Canadian Family Physician* **40**, 2105–2113.

Holroyd S, Snustad D, Zona C (1996) Attitudes of adults on being told the diagnosis of Alzheimer's disease. *Journal of the American Geriatrics Society* **44**, 400–403.

Hummert M, Morgan M (2001) Negotiating decisions in the aging family. In: Hummert M, Nussbaum J (eds) *Aging, Communication and Health: Linking Research and Practice for Successful Aging*. Lawrence Erlbaum Associates, London, pp. 177–203.

Irurita V (1999) Factors affecting the quality of nursing care: the patient's perspective. *International Journal of Nursing Studies* **5**, 86–94.

Jenkins V, Fallowfield L, Saul J (2001) Informational needs of patients with cancer: results from a large study in UK cancer centres. *British Journal of Cancer* **84**, 48–51.

Kendall M (1995) Truth-telling and collusion: the ethical dilemmas of palliative nursing. *International Journal of Palliative Care* **1**, 160–164.

Maestri-Banks A, Goseny M (1997) Nurses' responses to terminal illness in the geriatric unit. *International Journal of Palliative Care* **3**, 345–350.

Mead G (1934) *Mind, Self and Society*. University of Chicago Press, Chicago.

Miettinen T, Alaviuhkola H, Pietila AM (2001)The contribution of 'good' palliative care to quality of life in dying patients: family members' perceptions. *Journal of Family Nursing* **7**, 261–280.

Mystakikdou K, Parpa E, Tsilika E, Katsouda E, Vlahos L (2004) Cancer information disclosure in different cultural contexts. *Supportive Care Cancer* **12**, 147–154.

Nursing and Midwifery Council (NMC) (2008) *The Code: Standards of Conduct, Performance and Ethics for Nurses and Midwives*. NMC, London.

Nussbaum J (1990) Communication and the nursing home environment: survivability as a function of resident–staff affinity. In: Giles H, Coupland N, Wiemann J (eds) *Communication, Health and the Elderly*. Manchester University Press, London, pp. 151–171.

Nussbaum J (1991) Communication, language and the institutionalised elderly. *Ageing and Society* **11**, 149–165.

Nussbaum J (1993) The communicative impact of institutionalisation for the elderly: the admission process. *Journal of Aging Studies* **7**, 237–246.

Parathian AR, Taylor F (1993) Can we insulate trainee nurses from exposure to bad practices? A study of role play in communicating bad news to patients. *Journal of Advanced Nursing* **18**, 801–807.

Pfiffner J (1999) The contemporary presidency: presidential lies. *Presidents Studies Quarterly* **29**, 903–917.

Reeder J (1988) Should patients always be told the truth? *Association of Perioperative Registered Nurses Journal* **47**, 1306–1310.

Rosner F, Berger J, Kark P, Potash J, Bennett A (2000) Disclosure and prevention of medical errors. Committee on Bioethical Issues of the Medical Society of the State of New York. *Archives of Internal Medicine* **160**, 2089–2092.

Ross M, Dunning J, Edwards N (2001) Palliative care in China: facilitating the process of development. *Journal of Palliative Care* **17**, 281–288.

Sidgwick H (1966) *The Methods of Ethics*. Dover, New York.

Smith M, Sullivan J (1997) Nurses' and patients' perceptions of most important caring behaviours in a long-term care setting. *Geriatric Nursing* **18**, 70–73.

Sprigler G (1996) When the truth hurts. *Plastic Surgical Nursing* **16**, 56.

Strauss A, Corbin J (1998) *Basics of Qualitative Research: Techniques and Procedures for Developing Grounded Theory*. Sage Publications, Thousand Oaks, CA.

Surbone A (2004) Persisting differences in truth telling throughout the world. *Support Care Cancer* **12**, 143–146.

Tuckett A (2004) Truth-telling in clinical practice and the arguments for and against: a review of literature. *Nursing Ethics* **11**, 1–14.

Tuckett A (2005) The care encounter: pondering caring, honest communication and control. *International Journal of Nursing Practice* **11**, 77–84.

Tuckett A (2006) Registered nurses' understanding of truth-telling as practiced in the nursing-home: an Australian perspective. *Health Sociology Review* **15**, 179–191.

Tuckett A (2007) The meaning of nursing-home: 'Waiting to go up to St Peter, OK! Waiting house, sad but true'. An Australian perspective. *Journal of Aging Studies* **21**, 119–133.

Tuckett A, Hughes K, Schluter P, Turner C (2009) Validation of CARE-Q in residential aged-care. Rating of importance of caring behaviours from an e-cohort sub-study. *Journal of Clinical Nursing* **18**, 1501–1509.

United Nations (1991) General Assembly resolution 46/91 of 16 December 1991. Implementation of the International Plan of Action on Ageing and Related Activities, annex. Available at www.un.org/documents/ga/res/46/a46r091.htm (accessed 19 April 2010).

Wilmot W (1995) *Relational Communication*. McGraw-Hill, St Louis.

Wright L, MacRae S, Gordon D, Elliot E, Dixon D, Abbey S (2002) Disclosure of misattributed paternity: issues involved in the discovery of unsought information. *Seminars in Dialysis* **15**, 202–206.

Chapter 5

Delirium

Irene Schofield and Wolfgang Hasemann

Introduction

In Chapter 1 we highlighted that delirium, sometimes described by practitioners as acute confusion, is an important marker condition for changes in physical health status or a reaction to a stressful event for an older person. However, delirium in itself can be a seriously detrimental aspect of acute illness for an older person, as it can threaten their life or their continuing health and independence. Furthermore, at the service level, patients with delirium require more human, material and economic resources than those without delirium (Leslie *et al.* 2008). In this chapter we describe the clinical presentation of delirium and explain further why it is an undesirable development in the illness trajectory of an older person. We consider the impact of delirium from the perspective of the older person who develops delirium, from the perspective of a family member of a person with delirium, and from the perspective of nurses who have continuous contact with people who develop delirium. We address the challenges for nurses in caring for cognitively impaired patients in communal settings such as hospital wards. Next, we examine the nature and strength of evidence for delirium prevention and care. We include our own contributions to knowledge and practice development in the field of delirium care.

How delirium affects people

Delirium and dementia are common causes of altered cognition and whilst both are discrete conditions, people with dementia are up to five times more likely to develop delirium. When delirium occurs in the older person, it is frequently superimposed on an existing diagnosis of dementia and hence may be missed. It is important to consider too that delirium may be presenting in people with undiagnosed dementia. Delirium is a complex clinical syndrome characterised by disturbance of consciousness, cognitive function and perception, which comes on suddenly (within hours to days) and is fluctuating in its course. Most typically, prodromal symptoms, such as restlessness, anxiety, irritability, disorientation, distractibility or sleep disturbance, progress to full-blown delirium within 1–3 days (American Psychiatric Association 2000). Older people are at risk of developing

Evidence Informed Nursing with Older People, First Edition. Edited by Debbie Tolson, Joanne Booth and Irene Schofield.

Box 5.1 An older person's experience of hyperactive delirium

'There seemed to be a raid – loads of lorries coming in and dashing about...outside there seemed to be a lot of soldiers there. One of them says, "I'm the lieutenant Colonel." There was a lot of arguing amongst themselves and all of a sudden it finished ... I can distinctly see all this in front of me and what was going on and I can remember saying, "If you don't go away, I'll call the police." And the nurse said to me, "Shut up and go to sleep".'

Schofield (1997)

Box 5.2 An older person's experience of hypoactive delirium

'I must have been in [hospital] for a few days before I eventually came round to myself. I didn't know where I was ... I was eating ... they were looking after me, they were washing me. Apart from that I just didn't know where I was.'

Schofield (1997)

---

delirium because of an age-related impairment of cerebral metabolism, which results in a significant decrease in the synthesis of neurotransmitters, particularly acetylcholine. In contrast to delirium, dementia is a chronic condition which lasts at least 6 months and is in most cases progressive (World Health Organization 2004). The most common form of dementia, Alzheimer's disease, is associated with a chronic decline in acetylcholine. This explains the overlapping symptoms of dementia and delirium especially memory loss in both conditions and makes differentiation between the two conditions difficult, particularly when delirium is superimposed on dementia.

Acute confusion is a common presentation of physical illness in older people and sometimes it is the only visible sign of infection or physical and mental stress in this age group. It is important therefore for nurses to be aware of delirium and to regard its development as a signal to act quickly to identify the causative factors and begin treatment. Delirium has been described as 'a chameleon-like illness with a myriad of possible presenting symptoms' (Fann 2000, p. 64). Three discrete clinical presentations of delirium have been described (Lipowski 1990; O'Keeffe 1999). In the *hyperactive hyperalert* form, the person in hospital is on guard, restless, excitable and continuously on the move, searching, shouting, combative, leaving their bed or ward, and resisting when staff attempt to calm them. The person can experience frightening and vivid illusions and hallucinations, leading to paranoia, intense fear and outbursts of anger (Box 5.1).

In the *hypoactive hypoalert* form the person is less physically active and alert than usual. They are quiet and listless, and easily drift off to sleep during care, or lie with open eyes but seemingly indifferent to what is going on around them (Lipowski 1990) (Box 5.2). Patients with this presentation of delirium may be capable of responding to a simple

---

Box 5.3   Recognising delirium: what nurses look out for

'It can be obvious things like agitation, it can be you know undressing at inappropriate times or they're doing something odd, they're moving things around or they're continually trying to get up out of bed. Sometimes it's things like they're calling out for people who are not there or things like things around them you know drip stands or water jugs and things they'll try and it's like they don't appreciate them for what they're actually there and why they're there so they'll try to pull them over or pull them down or throw them away. But very often it can just be more subtle than that and it's not until you sort of speak to a patient that you realise that they're answering you inappropriately or they're not answering you at all. Yes with other folk it's a wee bit more subtle and it's not until you talk or sometimes it even it's not when you tell them something or speak to them about something it's when you try to ascertain whether or not they've taken on board what you've said and that's when you realise that they're confused.' (Medical ward nurse)

Schofield (2008)

---

greeting or brief questions and the condition may therefore not be diagnosed on a busy ward. The hypoactive form may mimic depression, in that the person appears withdrawn, has slowed speech, sleep disturbances and slowed movement. However, it is the features of inattention and slowed cognition that would differentiate delirium from depression.

A combination of the above two clinical presentations, known as the mixed type, has been found to be most common (O'Keeffe & Lavan 1997; Meagher *et al.* 2008). The patient alternates unpredictably between the two forms, either during the course of a day or during the course of a few days. A supposition might be that lack of awareness of the mixed type could lead professionals to believe that when the hypoactive form follows the hyperactive form that the patient's condition has improved when in fact it may have worsened. Pressure ulcers and infections are complications of delirium (O'Keeffe & Lavan 1997).

A description of how a person might behave when they develop delirium is illustrated in Box 5.3 The nurse describes patients with hyperactive and hypoactive forms of delirium.

A neglected aspect of delirium is its impact on relatives. It can be very shocking and anxiety provoking to visit a relative who has developed delirium, as illustrated in the account from an older person's daughter in Box 5.4

Box 5.4   A relative's perspective on delirium

'When we walked onto the ward I was not sure how bad mum was, we had been told that she was very poorly. We waited at the desk as I didn't know where her bed was and then I noticed a commotion down the end of the corridor and recognised her voice. It was mum shouting to be let out. She was rattling the fire doors with considerable force and shouting "get away from me". As I walked closer I was not prepared for her physical state or extreme state of panic. She was like a frightened animal trying to flee and so strong for her eighty four years. Everyone

> was looking at her and visitors were whispering and looking away. I found it shocking and I felt so unable to help her. As a nurse myself I suddenly realised how awful delirium is for the person and their relatives and I felt such an overwhelming anger that the GP had allowed her to get into that state before admitting her to hospital.' (Daughter of patient aged 84)

Causes and occurrence of delirium

There appears to be no single factor responsible for the onset of delirium. A useful and practical approach to understanding how delirium occurs is that predisposing factors interact with precipitating factors (Inouye 1999). Clinical judgement therefore plays an important role in recognising the interplay between the two as a means of identifying patients at high risk of developing delirium (Inouye 1999). Studies indicate that age over 65 years (Elie *et al.* 1998; Kalisvaart *et al.* 2006), dementia (Elie *et al.* 1998; Robinson *et al.* 2009), severe illness defined as a clinical condition that is deteriorating or is at risk of deterioration (Elie *et al.* 1998; National Institute for Clinical Excellence 2009), anticholinergic medications (Alagiakrishnan & Wiens 2004), and current hip fracture are consistent risk factors (Andersson *et al.* 2001). MacLullich *et al.* (2008) propose a new underlying mechanism, that of overreacting responses of the brain to psychological and illness stress. Their research has shown a clear systemic inflammation-induced exacerbation of neurodegenerative disease, with the likelihood that every episode of delirium will speed up the progression of dementia.

Delirium is mostly studied and described in the context of the acute hospital but with policy initiatives to provide care to people in their own homes or other settings, the research focus is shifting to include older people living at home, in care homes and hospices. In a typical UK acute hospital it is estimated that the mean prevalence of delirium in adult patients is 20% (range 7–61%); many more patients will have cognitive impairment for which the cause has not been ascertained. In concrete terms, this means that in a UK hospital of 500 beds, 330 beds are likely to be occupied by older people; 220 of these are likely to have a mental disorder, of whom 66 are likely to have delirium and 102 are likely to have dementia (Faculty of Old Age Psychiatry Royal College of Psychiatrists 2005). Epidemiological studies tend to focus on areas where older people comprise the main client group, i.e. general medical, geriatric, and surgical wards, particularly those where patients receive care for orthopaedic trauma and elective surgery for joint replacement. As the hospital population of very old people is projected to increase, it follows that there will be a corresponding rise in the incidence and prevalence of delirium. This trend is likely to occur globally in countries with ageing and aged populations.

Clinical outcomes of delirium

Delirium is often a transient phenomenon, and full recovery is a common outcome (Marcantonio *et al.* 2000). Recovery is influenced by a number of factors: age, morbidity, underlying cause, the effectiveness and timeliness of treatment, and management of the delirium symptoms. It is usual to recover from delirium within a week but there is increasing evidence to suggest that delirious episodes may recur for several weeks or months following initial onset (Marcantonio *et al.* 2000, 2003). Rather than being the benign and transient phenomenon it was once thought to be (Cole *et al.* 2008), it is now known that clinical outcomes can be serious, affecting quality of life and resulting in increased mortality (Pitkala 2005), especially for those people who develop delirium superimposed on dementia (Bellelli *et al.* 2007). Commonly delirium results in a slower rate of recovery (Marcantonio *et al.* 2003) and prolongs the time spent in hospital (Thomason *et al.* 2005). Increased functional decline at varying intervals up to 12 months after an episode of delirium has been demonstrated (Marcantonio *et al.* 2003). Older people who develop delirium in hospital are more likely to be admitted to a care home (McAvay *et al.* 2006) and more likely to be readmitted to hospital (George *et al.* 1997).

Types of evidence for delirium care

Knowledge underpinning the evidence base for delirium is provided by quantitative methods as a result of which researchers construct definitions and understandings of delirium from disease-led classification systems, thus supporting a biomedical understanding of delirium. Positivist scientific methods have been used to produce systematic sets of clinical observations in the form of diagnostic criteria and evidence based practice guidelines in order to assist clinicians in the diagnosis and treatment of delirium (American Psychiatric Association 1999; British Geriatrics Society 2005; Canadian Coalition for Seniors' Mental Health 2006; National Institute for Clinical Excellence 2009). Studies which contribute the perspectives of older people who develop delirium, their families, and nurses' day-to-day challenges of caring for patients with delirium have yet to feature in most guidelines. However, there is a growing body of qualitative research led by nurses that provides insights into how delirium is experienced by patients. Irrespective of differences in methodology a review of studies of patients' experience of delirium demonstrates some consensus around the experience and its after-effects (O'Malley *et al.* 2008). For example, findings are compatible with the seminal writing of Lipowski (1990), whereby patients experienced events that were frequently vivid and threatening and sometimes linked to past life experiences, causing a state of suspicion, paranoia and fear, loss of control and a need to escape; patients might be combative in their attempt to do so. Afterwards patients could feel guilt, remorse and humiliation for behaving 'badly'. In one study nurses were reticent to inform patients how they had behaved in their delirium. The nurses indicated that they would leave it up to patients to enquire about their resolved delirium, in which case nurses said that they would give a selective version of events to protect patients from embarrassment and to preserve their dignity (Schofield 2008). The nurses' approach reflects the notion of 'truth omitted' as described by Tuckett and Tolson in the study on truth-telling (Chapter 4). The findings from these qualitative studies suggest that patients could benefit if nurses had some understanding of what individuals might be going through when they experience delirium.

Interventions in delirium care

In order to test the effectiveness of an intervention to prevent or reduce the effects of delirium, the randomised controlled trial is the method that confers the highest rigour. It is the only way of demonstrating a causal inference, in this case that a specific intervention or interventions prevents the development of delirium or lessens the severity or duration of delirium. In real world situations, however, many factors such as ethical considerations and health service organisational factors mitigate against the use of the randomised controlled trial as a research method. Most intervention studies within delirium research therefore are quasi-experimental, in that patients are not randomised to control and interventions groups.

The care and treatment of people with delirium is a multidisciplinary endeavour (British Geriatrics Society 2005; Canadian Coalition for Seniors' Mental Health 2006; National Institute for Clinical Excellence 2010). Both nursing and medical staff can be responsible for the identification of delirium and preliminary examination of the patient in order to begin the search for the underlying cause of delirium. Evidence based guidelines on delirium reinforce the role of nurses in providing physical and psychological support from its onset to resolution. A comprehensive review of guidelines and their strength of evidence has been conducted by Michaud *et al.* (2007). Support with activities of daily living, effective communication strategies, and use of the correct environment to counteract the remediable predisposing factors that contribute to the development of delirium are recommended. However, guideline recommendations can be limited in their application depending on how health services are organised and delivered and according to whether recommendations are regarded as practicable (Day *et al.* 2009). For example, it has been recommended that people who develop delirium should be cared for in single rooms (Rapp and Iowa Veterans Affairs Nursing Research Consortium 2001) but the evidence is not strong. A methodologically weak study identified more sensory disturbances for patients in single bedrooms than in shared two-person rooms (Wood 1997). In contrast, McCusker *et al.* (2001) could not find a significant relationship between the development of delirium symptoms and being in a single room. However, there are few single rooms in UK acute hospitals and where these exist, they tend to be used to isolate patients with healthcare-associated infection or allocated to patients who require end-of-life care. Patients with delirium are therefore cared for mostly in multiple occupation wards where their needs are often in conflict with patients who do not have cognitive impairment. An environmental recommendation is that room changes should be avoided, although this is not always feasible in UK hospitals where patients may need to be moved in order to fulfil UK policy commitments to maintaining single sex wards.

The effectiveness of interventions to prevent or treat delirium tends to be investigated separately and they are further divided into those interventions that do not involve the use of drugs (non-pharmacological intervention) and those which do (pharmacological intervention). We now use these divisions to present the current evidence base for the interventions to prevent or treat delirium once it has been diagnosed.

Prevention of delirium

Approaches to delirium prevention have been studied on the premise that interventions to reduce known risk factors should reduce the impact of delirium.

Non-pharmacological approaches

The limited evidence for the prevention of delirium focuses on non-pharmacological approaches. Single component interventions have been targeted at preventing dehydration (a potential precipitating factor for the development of delirium) in long-term care residents (Mentes & Culp 2003) and the use of music therapy postoperatively with elective orthopaedic patients (McCaffrey & Locsin 2006). However, both studies are methodologically weak. The evidence for the prevention of delirium is provided from studies in which combinations of interventions such as training and education, multidisciplinary clinical management and structured treatment protocols are used to reduce the effects of known risk factors. A well-known multi-component intervention known as the Elder Life Program in the USA consisted of a protocol based on reducing the effects of six previously determined modifiable risk factors for the development of delirium: cognitive impairment, sleep deprivation, immobility, visual impairment, hearing impairment and dehydration (Inouye *et al.* 1999a). Inouye and colleagues recorded adherence to specific interventions as a means of demonstrating their contribution to overall effectiveness. Delirium developed in 9.9% of the intervention group compared with 15% in the control group and delirium episodes reduced by 34%. However, severity and recurrence rates were not significantly different in the intervention group. There was good adherence (87%) to the interventions and prevention was most effective with patients designated on admission as being at intermediate risk (the presence of one or two risk factors). Six-month follow-up of participating patients did not demonstrate a lasting beneficial effect for the interventions in terms of people's functional, cognitive and general health status (Bogardus *et al.* 2003). The Elder Life team is now part of a continuing programme to improve the care of older people in hospital (Inouye *et al.* 2000) and a study to replicate the programme has begun in the UK. However, its success in influencing care is dependent on senior management support and the allocation of dedicated financial resources.

Marcantonio *et al.* (2001) caried out a randomised controlled trial of hip fracture patients, who received proactive preoperative assessment and daily clinical management by a geriatrician. The intervention consisted of 10 recommendations: improving oxygenation, preventing postoperative complications, preventing dehydration, preventing severe pain, reducing polypharmacy, promoting nutrition, regulation of bladder and bowel function, promoting early mobility, preventing sensory impairment, and modification of the clinical environment. With a 77% adherence rate to the recommended interventions, the orthopaedics team reduced the incidence of delirium by one-third and severe delirium by half.

The evidence provided by other studies is less strong and suggests that the following interventions used in combination could by useful. Firstly, assess patients within 24 hours of admission to hospital and ongoing, or routinely monitor care home residents to determine whether they have or are developing risk factors that might contribute to delirium. Secondly, based on the assessment, tailor interventions towards the following risk factors (National Institute for Clinical Excellence 2010):

- Maintain stability of the care environment by avoiding room changes and maintaining continuity with care staff.
- Prevent disorientation by providing clear signage, lighting without glare, easily visible accurate clock and calendar. Use reorientating communication and stimulating cognitive activity such as structured reminiscence. Encourage regular visits from family and friends. Support visitors by providing them with brief information on delirium and support their communication.
- Address sensory impairment by ensuring that patients are wearing their spectacles or hearing aids.
- Prevent dehydration by ensuring adequate fluid intake, managing intake compatible with comorbidities.
- Prevent poor nutrition by ensuring that patients are wearing their dentures and that staff are following established nutritional guidelines for older adults.
- Prevent infection by adhering to infection control policies, avoiding unnecessary catheterisation or removing catheters at the earliest opportunity and looking out for and treating infection.
- Prevent or minimise pain by checking whether the person has pain or observe for nonverbal cues. Ensure that the person is given their prescribed analgesia.
- Prevent the effects of polypharmacy by carrying out regular medication reviews.
- Address limited mobility by encouraging patients to walk around. After surgery encourage early mobilisation or help the person to carry out range of motion exercises.
- Minimise sleep disturbance by finding out and promoting person-centred sleep routines, and by reducing noise.

If delirium can be prevented through attention to the above factors, it would seem logical that they should be extended to patients who develop delirium.

Pharmacological approaches

The prevention of delirium by prophylactic medication is a repeated and so far unsuccessful undertaking with the exception of alcohol withdrawal, where benzodiazepines are the first-line medication (Lonergan *et al.* 2009). None of the other 13 identified studies showed evidence that neuroleptics, atypical neuroleptics, gabapentin, benzodiazepines, platelet activating factor or piracetam given preoperatively are able to prevent postoperative delirium. In specified risk groups such as patients with vascular dementia, cholinesterase inhibitors may reduce the incidence of delirium (Moretti *et al.* 2004).

Treatment of delirium

The treatment of delirium symptoms involves a search for the underlying cause or causes and concurrent management of the delirium. There is weak evidence to suggest that the treatment of delirious patients with neuroleptics or atypical neuroleptics is of more benefit than not giving antipsychotic medication (Hu *et al.* 2004).

> **Box 5.5**   A nurse's perspective on caring for a patient with hyperactive delirium
>
> 'Eventually we did have to give him haloperidol but that was after around I would say 25 minutes out in the corridor. So I let it go that far. I let him come out of his base and walk up and down the ward a few times shouting that he was leaving and I let him go out into the main corridor. But then he was trying to get down the stairs and he kept saying "Somebody's going to get hurt here. I'm going to hit somebody if you don't let me go" and we did have to give him something then because he was actually becoming so aggressive. And he was out in the main corridor. We do try to keep people within the ward environment because it can be very distressing for the people walking by who maybe don't know what's going on. People can think that the person's being very rational and at the same time the patient may be acting like they're rational. But you actually know the patient and you know that this isn't their normal behaviour.' (Orthopaedic ward nurse)
>
> Schofield (2008)

Non-pharmacological approaches

The evidence base for the treatment of delirium is similarly not robust. A small number of multi-component intervention studies to treat delirium consist of combinations of consultation by a geriatrician, follow-up by a liaison nurse, intervention protocols targeted at risk factors, orientation and attention to environmental factors, an education component and medical treatment of symptoms (Naughton *et al.* 2005; Pitkala *et al.* 2006).

The limited evidence suggests that it may be helpful in the alleviation of the symptoms to practise effective communication and reorientation. Family and friends may be able to help with this if they are first briefed on the person's condition, the nature of delirium and how they can help. If the person is distressed and at risk of harming themselves or others, it is suggested that verbal and non-verbal techniques are used to calm the person and to de-escalate the situation. This should be done prior to considering the use of pharmacological interventions. Readers will undoubtedly recognise the scenario in box 5.5. The nurse tried her best to employ de-escalation techniques, but in the end it was necessary to administer medication. The scenario in Box 5.5 illustrates the powerful prolonged effects of severe agitated delirium on a patient's behaviour. This is often not appreciated by those who believe that effective communication is the universal panacea.

Pharmacological treatment

The neuroleptic haloperidol is the only substance which reduced the severity and the duration of delirium given preoperatively in hip fracture patients (Kalisvaart *et al.* 2005).

Key challenges for nurses

A nurse in the study by Dahlke and Phinney (2008) aptly sums up caring for older people with delirium in hospital as the 'silent, unspoken piece of what our business is really about' (p. 46), suggesting that nurses' work is neither recognised nor valued. Delirium often presents as an emergency situation at night when nurses bear the major responsibility for caring for very disturbed patients in settings little suited to their care, such as in multiple occupation wards and wards from which patients have easy access to busy thoroughfares. Feelings of paranoia that staff and other patients wish to cause them harm can lead people with delirium to take steps to defend themselves and in doing so frighten or injure other people in the vicinity. Patients with delirium may not realise that they are in hospital and/or feel the need to make their getaway from the place where they feel threatened. Nurses have commented on the physical strength and capacity to cover distances by patients with delirium, which are unanticipated in ill older people (Schofield 2008). Once the delirium has resolved, some people remember their strong feelings of the need to fight or flee and experience shame and regret for their behaviour, albeit that they were unable to control it at the time (Andersson *et al.* 2002). Self-injury can occur as a result of tearing open sutures, pulling at intravenous lines or drainage tubes, or falling and sustaining a fracture and/or head injury. Evidence is accumulating to suggest that people who develop delirium in hospital are more likely to have a fall (Lakatos *et al.* 2009), particularly if they have been given benzodiazepines in an attempt to control their behaviour (Fick *et al.* 2004). The care of patients with delirium can be highly challenging and stressful for nursing staff and other patients, especially at night when there are fewer staff on duty than during the day and both staff and other patients are fearful of being hurt. In addition, delirium affects essential self-care ability, putting the person at risk of dehydration, incontinence and urinary tract infection, and ultimately threatens dignity. The phenomenon that one geriatric syndrome can lead to another in a cascade effect is well illustrated in the development of delirium.

Inouye *et al.* (1999b) have suggested that since delirium is common and closely linked to the processes of care, it can serve as a marker for the overall quality of care delivered. Key issues for nurses caring for older people with delirium are to be able to recognise the phenomenon and to appreciate its seriousness in terms of bringing undesirable outcomes for both individuals and health services. Evidence shows that recognition of delirium is poor amongst nurses (Voyer *et al.* 2008) and healthcare professionals in general (Fick *et al.* 2007). A first step is to be aware of the risk factors, to have a high index of suspicion in patients at high risk and then to carry out diagnostic screening. There are some well-validated tools for the identification of delirium available for use amongst different patient populations and the Confusion Assessment Method (Inouye *et al.* 1990) is the most widely used of these. Clinical guidelines recommend that screening be carried out within the first 24 hours of admission to hospital. In the care home setting it is suggested that staff monitor residents on a daily basis for sudden changes in behaviour or behaviour that is different from usual as this might indicate that the resident is developing delirium (National Institute for Clinical Excellence 2010).

Applying the evidence base in practice

The following study, led by one of the authors (W.H.), illustrates the challenges and successes in terms of developing nurses' practice in delirium care. The study was part of a wider project, the Swiss Basle Dementia Delirium Programme, which started in 2004. The work began as a result of nurses expressing their concerns about the pressures of caring for several patients at one time with cognitive impairment and balancing their needs alongside those of other patients. It was initially planned solely as a delirium prevention project but the need to address early recognition and nursing interventions for all patients with cognitive impairment became a priority.

The first phase lasted 2 years and consisted of a practice development programme implementing preventive nursing measures (Inouye *et al.* 1999a), preventive interdisciplinary measures, and the principles of early recognition of delirium (Milisen *et al.* 2001; Schuurmans *et al.* 2003). The second phase of the programme consisted of a study to identify an appropriate screening instrument for patients with cognitive impairment, as a means of early identification of individuals at risk for delirium. It was anticipated that recognition of the early signs of delirium would reduce the incidence of full-blown delirium and that it would be less severe and of shorter duration than without any intervention.

Patients on four medical wards of a Swiss university hospital were included in the study if they scored less than 27/30 in the Mini Mental Status Examination (Folstein *et al.* 1975) or less than 5/7 in the Clock Drawing Test (Thalman *et al.* 2002). At the outset 200 (42%) declined to take part in the preliminary cognitive screening, leaving a study group of 275. Older people either did not want to sign a written consent form or they did not want to be troubled by taking part in a study. Of the remaining group, 147 (53%) had normal scores and 128 had scores less than the cut-off in the cognitive tests; they were assessed daily for delirium. Thirty-four people (28%) developed delirium. This corresponded with the reported mean incidence rate for comparable settings (Edlund *et al.* 2006).

The study continued with a compulsory training day for the entire nursing team from the four medical wards. The training consisted of delirium prevention and management, the introduction of systematic screening for cognitive impairment and delirium, and what nurses can do to provide a rapid response when patients first present with delirium symptoms. Nurses were taught to look out for the causes of delirium and to give the most appropriate care. For example to identify when a patient has significant urinary retention and to carry out catheterisation rather than immediately resort to giving psychoactive medication. It was emphasised that the use of psychoactive medication in such circumstances would be regarded as unsafe practice as this class of drugs can exacerbate the problem of urinary retention. As patients who have dementia are the main risk group for developing delirium, attention was given to people with underlying cognitive impairment. The nurses were taught how to adapt their communication to the special needs of those with memory impairment. For example, they learnt validation techniques to avoid confrontation with people who might not respond to reality orientation. In evaluating the training days the nurses reported that they had a better understanding of the pathological mechanisms underlying acute and chronic confusion and appropriate nursing interventions. They also felt more confident in putting forward their views on what they believed to be appropriate care in discussions with medical staff.

Ward nurses performed further screening for people identified with cognitive impairment using the Mental Status Questionnaire (Kahn *et al*. 1960) and the Clock Drawing Test (Thalman *et al*. 2002). The nurses used both the Delirium Observation Screening Scale (Schuurmans *et al*. 2003) and the Confusion Assessment Method (Inouye *et al*. 1990) to detect delirium. We decided not to use the Confusion Assessment Method as a single delirium screening instrument because it was challenging for the nurses to interpret signs of attention and inattention. The nurses preferred to use the Delirium Observation Screening Scale because they felt confident about recognising changes in a person's behaviour. This resonated with the findings of Inouye *et al*. (2001) who showed that the sensitivity for nurses recognising inattention in older people was low at 15%, in comparison to their recognition of altered behaviour, which gave a sensitivity of 47%. When the nurses identified a person with delirium they gave the prescribed psychoactive medication according to protocol and discussed further treatment with medical staff the next day. Most often the medication prescribed was the atypical neuroleptic quetiapine, rarely haloperidol or lorazepam.

The study continues, and over a period of 8 months the research team plan to carry out daily cognitive assessment with a total of 124 patients in order to ascertain the effect of the interventions (early recognition and early treatment of the delirium). We also plan to carry out qualitative interviews with nurses and older people to find out their views and experiences of cognitive screening and delirium care.

Summary

Delirium is an important geriatric syndrome that is poorly recognised and not well understood by many healthcare professionals including nurses. The evidence base for delirium resulting from research on the neurobiology, epidemiology, clinical outcomes, risk factors and interventions has increased steadily over the past two decades. However, more research is needed to strengthen the evidence base. There are clinical guidelines or protocols originating in the UK, USA, Canada and Europe that *healthcare* staff can draw on to guide their practice in the care of older people who develop delirium. However, guidelines are just that and not a definitive statement for what must be done. Practitioners will ultimately make care decisions about this complex phenomenon that are mediated by context, immediacy and their personal and professional values.

Key messages

- Delirium is an undesirable abrupt change in mental status resulting in personal loss of control and a threat to dignity.
- Older people who develop delirium are likely to have an increased length of stay in hospital, to be discharged to a care home and to be at risk of increased mortality.
- Delirium can be prevented or its effects reduced by using interventions that address known risk factors.
- Effective interventions are multifactorial, context appropriate and require the support of organisational managers and members of the multidisciplinary team.

References

Alagiakrishnan K, Wiens CA (2004) An approach to drug induced delirium in the elderly. *Postgraduate Medical Journal* **80**, 388–393.

American Psychiatric Association (1999) *Practice Guideline for the Treatment of Patients with Delirium*. American Psychiatric Association, Washington, DC.

American Psychiatric Association (2000) Delirium, dementia and amnestic and other cognitive disorders. In: *Diagnostic and Statistical Manual of Mental Disorders: DSM-IV Text Revision*, 4th edn. American Psychiatric Association, Washington, DC, pp. 135–147.

Andersson EM, Gustafson, L, Halberg IR (2001) Acute confusional state in elderly orthopaedic patients: factors of importance for detection in nursing care. *International Journal of Geriatric Psychiatry* **16**, 7–17.

Andersson EM, Hallberg IR, Norberg, A, Edberg, A (2002) The meaning of acute confusional state from the perspective of elderly patients. *International Journal of Geriatric Psychiatry* **17**, 652–663.

Bellelli G, Frisoni GB, Turco R, Lucchi E, Magnifico F, Trabucchi M (2007) Delirium superimposed on dementia predicts 12-month survival in elderly patients discharged from a postacute rehabilitation facility. *Journals of Gerontology A: Biological Sciences and Medical Sciences* **62**, 1306–9.

Bogardus ST, Desai MM, Williams CS (2003) The effects of a targeted multicomponent delirium intervention on postdischarge outcomes for hospitalized older adults. *American Journal of Medicine* **114**, 383–390.

British Geriatrics Society (2005) *Guidelines for the Prevention, Diagnosis and Management of Delirium in Older People in Hospital*. British Geriatrics Society, London.

Canadian Coalition for Seniors' Mental Health (2006) *National Guidelines for Seniors' Mental Health: The Assessment and Treatment of Delirium*. Available at www.ccsmh.ca/en/guidelinesdownload.cfm (acessed 23 October 2010).

Cole M, Ciampi A, Belzile E, Zhong L (2008) Persistent delirium in older hospital patients: a systematic review of frequency and prognosis. *Age and Ageing* **38**, 19–26.

Dahlke S, Phinney A (2008) Caring for hospitalized older adults at risk for delirium. *Journal of Gerontological Nursing* **34**, 41–47.

Day J, Higgins I, Koch T (2009) The process of practice redesign in delirium care for hospitalised older people: a participatory action research study. *International Journal of Nursing Studies* **46**, 13–22.

Edlund A, Lundstrom M, Brannstrom B, Karlsson S, Bucht G, Gustafson Y (2006) Delirium in older patients admitted to general internal medicine. *Journal of Geriatric Psychiatry and Neurology* **19**, 83–90.

Elie M, Cole MG, Primeau FJ, Bellevance F (1998) Delirium risk factors in elderly hospitalized patients. *General Internal Medicine* **13**, 204–212.

Faculty of Old Age Psychiatry Royal College of Psychiatrists (2005) *Who Cares Wins*. Royal College of Psychiatrists, London.

Fann JR (2000) The epidemiology of delirium: a review of studies and methodological issues. *Seminars in Clinical Neuropsychiatry* **5**, 64–74.

Fick D, Maclean JR, Rodriguez NA, Short L, Heuvel R, Waller JL (2004) A randomized study to decrease the use of potentially inappropriate medications among community-dwelling older adults in a southeastern managed care organization. *American Journal of Managed Care* **11**, 761–768.

Fick D, Hodo D, Frank L, Inouye SK (2007) Recognizing delirium superimposed on dementia: assessing nurses' knowledge using case vignettes. *Journal of Gerontological Nursing* **33**, 40–47.

Folstein MF, Folstein SE, McHugh PR (1975) The Folstein Mini-Mental State Examination. *Journal of Psychiatric Research* **12**, 189–198.

George J, Bleasdale S, Singleton SJ (1997) Causes and prognosis of delirium in elderly patients admitted to a district general hospital. *Age and Ageing* **26**, 423–427.

Hu H, Deng W, Yang H (2004) A prospective random control study comparison of olanzapine and haloperidol in senile delirium. *Chongging Medical Journal* **8**, 1234–1237.

Inouye SK (1999) Predisposing and precipitating factors for delirium in hospitalized older patients. *Dementia and Geriatric Cognitive Disorders* **10**, 393–400.

Inouye SK, Van Dyck CH, Alessi CA, Balkin S, Siegal AP, Horwitz RI (1990) Clarifying confusion: the Confusion Assessment Method, a new method for the detection of delirium. *Annals of Internal Medicine* **113**, 941–948.

Inouye SK, Bogardus S, Charpentier P *et al.* (1999a) A multicomponent intervention to prevent delirium in hospitalized older patients. *New England Journal of Medicine* **340**, 669–676.

Inouye SK, Schlesinger MJ, Lydon TJ (1999b) Delirium: a symptom of how hospital care is failing older persons and a window to improve quality of hospital care. *American Journal of Medicine* **106**, 565–573.

Inouye SK, Bogardus ST, Baker DI, Leo-Summers L, Cooney LM (2000) The Hospital Elder Life Programme: a model of care to prevent cognitive and functional decline in older hospitalised patients. *Journal of the American Geriatrics Society* **48**, 1697–1706.

Inouye SK, Foreman MD, Mion LC, Katz KH, Cooney LM (2001) Nurses recognition of delirium and its symptoms. *Archives of Internal Medicine* **16**, 2467–2473.

Kahn RL, Goldfarb AI, Pollack M, Peck A (1960) Brief objective measures for the determination of mental status in the aged. *American Journal of Psychiatry* **117**, 326–328.

Kalisvaart KJ, de Jonghe JF, Bogaards MJ, Vreeswijk R, Egberts TC, Burger BJ (2005) Haloperidol prophylaxis for elderly hip-surgery patients at risk for delirium: a randomized placebo-controlled study. *Journal of the American Geriatrics Society* **49**, 516–522.

Kalisvaart KJ, Vreeswijk R, de Jonghe JF, van der Ploeg T, van Gool WA, Eikelenboom P (2006) Risk factors and prediction of post operative delirium in elderly hip surgery patients: implementation and validation of a medical risk factor model. *Journal of the American Geriatrics Society* **54**, 817–822.

Lakatos BE, Capasso V, Mitchell MT *et al.* (2009) Falls in the general hospital: association with delirium, advanced age, and specific surgical procedures. *Psychosomatics* **50**, 218–226.

Leslie DL, Marcantonio ER, Zhang Y, Leo-Summers L, Inouye SK (2008) One-year health care costs associated with delirium in the elderly population. *Archives of Internal Medicine* **168**, 27–32.

Lipowski ZJ (1990) *Delirium: Acute Confusional States*. Oxford University Press, New York.

Lonergan E, Luxenberg J, Areosa Sastre A, Wyller T (2009) Benzodiazepines for delirium. *Cochrane Database of Systematic Reviews* (1), CD006379. Update 2009 (4), CD006379.

McAvay GJ, Van Ness PH, Bogardus ST, Zhang DL, Leo-Summers LS, Inouye SK (2006) Older adults discharged from the hospital with delirium: 1-year outcomes. *Journal of the American Geriatrics Society* **54**, 1245–1250.

McCaffrey R, Locsin R (2006) The effect of music on pain and acute confusion in older adults undergoing hip and knee surgery. *Holistic Nursing Practice* **20**, 218–226.

McCusker J, Cole M, Abrahamowicz M, Han L, Podoba JE, Ramman-Haddad L (2001) Environmental risk factors for delirium in hospitalized older people. *Journal of the American Geriatrics Society* **49**, 1327–1334.

MacLullich A, Ferguson KJ, Miller T, de Rooij S, Cunningham C (2008) Unravelling the pathophysiology of delirium: a focus on the role of aberrant stress responses. *Journal of Psychosomatic Research* **65**, 229–238.

Marcantonio ER, Flacker JM, Michaels M, Resnick NM (2000) Delirium is independently associated with poor functional recovery after hip fracture. *Journal of the American Geriatrics Society* **48**, 618–624.

Marcantonio ER, Flacker JM, Wright R, Resnick NM (2001) Reducing delirium after hip fracture: a randomized trial. *Journal of the American Geriatrics Society* **49**, 516–522.

Marcantonio ER, Simon SE, Bergmann A, Jones RN, Murphy KM, Morris JN (2003) Delirium symptoms in post-acute care: prevalent, persistent, and associated with poor functional recovery. *Journal of the American Geriatrics Society* **51**, 4–9.

Meagher DJ, Moran M, Raju B, Leonard M, Donnelly S, Saunders J (2008) A new data-based motor subtype schema for delirium. *Journal of Neuropsychiatry and Clinical Neuroscience* **20**, 185–193.

Mentes J, Culp K (2003) Reducing hydration-linked events in nursing home residents. *Clinical Nursing Research* **12**, 210–225.

Michaud L, Bula C, Berney A *et al.* (2007) The Delirium Guidelines Development Group. Delirium: guidelines for general hospitals. *Journal of Psychosomatic Research* **62**, 371–383.

Milisen K, Foreman MD, Abraham IL, Godderis J, Delooz HH, Broos P (2001) A nurse-led inter-disciplinary intervention program for delirium in elderly hip-fracture patients. *Journal of the American Geriatrics Society* **49**, 523–532.

Moretti R, Torre P, Antonello RM, Cattaruza T, Cazzato G (2004) Cholinesterase inhibition as a possible therapy for delirium in vascular dementia: a controlled, open 24-month study of 246 patients. *American Journal of Alzheimer's Disease and Other Dementias* **19**, 333–339.

National Institute for Clinical Excellence (2010) Delirium: diagnosis, prevention and management. Available at http://www.nice.org.uk/guidance/CG103 (accessed 7 December 2010).

Naughton B, Saltzman S, Ramadan F, Chadha N, Priore R, Mylotte J (2005) A multifactorial inter-vention to reduce prevalence of delirium and shorten hospital length of stay. *Journal of the American Geriatrics Society* **53**, 18–23.

O'Keeffe ST (1999) Clinical subtypes of delirium in the elderly. *Dementia and Geriatric Cognitive Disorders* **10**, 380–385.

O'Keeffe S, Lavan J (1997) The prognostic significance of delirium in older hospital patients. *Journal of the American Geriatrics Society* **45**, 174–178.

O'Malley G, Leonard M, Meagher D, O'Keeffe ST (2008) The delirium experience: a review. *Journal of Psychosomatic Research* **65**, 223–228.

Pitkala KH (2005) Prognostic significance of delirium in frail older people. *Dementia and Geriatric Cognitive Disorders* **19**, 177–183.

Pitkala KH, Laurila JV, Strandberg TE, Tilvis RS (2006) Multicomponent geriatric intervention for elderly inpatients with delirium: a randomized controlled trial. *Journals of Gerontology A: Biological Sciences and Medical Sciences* **61**, 176–181.

Rapp CG and Iowa Veterans Affairs Nursing Research Consortium (2001) Acute confusion/delirium protocol. *Journal of Gerontological Nursing* **28**, 21–33.

Robinson TN, Raeburn CD, Tran ZV, Angles EM, Brenner LA, Moss M (2009) Post-operative delirium in the elderly: risk factors and outcomes. *Annals of Surgery* **249**, 173–178.

Schofield I (1997) A small exploratory study of the reaction of older people to an episode of delir-ium. *Journal of Advanced Nursing* **25**, 942–952.

Schofield I (2008) *A critical discourse analysis of how nurses understand and care for older patients with delirium in hospital.* Unpublished PhD thesis. Glasgow Caledonian University, Glasgow.

Schuurmans M, Shortridge-Bagget L, Duursma S (2003) The Delirium Observation Screening Scale: a screening instrument for delirium. *Research and Theory for Nursing Practice: An International Journal* **17**, 31–50.

Thalman B, Spiegel R, Stahelin HB, Brubacher D, Ermini-Funfschilling D, Blasi S (2002) Dementia screening in general practice: optimized scoring for the Clock Drawing Test. *Brain Aging* **2**, 36–43.

Thomason JW, Shintani A, Peterson JF, Pun BT, Jackson JT, Ely EW (2005) Intensive care unit delirium is an independent predictor of longer hospital stay: a prospective analysis of 261 non-ventilated patients. *Critical Care* **9**, R375–R381.

Voyer P, Cole MG, McCusker J, St-Jacques S, Laplante J (2008) Accuracy of nurse documentation of delirium symptoms in medical charts. *International Journal of Nursing Practice* **14**, 165–77.

Wood M (1997) Clinical sensory deprivation: a comparative study of patients in single care and two-bed rooms. *Journal of Nursing Administration* **7**, 28–32.

World Health Organization (2004) *The ICD-10 Classification of Mental and Behavioural Disorders: Clinical Descriptions and Diagnostic Guidelines.* Available at www.Who.Int/Entity/Classifications/Icd/En/Bluebook.Pdf (accessed 29 March 2010).

Chapter 6

Palliative Care with Older People

Deborah Parker and Katherine Froggatt

Introduction

This chapter focuses on palliative care for older people. Palliative care in developed countries such as the UK and Australia originally centred on the needs of people with cancer. In the past two decades, the increasing recognition of the palliative care needs of people with non-cancer disease has highlighted that many people with chronic conditions associated with increasing age would benefit from palliative care. However, at present there is inequitable access to specialist palliative care services for older people and failure to address the complex needs of older people with advanced chronic and life-limiting conditions can increase the risk of hospital admission (Burt & Raine 2006). A report in the UK by the National Confidential Enquiry into Patient Outcome and Death (2009) identified that the majority of people who die in acute hospitals are over the age of 75. The enquiry found that up to 40% of people who were nearing the end of their life were inappropriately admitted to hospital to die.

Palliative care for older people is an important issue to be addressed and will emerge as a priority health issue in countries faced with an ageing population. In this chapter we focus on the palliative care needs of older people. Firstly, we define palliative care and then examine the leading causes of death for older people and where these deaths occur. Secondly, we identify the main palliative care needs for older people and, drawing on current evidence, discuss how these care needs can be addressed. Finally, we conclude the chapter with a case study of translating evidence into practice for older people living in residential aged-care facilities in Australia.

What is palliative care?

Palliative care is defined by the World Health Organization (2003) as:

> *an approach that improves the quality of life of patients and their families facing the problem associated with life threatening illness, through the prevention and relief of*

Evidence Informed Nursing with Older People, First Edition. Edited by Debbie Tolson, Joanne Booth and Irene Schofield.

© 2011 Blackwell Publishing Ltd. Published 2011 by Blackwell Publishing Ltd.

suffering by means of early identification and impeccable assessment and treatment of pain and other problems, physical, psychosocial and spiritual. Palliative care affirms life and regards dying as a normal process, and intends neither to hasten nor to prolong death. Using a team approach, palliative care addresses the needs of patients and their families, including bereavement counselling if necessary.

The essential elements of providing palliative care for a person who has a life-threatening illness include the prevention and relief of suffering, using a team approach, that will include not only physical symptoms but also problems related to psychosocial, spiritual and family issues. For older people a life-threatening illness may be related to cancer, heart disease, cerebrovascular disease, respiratory disease and dementia. Older people may have more than one life-threatening illness contributing to the physical, psychosocial and spiritual issues they may experience.

From this definition there is a clear alignment between relationship-centred care and palliative care. As discussed in detail in Chapter 3, the Senses Framework identifies the importance of relationships which promote security, belonging, continuity, purpose, achievement and significance. Like palliative care it is about partnerships with each group – practitioners, older people and families being valued. However, the Senses Framework is more overt in regard to the interface between place, people and processes. This has important implications for practitioners providing palliative care, particularly for older people in long-term care settings.

What do older people die from?

In Australia, the leading causes of death for males and females aged 65 and over are ischaemic heart disease, followed by cerebrovascular disease. For males, the next leading causes of death are lung cancer, chronic obstructive pulmonary disease (COPD), other heart diseases and dementia, while for females the pattern is other heart diseases, dementia, COPD and lung cancer (Australian Institute of Health and Welfare 2007) (Table 6.1). For older people in the UK, circulatory disease, cancer and respiratory disease are the three main causes of death (Office for National Statistics 2005).

Details on the leading causes of death for older people provides information for policy planners and service providers of the type and number of services that may be required to meet these population needs. Awareness of the way in which illnesses progress for common types of diseases is another way of illustrating what and where people will require services throughout their illness or at certain critical junctures. Trajectories of illness have been identified for three of the common types of life-threatening illnesses: cancer, organ failure such as heart failure, and dementia (Lynn & Adamson 2003).

Cancer

Cancers of the breast, lung, prostate and colorectum are most common in people over the age of 65. Prognosis varies with the type of cancer; however, notwithstanding other comorbidities, the trajectory of illness due to cancer is one of maintenance of

Table 6.1   Leading causes of death in Australia 2004, males and females aged 65 and over.

Cause of death	Males (%)	Females (%)
Ischaemic heart disease	20.9	20.0
Cerebrovascular diseases	8.6	12.7
Lung cancer	6.9	3.4
Chronic obstructive pulmonary disease	5.3	3.7
Other heart diseases	5.3	7.3
Dementia	3.0	5.9

physical function until a short time prior to death. Common symptoms are pain, nausea and vomiting, fatigue and shortness of breath (Lynn & Adamson 2003; Davies & Higginson 2004).

End stage organ failure

Ischaemic heart disease and other heart diseases are leading causes of death for people aged 65 and over. In contrast to cancer, people with heart failure have an illness trajectory of intermittent exacerbations of symptoms which may affect physical function, but with treatment a gradual return to either a previous level of function or slightly decreased function is possible. For people with ischaemic heart disease compared to those with cancer death is more likely from a sudden event. Common symptoms of heart failure are pain, breathlessness and fatigue (Lynn & Adamson 2003; Davies & Higginson 2004).

Dementia

In Australia, it is estimated that the number of people with dementia will grow from over 175 000 in 2003 to almost 465 000 in 2031. After the age of 65 the likelihood of living with dementia doubles every 5 years and it affects 24% of those aged 85 and over (Australian Institute of Health and Welfare 2006). The trajectory of illness for dementia is one of gradual loss of physical and mental function. Unlike heart failure there is no return to a previous level of function following an acute exacerbation. Common symptoms are mental confusion, incontinence, pain, loss of appetite and constipation (Lynn & Adamson 2003; Davies & Higginson 2004).

An obstacle in providing palliative care for older people is 'prognostic paralysis', i.e. if the prognosis is not clear, discussions of dying are not initiated. As predictions of prognosis are more difficult for end-stage organ failure or dementia than cancer, it is necessary to combine active and palliative management. Palliative management predominates as exacerbations are not reversible and death appears more likely (Australian and New Zealand Society for Geriatric Medicine 2009).

Where do older people die?

While a core value for palliative care is enabling people to die in the place they choose, the reality for most older people is that death will be determined by what services are available and in particular whether informal care from family members is an option. In England, only 18% of people over 65 years die at home, the rest occurring in hospitals (56.4%), 19.6% in long-term care settings such as nursing homes and residential care homes, 4% in hospices and 2% elsewhere (Office for National Statistics 2008).

In Australia, population-based data on place of death is not routinely reported. However, McNamara & Rosenwax (2007) using a population-based cohort design study for deaths in Western Australia report that 48.6% died in hospital, 20.2% died at home, 15.6% died in residential aged-care facilities, 5.5% in a hospice and 6.3% elsewhere. Their data indicate variability of place of death by age group: for those aged 65–74 death in hospital, followed by death at home, hospice and residential aged-care facility is most likely. With increasing age, death in hospital decreases and death in residential aged care increases.

Evidenced based palliative care for older people

Both the UK and Australia have national approaches to providing palliative care. In England the National End of Life Strategy advocates palliative care for everyone regardless of diagnosis and care setting. This strategy promotes three main tools that may help plan appropriate care for older people with palliative care needs: the Gold Standards Framework (GSF), the Liverpool Care Pathway (LCP) and the Preferred Priorities for Care (advance care planning) (Department of Health 2008). These tools were initially developed for people with cancer in hospitals (LCP) and primary care (GSF), so ongoing work is being undertaken to adapt them for older people living in other settings (Hockley *et al.* 2005; Badger *et al.* 2009).

In Australia, the National Palliative Care Strategy like the End of Life Care Strategy in England does not restrict palliative care to those with cancer and has over the last decade promoted a range of programmes across four broad areas: support for patients, families and carers in the community; increased access to medicines in the community; education, training and support for the workforce; and research and quality improvement for palliative care services. Many of these support palliative care for older people and in particular the programmes under education, training and support for the workforce. This has included the development of evidence based guidelines, including *Guidelines for a Palliative Approach for Residential Aged Care Facilities* (Commonwealth of Australia 2006) and, most recently, *Guidelines for a Palliative Approach for Aged Care in the Community Setting* (Australian Government Department of Health and Ageing 2010). In addition, like the UK, there has been a focus on advance care planning and the use of end-of-life care pathways.

The palliative care needs of older people are complex. The *Guidelines for a Palliative Approach for Residential Aged Care Facilities* (Commonwealth of Australia 2006)

Table 6.2 Level of evidence categories of the National Health and Medical Research Council (1999).

Level of evidence	Criteria
I	Systematic review of all relevant randomised controlled trials (RCTs)
II	At least one properly designed RCT
III-1	Well-designed pseudo-RCT
III-2	Comparative studies with concurrent controls and allocation not randomised, case–control studies or interrupted time series with a control group
III-3	Comparative studies with historical control, two or more single-arm studies, or interrupted time series without a parallel control group
IV	Case series, either post-test or pre-test and post-test

identified 14 areas of need and synthesised the best available evidence to develop 79 evidence based guidelines. The areas of palliative care identified for older people in residential aged care include:

(1) a palliative approach
(2) dignity and quality of life
(3) advance care planning
(4) advanced dementia
(5) physical symptom assessment and management
(6) psychological support
(7) family support
(8) social support, intimacy and sexuality
(9) Aboriginal and Torres Strait Islander issues
(10) cultural issues
(11) spiritual support
(12) volunteer support
(13) end-of-life (terminal) care
(14) bereavement support.

For each of the 79 guidelines, a rating of the level of evidence supporting the guideline was developed using the National Health and Medical Research Council levels of evidence (National Health and Medical Research Council 1999) (Table 6.2).

For guidelines where evidence using this rating was not available, qualitative studies were systematically examined for quality and for those assessed as appropriate a qualitative rating (QE) was assigned. Further details of this rating are available in the guidelines document (Commonwealth of Australia 2006). All guidelines were reviewed by an expert panel for consensus.

The *Guidelines for a Palliative Approach for Aged Care in the Community* (Australian Government Department of Health and Ageing 2010) is a companion document to the residential aged-care guidelines. The guidelines contain eight evidence based recommendations derived from systematic literature reviews regarding palliative care service delivery for older adults in the community and support for families. The systematic review used the same levels of evidence as the residential aged-care guidelines (Commonwealth of Australia 2006). Further narrative literature reviews were conducted in relation to:

(1) advance care planning and advance health directives
(2) symptom assessment and management
(3) cultural issues
(4) Aboriginal and Torres Strait Islander people
(5) psychosocial care
(6) spiritual support
(7) older adults with special needs.

From these narrative reviews 146 good practice points were derived for these seven areas.

Identifying the palliative care needs of older people

The remaining section of this chapter will focus on the evidence available for providing palliative care for older people in the following key areas:

(1) advance care planning
(2) symptom management
(3) spiritual support
(4) psychosocial care
(5) family care.

Whilst it is acknowledged that this does not cover all issues pertinent to providing palliative care, within the constraints of the chapter we feel these are important aspects in providing relationship-centred palliative care for older people. Evidence from the guidelines referred to above will be incorporated as will other evidence that supports best practice.

Advance care planning

Advance care planning is not a single event, but rather an interactive process of communication between a competent person and the healthcare team (Henry & Seymour 2008). It does not have to be a legalised formal process but rather should focus on ongoing communication with the person and/or family, as communication is the fundamental principle of advance care planning. The outcome of this process is an advance care plan, which makes clear the person's wishes regarding treatment decisions (which will often include decisions relating to their impending death), to extend their autonomy, and to guide decision-making when the person may be rendered incompetent of doing so (Australian Government Department of Health and Ageing 2010). This advance care plan may be a non-legal document or result in the completion of legal documents (advance directives) that formalise a person's wishes when they are no longer able to participate in decisions.

In Australia there are two options for advance directives. The first is the completion of a written advance health directive. These documents provide an opportunity for the person to stipulate what to do in the event of cardiopulmonary resuscitation, mechanical ventilation, artificial hydration and feeding. In Australia, different states and territories have different legislation and the documents vary slightly. A written advance health directive is only valid if made voluntarily and with information provided about what options are available. This is an important issue in palliative care. However, as highlighted in Chapter 4, not everyone desires to have all the information required to make informed treatment decisions. Or even for older people who do, families may block the disclosure of certain information. The second option is to appoint a proxy decision maker. This person, who does not necessarily need to be a family member, can provide guidance on issues that are not expressly covered in an advance health directive or in the absence of an advance health directive can make decisions in consultation with the medical team. It is possible to have both a proxy decision maker and a written advance health directive. In these instances, the proxy decision maker must abide by the decisions written in the advance health directive (Commonwealth of Australia 2006; Australian Government Department of Health and Ageing 2010). In the UK, the different countries have different legal frameworks, but overall similar options are available with a framework that addresses the nomination of proxies, advance directives and less formal setting out of values and wishes.

The use of advance directives in Australia is not yet routine and there is some debate about their role in advance care planning (Australian and New Zealand Society for Geriatric Medicine 2009). A number of barriers exist that have impacted on the success of people either completing an advance health directive or appointing a proxy decision maker. These include literacy, visual acuity, the perception of cost associated with seeking legal or medical advice, the inability to describe all situations that may confront a person, and the limited educational support for health professionals in the process of advance care planning (Baker 2002; Brown 2003). At present in Australia a number of initiatives – 'Let me decide' and 'Respecting patient choices' (Australian Government Department of Health and Ageing 2010) – are gaining momentum. In England, the Preferred Priorities for Care (Advance Care Planning) is promoted in the national End of Life Care Strategy (Department of Health 2008).

Symptom management

Symptom management for older people who require palliative care is complex and three key issues, pain, dyspnoea and fatigue, are addressed.

Pain

Pain is defined is a subjective experience, occurring when and where the individual says it does. Older people are often reluctant to report unrelieved pain, perhaps due to stoicism (with reluctance to report pain until it is moderate or severe) or because they do not wish to bother busy health professionals. They may also deny 'pain', instead using other terms such as 'ache', 'soreness' and 'stabbing' to describe what they are feeling. This results in poor pain control when medications are prescribed on an 'as necessary' basis (Commonwealth of Australia 2006).

Impeccable pain assessment is important in providing palliative care. A barrier to effective pain management is inadequate knowledge or failure to use assessment tools.

A thorough assessment of pain is necessary before a management strategy can be developed. Pain assessment should include:

- pain history
- general medical history
- physical examination
- physical impact of the pain
- social impact of the pain
- psychosocial factors related to the pain
- a review of medications and treatments
- severity and intensity of the pain
- prognosis.

The use of valid and reliable pain assessment tools can assist in pain assessment. The Australian Pain Society (2005) recommends the use of the Modified Residents' Verbal Brief Pain Inventory (M-RBVPI) (Auret *et al.* 2008). For some older people with cognitive impairment, reporting of pain may be difficult and the use of behavioural rating tools is necessary. The Australian Pain Society (2005) recommend the Pain Assessment in Advanced Dementia (PAINAD) Scale (Warden *et al.* 2003) or the Abbey Pain Scale (Abbey *et al.* 2004).

An understanding of the different types of pain is important in identifying appropriate pharmacological and non-pharmacological treatment. There are two major types of pain: nociceptive and neuropathic. Nociceptive pain is related to the stimulation of pain receptors. This type of pain can be further classified as visceral or somatic. Visceral pain is related to organs such as the liver, heart and gut. Visceral pain is often described as deep, squeezing or a dull ache. Somatic pain is related to pain stimuli in the skin, muscles or bones. Somatic pain is generally well localised, and may be described as aching, gnawing or sharp. Somatic pain can include arthritis and musculoskeletal conditions. Neuropathic pain is related to damage to the nervous system. This sort of pain is often described as burning, shooting or tingling. Neuropathic pain can be related to diabetic neuropathy, cerebrovascular accident, phantom limb pain and sciatica (Australian Pain Society 2005).

Pain management should include pharmacological and non-pharmacological strategies tailored to the individual. The World Health Organization has an analgesic ladder which recommends a three-step pharmacological approach for pain management: the first step is for mild pain, for which non-opioids are recommended; the second step is for moderate pain, for which weak opioids and a non-opioid adjuvant are recommended; and the third step is for strong pain, for which strong opioids and a non-opioid adjuvant are advocated. Common non-opioid adjuvants include paracetamol (acetaminophen) and non-steroidal anti-inflammatory drugs (Australian Government Department of Health and Ageing 2010).

Non-pharmacological strategies used in conjunction with pharmacological treatments are most effective. These may include cognitive behavioural strategies, application of heat or cold, exercise, transcutaneous electrical nerve stimulation (TENS) and complementary therapies (Australian Pain Society 2005; Australian Government Department of Health and Ageing 2010).

Dyspnoea

Dyspnoea is the sensation of uncomfortable breathing and has been estimated to affect between 50 and 70% of people at the end of life (Thomas & von Gunten 2003). It is a distressing and frightening symptom. A thorough assessment of dyspnoea should include a thorough history including pre-existing illnesses, associated symptoms, what makes it better or worse and a severity rating. The use of a visual analogue scale is generally the best measure of severity (Commonwealth of Australia 2006).

Pharmacological treatment options for dyspnoea include opioids, sedatives and oxygen. Opioids reduce the perception of dyspnoea and decrease oxygen consumption and as such are the main pharmacological treatment option. Sedatives may be useful for relieving anxiety related to dyspnoea. Oxygen may not be beneficial and a thorough assessment should be undertaken prior to oxygen being used (Commonwealth of Australia 2006). Non-pharmacological management includes advice and support about the management of dyspnoea, as well as reassurance and a calm presence. Provision of counselling, use of relaxation and breathing control techniques have also been found to be effective (Commonwealth of Australia 2006).

While some individuals such as those with COPD may experience dyspnoea over a prolonged period of time, for many individuals change in breathing may occur more in the final hours of life. Noisy or rattly breathing may be distressing particularly for family members. The cause is usually an accumulation of secretions in the oropharynx and management including the use of antimuscarinic drugs is recommended (Bennett *et al.* 2002).

Fatigue

Fatigue is one of the most common palliative care symptoms but like pain it is often under-treated. It is a sense of exhaustion, loss of strength, or tiredness that occurs without exertion and is not relieved by rest (Liao & Ferrell 2000). Fatigue may have many causes such as pre-existing disease, comorbidities, the disease process or treatment effects (Commonwealth of Australia 2006).

Assessment is based on self report; although some tools have been developed, these have not been used with older people. There are no pharmacological interventions specifically for fatigue, although underlying conditions should be investigated and treated. Non-pharmacological strategies that may be useful include exercise programmes and energy conservation (Commonwealth of Australia 2006). Guidelines for cancer-related fatigue are available but these are not specifically formulated for older adults with non-cancer disease (Australian Government Department of Health and Ageing 2010).

Spiritual support

Determining the spiritual needs of an older person requiring palliative care is important. While for many older people spirituality is partly manifested through religious beliefs, this may be one aspect of spirituality. Ascertaining if a person has religious beliefs alone is not an adequate mechanism of assessing spiritual needs. Some possible questions to consider include the following (Hicks 1999).

- How are you in yourself?
- What is your source of hope and strength?
- What are your spiritual needs?
- Are there ways we might help with your spiritual needs or concerns?

Spirituality should be routinely included in assessment, planning and delivery of care and is a key dimension of the provision of relationship-centred palliative care. Spiritual or religious issues may become more pronounced when people have a life-limiting illness. Health professionals should provide opportunity for individuals to discuss any fears or wishes to be completed prior to their death. Similarly, some individuals may not want to discuss these issues with a health professional or family and these wishes should be respected (Chan & McConigley 2006). Spiritual care involves coordinating services and people as requested by the person such as active and sensitive listening, access to services or other related items such as rosaries.

Psychosocial care

Psychosocial assessment is important in relationship-centred palliative care, particularly screening for depression. Depression is one of the commonest psychiatric disorders in older people and under-diagnosis is common. Rates of depression for people requiring palliative care range from 25 to 40% (Lloyd-Williams 2002) but the rate of treatment is lower, indicating that older people are not receiving appropriate psychological support (Watts *et al.* 2002).

Symptoms of depression include:

- lack of interest or pleasure
- depressed mood
- sleep disturbance
- poor pain and symptom control
- suicidal thoughts
- inability to think or concentrate
- feelings of worthlessness, hopelessness, or helplessness, inappropriate guilt and/or persistent negativism
- agitation or retardation
- fatigue
- altered appetite
- flattened mood
- frequently expressing a death desire
- social withdrawal.

Screening for depression is effective using brief scales and there are specific scales that have been developed for older people, such as the Geriatric Depression Scale (Soon & Levine 2002). However, this scale is not suitable for people with cognitive impairment and an alternative, the Cornell Scale for Depression in Dementia, is recommended (Camus *et al.* 1993). A combination of pharmacological and non-pharmacological management for depression in older people is the ideal. Consideration for pharmacological management is the prognosis of the person. For those with a life expectancy of more than 2 months, antidepressants are appropriate. For those with a shorter life expectancy a psychostimulant may relieve symptoms within the time available (MacLeod 1998; Martin & Jackson 2000). Non-pharmacological management should include emotional and social support.

Delirium is a disturbance of consciousness and is characterised by disordered attention, thinking and perception. It has been estimated to occur in up to 25% of hospitalised adults. Main causes are prescribed medications or infection. Management requires identification and treatment of the underlying cause, providing a quiet environment and medications to manage the symptoms (Brown & Boyle 2002). No assessment tool distinguishes between depression and delirium and therefore screening for each should occur. The Confusion Assessment Method is a valid and reliable screening tool for delirium (Australian Government Department of Health and Ageing 2010).

Family care

Family care is complex and comprises four key issues: communication, information/education, respite, and grief and bereavement.

Communication

Families appreciate good communication, particularly being informed about the person's condition. Family conferences provide opportunities to obtain and share information and set goals of care (Rutman & Parke 1992). For older people admitted to a residential aged-care facility, consideration of the effect of a transfer into this care setting either from home or often after admission to hospital or hospice is required (Maccabee 1994). Understanding the social relationships between family members is crucial and the use of tools such as a genogram or an ecomap helps document formal and informal support and assists health professionals to understand who may be affected by the death of the older person (Hockley 2000).

Information and education

Information and education support is important to families (Osse *et al.* 2006), particularly in relation to:

- physical problems and symptoms
- treatment and side effects
- alternative healing methods
- skills needed to provide care
- how to provide nourishment
- what will happen.

Active education refers to education combined with skills training and this has shown to be effective for carers providing support for people across a range of diseases. It may include how to assess symptom intensity or how to cope with the stress of being a carer (Meuser & Marwit 2001).

Respite care

Respite care is often under-utilised by those caring for older people in the community. This reluctance may come from a sense of duty, concern that the care recipient will be stressed by respite, or the carers not recognising that they could benefit from a break in providing care. In particular carers who are providing high levels of physical care or caring for someone with challenging behaviours associated with dementia or other mental health concerns should be encouraged to use respite services. The use of respite, particularly for people caring for someone with dementia, can improve outcomes such as reduced burden, depression, stress and increased well-being (Australian Government Department of Health and Ageing 2010).

Grief and bereavement

Grief is the normal response to loss and may be exhibited as emotional, physical. mental, behavioural and spiritual reactions. Bereavement is the total reaction to a loss and includes a period of recovery from the loss (Australian Government Department of Health and Ageing 2010). Caring for an older person who requires palliative care means providing care while coping with grief. For people caring for someone with dementia grief can occur as the person with dementia loses cognitive function (Meuser & Marwit 2001).

Risk factors that may indicate the need for professional bereavement support for families include (Australian Government Department of Health and Ageing 2010):

- a death that was traumatic;
- being unable to attend the death or funeral;
- believing the death was preventable;
- ambivalence towards the person who died;
- a death that impacts on the person's social support;
- a bereaved person who has a pre-existing psychiatric disorder;
- a prolonged death;
- other crises occurring simultaneously.

Whilst most family members will be supported by family and friends, for those who require assistance, community bereavement programmes offer counselling and support groups; some of these offer assistance in learning new skills (e.g. cooking), self-care activities and social opportunities (Caserta *et al.* 2004).

Case study 6.1   Translating evidence into practice

This case study reports on a project which developed and evaluated a model of multidisciplinary palliative care for residents with end-stage dementia in two residential aged-care facilities (Abbey *et al.* 2008). The model of care was based on the *Guidelines for a Palliative Approach in Residential Aged Care* (Australian Government Department of Health and Ageing 2010). The model of care included the following:

- Education for all facility staff on the palliative approach, terminal care, dysphagia, nutrition and hydration, bowel care, skin integrity, fatigue, pain, bereavement support, case conferences and care planning.
- Convening a multidisciplinary case conference with the family, nursing, medical and allied health staff to review goals of care and identify appropriate palliative care interventions.
- Clinical support from a specialist palliative care service for both the facility staff and general practitioner.

The model of care was evaluated using a pre- and post-study design. Care was compared for 25 residents prior to the implementation of the model with care for 17 residents who received care as part of the model. Outcomes were measured by chart audits, the Symptom Management at the End-of-Life in Dementia (SM-EOLD) and the Satisfaction with Care at the End-of-Life in Dementia (SWC-EOLD) (Volicer *et al.* 2001) scales. The SM-EOLD records the occurrence of nine common symptoms in the 90 days prior to the person's death: fear, anxiety, shortness of breath, depression, agitation, resistiveness to care, pain, skin breakdown and calm. These audits were completed by a research nurse with experience in dementia care. The SWC-EOLD is a 10-question scale which focuses on satisfaction with care, involvement in decision-making and care planning. This scale was administered by the research nurse with the resident's closest relative.

The main findings before intervention were:

(1) limited use of case conferencing (12%) to discuss a palliative approach;
(2) limited use of advance health directives (8%);
(3) documentation of the recognition of palliative care was limited to a few days prior to death;
(4) common symptoms as measured by the SM-EOLD were agitation, resistance to care, pain and skin breakdown;
(5) carer concerns as measured by the SWC-EOLD indicated there was some dissatisfaction with medical care, knowing who was in charge of care and medications not being explained.

The main findings after intervention were as follows.

(1) An increase in the use of palliative care case conferences (71%) and a slight increase in the use of advance health directives (12%).
(2) Ratings on the SM-EOLD indicated that after intervention, shortness of breath, pain, anxiety, resistiveness to care and agitation were recorded more frequently. While this is counter to what was expected, the education raised awareness of the importance of documentation and of key symptoms. Therefore more symptoms were reported after intervention.
(3) Ratings on the SW-EOLD were generally high both before and after intervention and there were no statistically significant improvements in satisfaction after intervention. However, four questions showed higher satisfaction. These concerned information to make decisions, measures to keep the resident comfortable, information about the end stage of dementia and satisfaction with medical care.

The study concluded that providing a structured multidisciplinary approach for residents with end-stage dementia shows promising results and more work in this area is required.

Summary

This chapter has highlighted the importance of relationship-centred palliative care for older people. As the world's population ages, understanding trajectories of illness and causes of death for older people will assist service providers and planners to meet the needs of older people. While not exhaustive we have identified some of the key issues that should be considered in providing relationship-centred palliative care for this population. In particular is the need for impeccable assessment of common symptoms such as pain, fatigue, dyspnoea, delirium and depression. Also crucial is incorporating advance care planning as early as possible with regular review. This will assist older people to receive the care they wish in the setting of their choice. Family care is integral to relationship-centred care and this should extend beyond the older person's illness into bereavement.

The case study illustrates how evidence based guidelines can be taken off the shelf and incorporated into practice. However, it does raise the interesting issue that in some instances providing education may lead to greater reporting of symptoms. While this may be seen as a negative effect and the intervention seemingly unsuccessful, a positive outcome is that an increase in the recognition of symptoms will highlight the need for treatment to be provided and follow-up evaluations to be conducted.

In the UK and Australia, palliative care is part of national policy and the palliative care needs of older adults are starting to receive the recognition required. The challenge for these and other countries with an ageing population is to ensure that flexibility and high-quality services are available for older people to access care when and where they need it.

Key messages

- Developing comprehensive advance care plans that include ongoing assessments and which respond to changes in a person's health increases the person and his/her family's satisfaction with care (Molloy *et al.* 2000) (Evidence Level II).
- A comprehensive assessment of pain and the use of evidence based analgesia decision-making provides enhanced pain management, thereby improving the individual's quality of life (Du Pen *et al.* 1999) (Evidence Level II).
- The use of sustained-release low-dose oral morphine administered orally or parenterally can benefit individuals with dyspnoea by reducing the severity of their symptoms and improving the quality of their sleep (Abernethy *et al.* 2003) (Evidence Level II).
- Fatigue is the most frequently reported physical concern by individuals nearing death. Therefore careful assessment of factors that may indicate or bring about fatigue will enhance early identification and management of fatigue (Liao & Ferrell 2000) (Evidence Level IV).
- Understanding a person's current or desired practices, attitudes, experiences and beliefs by obtaining a comprehensive history assists in meeting the spiritual needs of a person, as does a regular review (Koenig *et al.* 1997) (Evidence Level IV).
- The use of the Geriatric Depression Scale can increase the frequency with which treatment is provided for depression by prescription or via referral to appropriate healthcare providers (Soon & Levine 2002) (Evidence Level II).

- A thorough assessment of the symptoms of delirium is required, which includes consideration of the persistence of symptoms (e.g. inattention, disorientation and impaired memory)
  to accurately and quickly detect delirium in older persons. This increases resident's frequency of treatment and referral (McCusker *et al.* 2003) (Evidence Level III-2).
- Family conferences can provide emotional support to family members and an opportunity
  to discuss concerns about the resident's illness/ageing process. Such discussion benefits
  families and ultimately improves the quality of life for the resident (Dempsay & Pruchno
  1993; Kristjanson *et al.* 1996) (Evidence Level III-2).
- Active education should be made available for family carers of older adults who have
  moderate or severe dementia, disability and/or frailty due to a stroke and advanced cancer
  (Australian Government Department of Health and Ageing 2010) (Evidence Level I).
- Respite care should be routinely available to support family carers of older adults with
  non-specific and advanced life-limiting illness, frailty or extreme old age (Australian
  Government Department of Health and Ageing 2010) (Evidence Level I).
- The greater the level of social support that a family can access, the better their ability to
  cope with bereavement of their family member; however, it is the quality of the support
  rather than the quantity that enhances resilience (Kelly *et al.* 1999) (Evidence Level IV).

References

Abbey J, Piller N, Bellis A *et al.* (2004) The Abbey Pain Scale: a 1-minute numerical indicator for
people with end stage dementia. *International Journal of Palliative Nursing* **10**, 6–13.

Abbey J, Sacre S, Parker D (2008) *Develop, trial and evaluate a model of multidisciplinary palliative care for residents with end-stage dementia.* Queensland University of Technology,
Brisbane.

Abernethy A, Currow D, Frith P, Fazekas B, McHugh A, Bui C (2003) Randomised double-blind
placebo-controlled crossover trial of sustained-release morphine for the management of refrac-
tory dyspnoea. *British Medical Journal* **327**, 523–528.

Auret K, Toye C, Goucke R, Kristjanson L, Bruce D, Schug S (2008) Development and testing of
a modified version of the Brief Pain Inventory for use in residential aged care facilities. *Journal
of the American Geriatrics Society* **56**, 301–306.

Australian and New Zealand Society for Geriatric Medicine (2009) Position statement 16. *Palliative Care for the Older Person.* Australian and New Zealand Society for Geriatric Medicine,
Sydney.

Australian Government Department of Health and Ageing (2010) *Guidelines for a Palliative Approach
for Aged Care in the Community Setting. Best Practice Guidelines for the Australian Context.*
Office for an Ageing Australia, Canberra, Australia. Available at http://www.caresearch.com.au/
caresearch/ClinicalPractice/tabid/93/Default.aspx (accessed 9 December 2010).

Australian Institute of Health and Welfare (2006) *Dementia in Australia: National Data Analysis
and Development.* Cat. no. AGE 53. AIHW, Canberra, Australia.

Australian Institute of Health and Welfare (2007) *Older Australia at a Glance*, 4th edn. Cat. no.
AGE 52. AIHW, Canberra, Australia.

Australian Pain Society (2005) *Pain in Residential Care Facilities: Management Strategies.* North
Sydney, NSW, Australia. Available at http://www.apsoc.org.au/owner/files/9e2c2n.pdf (accessed
10 December 2010).

Badger F, Clifford C, Hewison A, Thomas K (2009) An evaluation of the implementation of a programme to improve end-of-life care in nursing homes. *Palliative Medicine* **23**, 502–511.

Baker M (2002) Economic, political and ethnic influences on end-of-life decision-making: a decade in review. *Journal of Health and Social Policy* **14**, 27–39.

Bennett M, Lucas V, Brennan M, Hughes A, O'Donnell V, Wee B (2002) Using anti-muscarinic drugs in the management of death rattle: evidence based guidelines for palliative care. *Palliative Medicine* **16**, 369–374.

Brown M (2003) The law and practice associated with advance directives in Canada and Australia: similarities, differences and debates. *Journal of Law and Medicine* **11**, 59–76.

Brown T, Boyle M (2002) Delirium. *British Medical Journal* **325**, 644–647.

Burt J, Raine R (2006) The effect of age on referral to and use of specialist palliative care services in adult cancer patients: a systematic review. *Age and Ageing* **35**, 469–476.

Camus V, Schmitt L, Ousset P (1993) A comparative study of Hamilton, Cornell, and Sunderland Depression Rating scales in dementia. *Journal of the American Geriatrics Society* **41** (Suppl. 10), SA42.

Caserta M, Lund D, Obray S (2004) Promoting self-care and daily living skills among older widows and widowers: evidence from the Pathfinders Demonstration Project. *Omega: Journal of Death and Dying* **49**, 217–236.

Chan V, McConigley R (2006) *Outline of Palliative Medicine*. Cabramatta, NSW, Australia.

Commonwealth of Australia (2006) *Guidelines for a Palliative Approach in Residential Aged Care Facilities: NHMRC Endorsed Edition*. Available at http://www.nhmrc.gov.au/publications/synopses/ac12to14syn.htm (accessed 10 December 2010).

Davies E, Higginson I (2004) *Better Palliative Care for Older People*. WHO Regional Office for Europe, Copenhagen.

Dempsay N, Pruchno RA (1993) The family's role in the nursing home: predictors of technical and non-technical assistance. *Journal of Gerontological Social Work* **21**, 127–145.

Department of Health (2008) *End of LIfe Care Strategy: Promoting High Quality Care for all Adults at the End of Life*. Department of Health, London.

Du Pen S, Du Pen A, Polissar N *et al.* (1999) Implementing guidelines for cancer pain management: results of a randomised controlled trial. *Journal of Clinical Oncology* **17**, 361–370.

Henry C, Seymour J (2008) *Advance Care Planning: A Guide for Health and Social Care Staff*. Department of Health, London.

Hicks T (1999) Spirituality and the elderly: nursing implications with nursing home residents. *Geriatric Nursing* **20**, 144–146.

Hockley J (2000) Psychosocial aspects in palliative care: communicating with the patient and family. *Acta Oncologica* **39**, 905–910.

Hockley J, Dewar B, Watson J (2005) Promoting end of life care in nursing homes using an 'integrated care pathway for the last days of life'. *Journal of Research in Nursing* **10**, 132–152.

Kelly B, Edwards P, Synott R, Neil C, Baille R, Battistutta D (1999) Predictors of bereavement outcome for family carers of cancer patients. *Psycho-Oncology* **8**, 237–249.

Koenig H, Weiner D, Peterson B, Meador K, Keefe F (1997) Religious coping in the nursing home: a biopsychosocial model. *International Journal of Psychiatry in Medicine* **27**, 365–376.

Kristjanson L, Sloan J, Dudgeon D, Akaskin E (1996) Family members' perceptions of palliative cancer care: predictors of family functioning and family members' health. *Journal of Palliative Care* **12**, 10–20.

Liao S, Ferrell B (2000) Fatigue in an older population. *Journal of the American Geriatrics Society* **48**, 426–430.

Lloyd-Williams M (2002) Is it appropriate to screen palliative care patients for depression? *American Journal of Hospice and Palliative Care* **19**, 112–114.

Lynn J, Adamson D (2003) *Living Well at the End of Life: Adapting Health Care to Serious Chronic Illness in Old Age*. Rand Health, Arlington.

Maccabee J (1994) The effect of transfer from a palliative care unit to nursing homes: are patients' and relatives' needs met? *Palliative Medicine* **8**, 211–214.

McCusker J, Cole P, Dendukuri N, Han L, Betzile E (2003) The course of delirium in older medical inpatients: a prospective study. *Journal of General Internal Medicine* **18**, 696–704.

MacLeod A (1998) Methylphenidate in terminal depression. *Journal of Pain and Symptom Management* **16**, 193–198.

McNamara B, Rosenwax L (2007) Factors affecting place of death in Western Australia. *Health and Place* **13**, 356–367.

Martin A, Jackson K (2000) Depression in palliative care patients. In: Jackson II KC, Lipman AG, Tyler LS (eds) *Evidence Based Symptom Control in Palliative Care: Systematic Reviews and Validated Clinical Practice Guidelines for 15 Common Problems in Patients with Life Limiting Disease*. Pharmaceutical Products Press, New York.

Meuser T, Marwit S (2001) A comprehensive, stage-sensitive model of grief in dementia caregiving. *Gerontologist* **41**, 658–670.

Molloy D, Guyatt G, Russo R *et al.* (2000) Systematic implementation of an advance directive program in nursing homes: a randomized controlled trial. *Journal of the American Medical Association* **283**, 1437–1444.

National Confidential Enquiry into Patient Outcome and Death (2009) *Caring to the End? A Review of the Care of Patients who Died in Hospital Within Four Days of Admission*. National Confidential Enquiry into Patient Outcome and Death, London.

National Health and Medical Research Council (1999) *A Guide to Development, Implementation and Evaluation of Clinical Practice Guidelines*. Commonwealth of Australia, Canberra.

Office for National Statistics (2005) *Focus on Older People*. Office for National Statistics, London.

Office for National Statistics (2008) *Mortality Statistics. Deaths registered in 2008*. Office for National Statistics, London.

Osse B, Vernooij-Dassen M, Schade E, Grol R (2006) Problems experienced by the informal caregivers of cancer patients and their needs for support. *Cancer Nursing* **29**, 378–390.

Rutman D, Parke B (1992) Palliative care needs of residents, families, and staff in long-term care facilities. *Journal of Palliative Care* **12**, 10–20.

Soon J, Levine M (2002) Screening for depression in patients in long-term care facilities: a randomised controlled trial of physician response. *Journal of the American Geriatrics Society* **50**, 1092–1099.

Thomas J, von Gunten C (2003) Pain in terminally ill patients: guidelines for pharmacological management. *CNS Drugs* **17**, 9.

Volicer L, Hurley A, Blasi Z (2001) Scales for evaluation of end-of-life care in dementia. *Alzheimer Disease and Associated Disorders* **15**, 194–200.

Warden V, Hurley A, Volicer L (2003) Development and psychometric evaluation of the Pain Assessment in Advanced Dementia (PAINAD) Scale. *Journal of American Medical Directors Association* **4**, 9–15.

Watts S, Bhutani G, Stout I *et al.* (2002) Mental health in older adult recipients of primary care services: is depression the key issue? Identification, treatment and the general practitioner. *International Journal of Geriatric Psychiatry* **17**, 427–437.

World Health Organization (2003) *WHO Definition of Palliative Care*. WHO, Geneva.

Chapter 7

Promoting Urinary Continence

Joanne Booth, Suzanne Kumlien and Yuli Zang

Introduction

Older people commonly experience lower urinary tract symptoms, including urinary incontinence. Urinary incontinence is one of the geriatric syndromes, together with falls and delirium, that is thought to occur when impairments in multiple domains accrue and interact. The resulting health deterioration and functional decline directly leads to frailty and dependency (Coll-Planus *et al.* 2008). Therefore intervening to maintain or promote continence is of benefit to the individual and contributes to their continued quality of life. Continence issues negatively impact on every aspect of an older person's life and often those of their family carers, being one of the key determinants of well-being and admission to institutional care (Thom *et al.* 1997; Brittain & Shaw 2007). The effects of difficulties with lower urinary tract symptoms and maintaining continence should not be underestimated as the costs are high psychologically, physically, socially and economically. Furthermore, with the global changes in demography towards an increasing number of older people, the absolute number of families affected by continence issues is expanding rapidly. Thus there is great potential for public health benefit in reducing the occurrence and impact of urinary incontinence and lower urinary tract symptoms. A recent proliferation of research is likely to provide evidence to assist nurses to move away from an over-reliance on strategies to contain urinary incontinence towards continence promotion and methods of active bladder rehabilitation. These will be illustrated in the case study, which focuses on the developing evidence to inform nursing management of incontinence following stroke.

What does urinary incontinence mean to older people?

Maintaining emotional well-being and quality of life among older people is the main concern of the person, their family and nurses alike. Difficulties with continence threaten this, disempowering the person and influencing every aspect of daily life (Norton 2006). The negative impact may be immense, affecting self-esteem, personal relationships,

Evidence Informed Nursing with Older People, First Edition. Edited by Debbie Tolson, Joanne Booth and Irene Schofield.
© 2011 Blackwell Publishing Ltd. Published 2011 by Blackwell Publishing Ltd.

Box 7.1 Views about continence issues expressed by older people

'I wear a pad during the night and then I wear another one during the day…they're horrible, horrible!' (Woman, aged 76)

'My oldest daughter's just phoned me saying, "Do you want to come down?" I do, and she's got a room there and she says, "That's yours, so just come down"…but I feel if I go there, I'm frightened anything happens to me…in case I wet…oh, it's terrible.' (Woman, aged 83)

'Constantly having to run to the loo…I feel as if people are watching me. When I'm out, I try and take different routes so they don't keep seeing me go.' (Man, aged 81)

'I have found I only go out when I have to…I am so frightened I smell. Do I smell hen?' (Woman, aged 75)

---

sexual and social activities and resulting in loneliness, isolation and depression (Brittain & Shaw 2007; Nicolson *et al.* 2008). Some examples of views expressed by older people are given in Box 7.1

It is particularly apparent in older people with cognitive impairment who may not demonstrate awareness of their urinary condition (DuBeau *et al.* 2006). Recent studies have highlighted anxiety, fear of leakage, depression and hopelessness when people have an overactive bladder and demonstrated that these effects are much worse for those who also experience incontinence (Nicolson *et al.* 2008). Thus for reasons of embarrassment and associated stigma urinary symptoms are often hidden by older people and their carers and self-managed. They are also under-reported to health services (Shaw *et al.* 2001; Horrocks *et al.* 2004; Booth *et al.* 2010). Many people see urinary incontinence as the final boundary, which once crossed makes it impossible to maintain societal roles and engagement (Twigg 2000). The suggestion has been made that the psychological costs to older people with hidden incontinence are much higher than for diagnosed chronic medical illnesses because there is no acknowledgement of the condition and thus no attempts made towards resolution (Nicolson *et al.* 2008). It can also be argued that the long-term demand for concealment requires effort and is thus detrimental to health and quality of life.

Physically, older people with continence difficulties may experience impaired mobility (Fonda *et al.* 2005), falls and fractures (Brown *et al.* 2000), poor skin integrity, and functional and cognitive decline (Huang *et al.* 2007). Incontinence can prevent discharge from hospital to home and heighten vulnerability to institutional placement (Thom *et al.* 1997). Symptoms associated with overactive bladder, urge and mixed urinary incontinence are more distressing than stress symptoms and are linked to poorer physical health and quality of life (Mons *et al.* 2005; Chiarelli *et al.* 2009). Thus what may at first be thought of as a relatively simple condition may in reality have numerous consequences for older people, triggering a cascade of unwanted events. Clearly urinary incontinence has a pivotal role in the development of syndromes of old age and should not be ignored, accepted or indeed hidden.

Causes of urinary incontinence in older people

The causes of urinary incontinence are many and frequently complex. Direct and indirect routes of development are found and recent evidence has highlighted the active role of urinary incontinence in the development of disability and frailty (Coll-Planus *et al.* 2008). A number of intrinsic and extrinsic influencing factors increase the likelihood of urinary incontinence occurring in older people, relative to younger populations, hence the perpetuation of the myth that incontinence is to be expected as part of normal ageing. Therefore, as incontinence is not an inevitable consequence of the ageing process, when it develops it should be investigated in full.

Maintaining urinary continence is a complex interaction of sensory, motor, cognitive and social skills to enable successful recognition, access to and use of toilet facilities. It involves both automatic and voluntary behaviour and is dependent on a fully functioning urinary tract, musculoskeletal competence and integrity of the central and peripheral nervous systems. Disturbances in any part of these systems can induce lower urinary tract symptoms resulting in difficulties with continence. Such disturbances are more likely as we age but not inevitable.

One key message to note is that urinary incontinence may be a *transient* or an *established* condition. Acute onset usually indicates a transient reversible cause and is common among acutely ill, hospitalised older people. Direct causes should be identified and treated immediately. These, together with effects on the bladder and urinary system, are shown in Box 7.2.

A typology of established urinary incontinence exists with globally recognised descriptors agreed by the International Continence Society (which can be found at www.icsoffice. org/). Each of these is the result of impairments caused by pathology in the systems controlling continence and for the purposes of revision are explored in Box 7.3.

Why do older people develop urinary incontinence?

Urinary incontinence is defined as the complaint of any involuntary loss of urine (Abrams *et al.* 2002) and is associated with frail older people in all societies. Despite the typology of urinary incontinence described in Box 7.2 which indicates specific aetiological pathways, it is rare to find a single identifiable cause for urinary incontinence among older people, particularly those who are frail. For this population urinary incontinence is a recognised syndrome of older age (Inouye *et al.* 2007) and in this respect is a clinical condition that does not fit any discrete disease category. Rather, urinary incontinence is the consequence of multiple risk factors some of which arise as normal changes that occur with ageing, affecting multiple organ systems and which increase the older person's vulnerability to health-related insults (Coll-Planus *et al.* 2008). Common examples of how this vulnerability manifests include a reduction in bladder capacity by 200–300 mL and urethral closure pressure leading to problems such as stress urinary incontinence, nocturia and frequency (Grimby *et al.* 1993; Ouslander *et al.* 1995). Similarly, post-void residual urine volume increases with ageing, which may stimulate involuntary detrusor contractions leading to urgency and increasing the risk of urinary tract infection (Lekan-Rutledge 2004).

Box 7.2   Transient causes of urinary incontinence

Urinary tract infection

Inflammation and toxin release irritate urothelium and induce detrusor overactivity (see Chapter 13).

Faecal impaction

Direct pressure on bladder neck and obstruction of urethra leads to retention of urine and overflow incontinence. Presence of 'foreign body' pressure can induce detrusor irritability and urge.

Medication effects, including polypharmacy

Diuretics cause polyuria, which can contribute to urge incontinence. Older people with reduced bladder capacity and a weakened pelvic floor may not have sufficient control to reach the toilet before stress leakage occurs. Anticholinergics/antispasmodics/narcotic analgesics dampen detrusor activity and bowel peristalsis, and thus may cause urinary retention, faecal impaction and overflow incontinence. Drug interactions are common: these impact on cognitive status leading to functional urinary incontinence as well as direct effects on the bladder, such as reduced sphincter and bladder tone.

Delirium

Disorientation may impact on ability to find a toilet; impaired conscious level and reasoning affects abilities to recognise and interpret bladder sensation and desire to void and initiate toilet activities (see Chapter 5).

Acute retention

Bladder fills to capacity and overflow leakage occurs. Risk of kidney damage increased through ureteric back pressure and reflux.

Depression

Mental status may lead to hypomanic condition; volition and motivation impaired which can result in voluntary incontinence. Drug treatment of depression may cause urinary retention and reduced sensation resulting in overflow incontinence, especially where bladder capacity is reduced (see Chapter 10).

Atrophic vaginitis/urethritis

Thinning of mucosa, dryness and increased friability as a result of decreased oestrogen in women leads to symptoms of irritation including frequency, burning when passing urine and urgency incontinence.

Acute exacerbations of illness

Heart failure and diabetes may cause polyuria, especially overnight leading to nocturia, urge and stress symptoms. Cough associated with chronic obstructive pulmonary disease increases stress symptoms.

Hyperplasia of the prostate gland which occurs in older men may lead to bladder outlet obstruction and voiding difficulties such as hesitancy, straining to void, intermittent flow and weak stream. Changes in diurnal and nocturnal urine production that accompany ageing result in nocturia, often in multiple episodes that disturb sleep and increase the risk of falls and social isolation (Stewart *et al.* 1992; Booth *et al.* 2010).

Box 7.3   Types of urinary incontinence: revision notes

Urge urinary incontinence (urge UI)
The complaint of involuntary leakage accompanied by or immediately preceded by urgency (International Continence Society 2009). The single most common type of urinary incontinence experienced by older people, particularly older women. Neurological deterioration associated with ageing or medical conditions such as stroke, Parkinson's disease and diabetes mellitus interferes with the higher centre control of the bladder. The ability to suppress automatic detrusor contractions is lost. These occur when provoked by physical or psychological triggers, such as standing up, the sound of running water or putting the key in the lock when arriving home. There is also reduced bladder capacity. Large amounts of urine loss are common with urge urinary incontinence.

Stress urinary incontinence (stress UI)
The complaint of involuntary leakage on effort or exertion, or on sneezing or coughing (International Continence Society 2009) This type of urinary incontinence is associated with younger women following childbirth and those who are overweight. Pure stress urinary incontinence is less common in older people than urge and mixed urinary incontinence.

Stress urinary incontinence arises from mechanical difficulties with pelvic floor muscles and urethral sphincter closure. Leakage of urine is brought about by an increase in bladder pressure that exceeds the urethral sphincter pressure and allows small bursts of urine to flow. A rise in intra-abdominal pressure is the main cause, occurring with activities such as coughing, sneezing and lifting. Equally, activities that increase the pressure and gravitational pull on the pelvic floor such as running, trampolining and other forms of rhythmic physical activity stretch the bladder support mechanisms. This is also the reason for the high levels of urinary incontinence found in women with obesity.

Mixed urinary incontinence (mixed UI)
The complaint of involuntary leakage associated with urgency and also with effort, exertion, sneezing and coughing (International Continence Society 2009). This type of urinary incontinence is commonly found in older populations, particularly older women. Features of urge urinary incontinence and stress urinary incontinence are found. Treatment is dependent on which type of incontinence is predominant.

Overflow urinary incontinence (overflow UI)
Involuntary leakage associated with inability of the bladder to empty completely, over-distension and overflow leakage of urine. The most common causes of this are bladder outlet obstruction in men with benign prostatic hyperplasia and reduced sensation in older people with neurological disease, such as multiple sclerosis and stroke whereby the bladder does not signal the brain when an urge to pass urine is felt and the bladder does not contract completely to fully empty and thus urinary retention is experienced. Tumours and stones may also cause overflow urinary incontinence.

Functional urinary incontinence (functional UI)
Involuntary leakage associated with the inability to reach or use toilet facilities. It is the result of physical, cognitive or communicative impairments. It is commonly found among older people often following an acute illness or event, or in those who are frail. It is characterised by factors outside the functioning of the urinary tract including the older person's environment, both physical and social that influences the development of incontinence.

A key challenge for nurses in all care contexts is identifying the predominant type of continence difficulty experienced by the older person. This is essential because the type of urinary incontinence will direct the approach to therapeutic intervention.

The association between urinary incontinence and falls

Maintaining continence involves more than the physiological ability to control bladder functioning. It also requires appropriate use of toilet facilities. The complexity of toileting activities is often under-recognised and given lower priority than many other aspects of function in rehabilitation programmes and falls services. It requires the combined activity and coordination of the cognitive, sensory, motor, balance and proprioceptive systems. Box 7.4 highlights the essential elements necessary for successful use of the toilet.

Given the range of physical demands made on an older person to successfully use the toilet, the links between urinary incontinence and falls in older people is unsurprising (Chiarelli *et al.* 2009). In the UK the Patient Safety Observatory (2007) reported that 15% of falls in acute hospitals were related to toilet use, 14% in community hospitals and 8% in mental health units. This was a high proportion of overall falls in relation to the fairly small part of each day patients are using the toilet. In contrast, less than 2% of falls took place in bathrooms and shower rooms, despite being occupied by patients for longer time periods. Urinary incontinence or urinary frequency were significant risk factors for falling in hospital identified in a meta-analysis (Oliver *et al.* 2004). A recent study of patients' views identified the urgent need to use the toilet as the most common reason for falls (Carroll *et al.* 2009).

In a study in three different residential settings for older people, Jenson *et al.* (2002) showed that over one-quarter of falls were related to visits to the toilet, with half of these occurring overnight during a toilet visit. The risks associated with night-time toilet use were also highlighted in a qualitative study exploring older people's experience of falls, where 5 of 27 interviewees reported falling at night when getting up to use the toilet (Roe *et al.* 2008).

Box 7.4   Elements of successful use of toilet

- Sensing, recognising and acknowledging the call to urinate
- Locating suitable toilet facilities
- Moving to and from toilet
- Negotiating access to toilet
- Management of clothing (and aids)
- Transfer onto and off toilet
- Control of elimination from bladder and bowel
- Perineal cleansing
- Washing and drying hands

Urinary incontinence was found to be one of four strong predictors for falls among older people living in the community (Tromp *et al.* 2001). In a large study of older women across four sites in the USA, urge urinary incontinence independently increased the risk of falls by 26% and risk of fractures by 34% (Brown *et al.* 2000). Thus the evidence indicates that it is not all types of urinary incontinence that are linked to falls. Chiarelli *et al.* (2009) undertook a meta-analysis of studies associating urinary incontinence and falls in older people. They showed that urge incontinence (and thus by definition mixed urinary incontinence) was associated with an increased risk of falling, whereas stress incontinence was not. This can be explained by the symptoms of urgency, where there is a need to rush to the toilet to prevent a sudden loss of a large amount of urine, as opposed to the minor leaks commonly found in stress incontinence. Similarly, the overactive bladder symptoms that occur with urge urinary incontinence include frequency, necessitating more regular trips to the toilet. This increases the risk of instability and toilet-related falls by the extra time spent in physical activity getting to and from the toilet.

In a study exploring lower urinary tract symptoms in community-living older people in a deprived and an affluent area, nocturia (85%), frequency (68%) and urgency (53%) were the most commonly reported symptoms. Together with weak urinary stream (43%) and feelings of incomplete bladder emptying (43%), all were more prevalent than actual urinary incontinence (42%) (Booth *et al.* 2010). These findings agree with Stewart *et al.* (1992) who showed that an increased risk of falls was associated with nocturia. However, Booth *et al.* (2010) also showed that older people in the deprived area experienced more falls than those in the affluent site, when getting up to use the toilet at night.

The evidence from these studies confirms that urinary incontinence and urinary symptoms are risk factors for falls among hospital inpatients, older people living at home and in various types of supported care environments. Moreover, it highlights the importance of considering all the syndromes of older age and the potential associations between them when planning and delivering effective care.

Evidence for continence promotion

Managing urinary incontinence is unquestionably a nursing responsibility in all care contexts (Cheater *et al.* 2008; Heckenberg 2008; Booth *et al.* 2009). Bladder-related activities comprise a significant proportion of nurses' work with older people, with 13% of staff time in a subacute care setting spent on continence care tasks (Morris *et al.* 2004). Despite the significance of their role, nurses have been found to be largely disinterested in working with older people to promote continence and activities relating to continence are seen as low priority (Dingwall & McLafferty 2006; Booth *et al.* 2009).

The reasons for the lack of attention to continence issues remain unclear and such attitudes are of concern as there is good evidence that lifestyle and behavioural interventions to promote continence in older people are effective. An estimated 70% of older people will significantly improve their urinary symptoms or recover continence with simple conservative approaches delivered by nurses (Williams *et al.* 2000; Borrie *et al.* 2002; Byles *et al.* 2005). This is a much higher therapeutic effect than is expected from most drug treatments but few nurses recognise the potential significance of their contribution.

Continence promotion is regarded as one of the fundamentals of nursing care that can appreciably increase an older person's dignity, well-being and quality of life (Crestodina 2007; Cheater *et al.* 2008). Despite this, urinary incontinence remains under-assessed and untreated in the older population (Wagg *et al.* 2008) with management focusing almost entirely on containment of urinary leakage, using absorbent pads and pants (Rodriguez *et al.* 2007; Godfrey 2008; Wagg *et al.* 2008).

Nurses working with older people are ideally placed to dispel the negativity associated with incontinence and instigate therapeutic activities. The latest international consultation on incontinence (International Continence Society 2009) certainly supports this view, recommending conservative advice and treatments as first-line management for all forms of incontinence, regardless of type or cause. Conservative approaches include lifestyle advice and behavioural therapies that can be provided by any gerontological nurse and are not reliant on referral to specialist services. Such approaches are dependent on comprehensive assessment, accurate identification of the type of continence difficulties and specific contributing factors followed by delivery of interventions that are tailored to the specific needs and experiences of the older person in their particular care context.

Models of continence promotion

Provision of best practice is an amalgam of the available evidence, interpreted through the lens of gerontological nursing values and combined with older people's and carers' preferences (see Chapters 1 and 2). It is these latter two aspects that determine the model of continence promotion used. Successful continence promotion with older people demands a practitioner with the knowledge and skills to flexibly utilise different approaches. It is a challenging enterprise, yet rewarding, with a high likelihood of success in impacting positively on an older person's quality of life.

Different models can be seen to underpin approaches to promotion of continence. In a traditional medical model the aim of the activities is to cure the problem. The older person is a passive recipient of treatment, which normally begins with prescription drug treatment and often ends with surgical intervention. The older person takes little part, being a passive recipient of treatment.

In contrast, the purely social model focuses only on palliation, seeking not to alter the person's continence status but rather to manage it in such a way that its impact on the individual is minimised. The mainstay of this approach is containment, which is usually achieved using absorbent products. This enables the older person to continue to engage with society and fulfil their social roles.

The third model, the rehabilitation model, is implicit in the literature yet poorly evidenced in practice. Its tenets are that urinary symptoms and incontinence are disabling and limit participation, but that the impact on the individual can be reversed or at least limited if the person engages with activities aimed at restoring control and function. Rehabilitative activities focus on enabling the older person to understand and change their continence behaviour using education and other supportive behavioural activities.

Each of these models has its place in directing the effective management of urinary incontinence in older people. However, we suggest there is an urgent need to shift the balance from a predominantly social model towards a much greater focus on the rehabilitation model. A number of reasons underlie this proposal.

(1) Bladder rehabilitation using lifestyle and behavioural modifications is likely to be successful.
(2) Continued reliance on the social model for the majority of older people wrongly implies that urinary incontinence is an accepted part of ageing and encourages the perpetuation of this myth.
(3) Avoidance of drug treatments is particularly important for older people in order to minimise drug interactions from polypharmacy and debilitating side effects such as the severe dry mouth and constipation associated with anticholinergics used to treat urgency and overactive bladder.

Applying different models of continence promotion depends on an understanding of the nature of the older person's specific continence difficulties in the context of their care situation, their beliefs and preferences for intervention. It will also depend on a thorough documented assessment and identification of type of incontinence. Continence assessment is globally highlighted as an area of poor practice (Leakin-Rutledge 2004; Wagg *et al*. 2008). However, there is a lack of validated assessment tools and decision aids to support practitioners to accurately identify types of urinary incontinence and hence inadequate treatment plans are developed, especially for the frail older population (Martin *et al*. 2006). Dingwall and McLafferty (2006) found that older people were labelled as incontinent without a full assessment and often after only one episode of urinary leakage. They described a social model of continence care where the assessment older people received in hospital aimed only to identify the most suitable products to adequately contain the leakage and odour. No specific continence promotion plan was developed.

If we are to make changes towards the delivery of best nursing practice in promoting continence with older people, a comprehensive assessment *must* form the basis of decision-making about therapeutic treatment plans appropriate to the particular type of urinary incontinence experienced. Box 7.5 indicates the components of such an assessment and for further information readers are referred to the paper by Lekan-Rutledge (2004).

Box 7.5   Components of a comprehensive assessment of older person's continence

History
- General health history: medical, surgical, obstetric, current medication
- Lower urinary tract symptoms: type, onset, duration, frequency, severity, timing, precipitating factors and associations
- Previous continence status
- Usual urinary habits and patterns of elimination including bowel habits, awareness of need to pass urine
- Functional status and presence of conditions of old age: immobility, falls, delirium, dementia, communication, vision and hearing status, skin condition

- Cognitive status: comprehension, planning and sequencing, memory, mood, orientation
- Environmental assessment: physical, social
- Fluid patterns: type, quantities, timings, self-modifications
- Lifestyle factors: physical activity, alcohol, smoking, nutritional status
- Older person's perceptions: cause and impact on quality of life, motivation for treatment and expectations of treatment effect

Clinical assessment
- Urinalysis
- 3-day bladder diary or frequency–volume chart
- Post-void residual urine

Physical examination
- Abdomen, pelvis, urogenital: pelvic organ prolapse, hernias, atrophic vaginitis

Conservative techniques to promote continence with older people

Non-surgical, non-pharmacological approaches to continence promotion include working with the older person and their family where appropriate to enable lifestyle and behaviour changes to be made to facilitate restoration of function and support the person to self-manage their condition.

An individualised plan to promote continence in an older person will have two components (Figure 7.1). The first will comprise education on lifestyle factors that may cause or worsen urinary symptoms and leakage: enabling older people to understand their bladder and what influences their continence status is an effective aspect of continence promotion (Kincade *et al.* 2007). Lifestyle modifications are appropriate for all older people and focus on bladder health and preventative measures. An important element of lifestyle for older people is their fluid intake. Controlling the amount and type of fluids drunk is key to continence status and a significant feature of self-management programmes (Kincade *et al.* 2007). The first reaction of older people experiencing urinary leakage is often to restrict fluid intake, especially overnight when nocturia may be problematic. However, this strategy may be counterproductive, resulting in dehydration and worsening urgency symptoms and leakage, because concentrated urine irritates the urothelium. It may also lead to urinary tract infection as the incomplete emptying and increased residual volume that occurs with ageing is then more prone to microbial proliferation. Conversely, studies have indicated that some older people drink large volumes, often of caffeine-containing fluids. This then results in regular leakage due to increased urge and greater pressure on a weakened pelvic floor and sphincter (Dougherty *et al.* 2002). The advice is to maintain a fluid intake of between 1500 and 3000 mL each 24-hour period and reduce or avoid caffeine consumption, alcohol and carbonated drinks. Two studies where older women adjusted their fluid intake to within these parameters showed an improvement in urinary symptoms despite fears at the outset that urinary leakage would worsen (Tomlinson *et al.* 1999; Swithinbank *et al.* 2005).

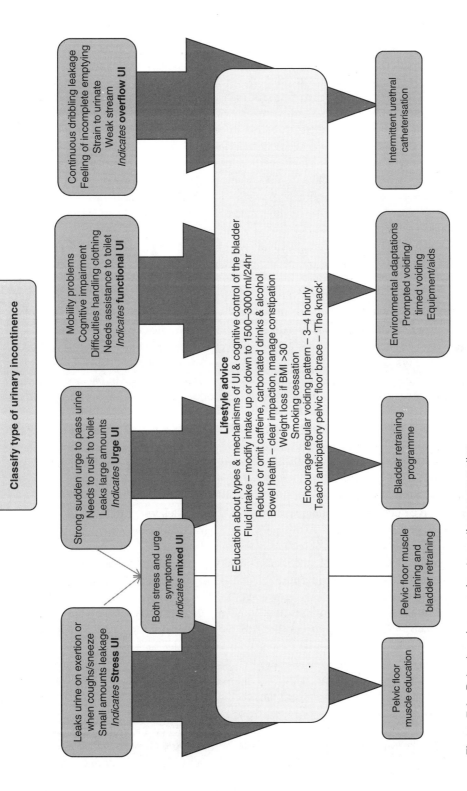

Figure 7.1 Behavioural approaches to continence promotion.

Self-monitoring of fluids together with appropriate dietary advice also helps to prevent constipation, which is a particular problem for many older people and contributes to urinary retention. A further component of initial self-management programmes is exercise and physical activity. Increases are possible even in very frail older people and have been shown to have a range of positive impacts, including improvements in bowel functioning (see Chapter 8). There is also some limited evidence that increases in physical activity may improve urinary incontinence (Peterson 2008) and enable frail older people to more easily use the toilet (Schnelle *et al.* 2002; Van Houten *et al.* 2007). Smoking cessation and weight control for those with a body mass index of 30 or more are further lifestyle measures that improve bladder health, as the chronic cough and extra weight strain the pelvic floor. Furthermore, active treatment of atrophic vaginitis or urethritis, which commonly occurs in older women, will alleviate irritative symptoms and potentially improve their continence status.

The second component in an individualised plan designed to enable the older person to achieve continence will focus on specific behavioural treatments. A range of non-invasive behavioural interventions is available for use by nurses, with evidence of positive effects. They include various voiding regimes, pelvic floor muscle training and intermittent self-catheterisation. Choice of particular approach is dependent on the identified type of urinary incontinence and the older person's capabilities and situation. It is important to note that such behavioural approaches are most effective when combined with lifestyle interventions (Figure 7.1).

Bladder retraining is a personalised voiding programme for use by older people with urge urinary incontinence or mixed urinary incontinence who are cognitively able and motivated. The approach helps the older person to improve control over their overactive bladder by gradually increasing the intervals between voids while at the same time enabling them to suppress their urge to void. One reason for its success is that it is thought to increase the person's functional bladder capacity. Retraining programmes are individualised, based on a 3-day voiding diary or frequency–volume chart. The intervals between voids are agreed with the person, together with the graduated increases. The person is taught urge suppression techniques to enable them to delay going to the toilet for the specified period of time.

An important part of bladder retraining and other voiding programmes is *urge suppression* techniques. These enable the older person to take control of their bladder function and resist a sudden compelling urge to void. These techniques are important for falls prevention as well as preventing incontinence. The person is taught to 'listen' to their bladder urges and when they experience urgency to stop whatever they are doing and concentrate on controlling the urge. They are taught to do five rapid pelvic floor contractions and distract themselves using a method of their choice such as counting backwards, reciting poetry or other mental activities that demand concentration. They continue this until the urge subsides. At that point they are in control of their bladder and can proceed to the toilet at their own pace rather than reacting to an overwhelming desire to void that puts them at risk.

Prompted voiding is an active approach to continence promotion that has been shown to be useful for older people with cognitive impairment and is particularly useful where functional urinary incontinence is the type of continence problem experienced. The technique involves teaching the older person to initiate their own toileting through requests for help. They receive praise and positive reinforcement for their appropriate behaviour from carers when they do this. Although considered a resource intensive approach, there is some evidence of short-term effectiveness (Eustice *et al.* 2000).

Habit training is a voiding approach whereby the older person's usual micturition pattern is identified using a bladder diary or frequency–volume chart and they are assisted to use the toilet at these times. It is a nurse-initiated approach using the social model to effect containment of leakage, rather than restoration of bladder function. It is similar to *timed voiding*, which is a fixed time interval toileting assistance programme designed to manage urinary incontinence in older people who cannot participate in independent use of the toilet. Both habit training and timed voiding, like prompted voiding, are useful behavioural approaches for functional urinary incontinence.

Pelvic floor muscle therapy is an effective inexpensive treatment approach used to treat stress urinary incontinence and may be combined with bladder training for urge urinary incontinence or mixed urinary incontinence in older people (Wyman *et al.* 1998). Although most would associate pelvic floor muscle therapy with women, it has been successfully used to treat men who experience urinary incontinence following prostatectomy. The programmes work by strengthening the pelvic floor muscles through regular intensive exercise in order to support the pelvic organs, bladder and particularly the bladder neck. The stronger muscles and increased muscle bulk increase urethral resistance. These exercises are not known to have any adverse effects, although an improvement in symptoms might not be apparent for several weeks. There is a need to maintain the exercise approach if sustained benefit is to be achieved. A single pelvic floor muscle contraction may be made immediately prior to activity (known as 'the knack'), and is an effective part of self-management (Kincade *et al.* 2007).

Intermittent self-catheterisation is increasingly used in practice for incomplete emptying, urinary retention and overflow urinary incontinence. It is suitable for those with urinary outflow obstruction, neurological disorders such as multiple sclerosis or stroke, and following surgery and spinal injuries. The catheter is inserted at agreed intervals throughout the day depending on the volume of retention and other symptoms. To learn intermittent self-catheterisation, the person must have sufficient manual dexterity, cognitive ability and eyesight to perform the procedure plus good hygiene, which is essential to reduce the risk of infection. This type of catheterisation is increasingly favoured over indwelling catheterisation as it is associated with lower infection risk, although not every person is able or willing to carry out the technique.

An overview of current evidence on behavioural techniques associated with particular types of urinary incontinence is provided in Figure 7.1.

The following case study does not focus on a patient or practice development project. Rather it explores evidence to inform nurses' management of urinary incontinence following stroke. Gaps in the knowledge base and how contemporary continence research is attempting to answer the specific questions about continence needs following stroke are presented.

Case study 7.1   Best nursing practice for post-stroke urinary incontinence

What is the need?

Urinary incontinence is very common following stroke, with 40–60% of hospitalised patients experiencing it in the acute phase, 25% on discharge and one-third of survivors experiencing ongoing problems at 1 year (Barrett 2002; Kolominsky-Rabas *et al.* 2003). A large proportion of these people live in long-term care. The Leicester Medical Research Council Incontinence Study, a large epidemiological survey of 14 600 people, 423 of whom reported stroke, showed that the prevalence of urinary symptoms following stroke was twice that of a non-stroke population (64% vs. 32%). People with stroke reported more severe symptoms and significantly greater impact on lifestyle (Brittain *et al.* 2000). Despite knowledge of the prevalence and impact of urinary incontinence following stroke, there is a poor understanding of why urinary incontinence occurs. This influences our understanding of the most effective approaches to bladder rehabilitation. Urge and functional incontinence are common following stroke (Barrett 2002), although the exact mechanisms have not been clarified. Stress incontinence is not directly associated with stroke but may feature in pre-stroke urinary incontinence. A Cochrane review demonstrated the lack of evidence to guide nurses' practice (Thomas *et al.* 2008). A number of national audits have confirmed the lack of attention paid by nurses to managing urinary incontinence following stroke (Royal College of Physicians Healthcare of Older People Programme 2006, 2010). There are many gaps in our understanding of how best to promote urinary continence and rehabilitation of the bladder after stroke. Some of these are highlighted in Box 7.6.

Nurses and urinary incontinence after stroke

Our understanding of nurses' perceptions of their role and contribution to post-stroke urinary incontinence is limited and reliant on a small number of old studies, case reports and clinical experience. A seminal study of the role of the nurse in rehabilitation identified bladder and bowel management as one of nursing's specialist functions (Waters & Luker 1996). Others have reached similar conclusions (O'Connor 1993; Kirkevold 1997). However, negative descriptions of reactive 'toileting' as being time-consuming (Long *et al.* 2002) and a lack of positive descriptions of proactive bladder rehabilitation in the literature prompted a study to explore the details of nursing practice in relation to continence following stroke. The purpose of the research was to better understand current management techniques and influences.

Thirty interviews with nurses from 14 stroke units in Scotland, China and Sweden were undertaken and analysed thematically. Findings showed that promoting continence was not a priority for stroke nurses. Recovery of mobility, swallowing, speech and the provision of psychological support were all considered to be of greater importance in all three countries than recovery of urinary continence.

Care provision focused on containing urine loss, with the purpose of achieving social continence so that the person could be discharged home. An institutionalised care process was described where a core group of activities sought to eliminate infection and urinary retention and then provide emotional support and a 'regular toileting regime'. The nurses believed that urinary incontinence was not a target for rehabilitation effort and that it would resolve spontaneously, or require ongoing containment. There was no evidence of any efforts to proactively promote recovery of bladder function and the study concluded that nurses' management of urinary incontinence following stroke is reactive. A routinised approach is adopted based on local custom and practice rather than robust evidence (Booth *et al.* 2009).

It is not clear why stroke-related bladder dysfunction is viewed differently to stroke-related swallowing dysfunction or post-stroke hemiparesis. A study is in progress to explore the reasons why stroke nurses contain urinary incontinence rather than actively promote continence. The study is designed to discover whether nurses intend to promote bladder recovery from the outset, or whether they only intend to contain the urinary incontinence. The Theory of Planned Behaviour (Ajzen 1985) provides the theoretical framework for the study. This theory suggests that a person's intention predicts their behaviour. Thus if nurses do not actually intend to promote bladder recovery but rather their intentions are to contain incontinence, this will explain their practice. Alternatively, if they do intend to use nursing techniques to promote recovery of continence other factors must be preventing them from doing so. Nurses will need to identify and overcome these factors in order to introduce changes to practice. Of course even if nurses intend to promote continence, it remains the case that there is a lack of evidence of specific behavioural techniques that are effective for promoting bladder rehabilitation following stroke.

It cannot be assumed that continence promotion techniques suitable for urinary incontinence in general are automatically appropriate for stroke patients. Thus a research programme is in progress to develop and test an evidence based continence promotion programme for use following acute stroke (Thomas *et al.* 2009). The programme includes bladder retraining and pelvic floor muscle exercises for cognitively intact stroke patients and a prompted voiding programme for those with cognitive impairment. The research programme, known as ICONS (Identifying Continence OptioNs after Stroke), includes a systematic review of the effectiveness of combined behavioural interventions for urinary incontinence (French *et al.* 2009). A standard intervention for use following stroke will be constructed from this, which will be tested in a randomised controlled trial of the programme's effectiveness in comparison with usual continence care. The initial results, available in 2012, will inform nurses' choice of approach for effective promotion of urinary continence following stroke.

A further area of research has been instigated by a review of issues considered to be of importance to stroke nurses in Scotland (Rowat *et al.* 2009). The review highlighted a number of practice questions around urinary catheter use (indwelling and intermittent) and incontinence, where evidence to inform practice is scarce. Furthermore, national audits undertaken in England and Wales showed an association between the development of a urinary tract infection and use of indwelling urinary catheters (16% vs. 6% incidence in non-catheterised patients; Intercollegiate Stroke Working Party 2009). Although apparently valid reasons for catheterisation were found for the majority of patients who were catheterised after stroke, in 17% of cases 'urinary incontinence' was the only reason cited. Given the risks associated with use of indwelling catheters, this was not considered acceptable practice. However, the rationale for catheterisation was not clear from the audit. If practice is to be changed we need to know more about how, when and why the decision to catheterise a stroke patient is made. We also need to know who makes the decision, where it is made and what factors influence the decision. To this end a study is underway to increase understanding of decision-making around the use of indwelling urinary catheters following stroke (Smith *et al.* 2009).

> **Box 7.6**   Gaps in evidence and knowledge around urinary continence following stroke
>
> - How nurses assess continence following stroke, and diagnose type of urinary incontinence.
> - Nurses' management and treatment strategies for urinary incontinence following stroke at all stages, i.e. acute stage, rehabilitation phases and in long-term survival.
> - Whether post-stroke urinary incontinence can be effectively treated and reversed.
> - Which specific treatments are most effective for each type of urinary incontinence following stroke.
> - Effects of specific treatment for urinary incontinence on overall stroke outcomes, e.g. survival, recovery, discharge destination.
> - Effects of treatment of urinary incontinence on quality of life for stroke survivors and carers.
> - Prevalence, consequences, associations and impact of lower urinary tract symptoms other than incontinence following stroke.

Summary

Urinary incontinence and lower urinary tract symptoms are commonly experienced by older people and are distressing and costly. Causes are complex but the majority of urinary incontinence and lower urinary tract symptoms may be ameliorated with therapeutic approaches involving lifestyle and behavioural changes. Such restorative treatment is initiated and applied by nurses in accordance with the type of urinary incontinence and symptoms experienced by the older person. These can only be identified by a comprehensive assessment. Current practice with older people favours a social model of containment and is largely palliative. It denies those with potential to recover independent bladder function. A shift by nurses towards emphasis on rehabilitative approaches is needed to overcome the negativity associated with this area of practice.

The evidence supporting techniques for proactive continence promotion is expanding, although some areas of practice remain unclear. This is particularly true for continence promotion with frail older people. Nonetheless, a great deal of research to answer specific practice questions is currently in progress, principally in the area of stroke.

Urinary incontinence continues to be investigated as a single entity with little evidence of studies associating urinary symptoms with other syndromes of older age such as falls and delirium, where interaction is known to be important for the person's wellbeing and continued functioning. Nor has any research yet focused on the importance of effective continence promotion as a potential treatment for the other conditions of older age, such as in prevention of falls and improved physical activity. An increased evidence base for all types of restorative approaches is essential to the improvement of practice. This should include therapeutic techniques suitable for meeting the needs of older people irrespective of care context. It is crucial that nurses develop their confidence and expertise in applying such techniques and engage further in proactive continence promotion with older people.

Key messages

- Incontinence is not an inevitable part of ageing.
- More than 70% older people with urinary symptoms, including incontinence, can be cured or significantly improved using simple lifestyle and behavioural measuers
- Promoting continence is a fundamental feature of gerontological nursing
- Every gerontological nurse should be competent and confident to utilise a range of continence promoting activities
- A paradigm shift to focus on bladder rehabilitation from the current emphasis on containment of incontinence is needed to promote continence effectively.

References

Abrams P, Cardozo L, Fall M *et al.* (2002) The standardisation of terminology of lower urinary tract function: report from the standardisation subcommittee on the International Continence Society. *Neurourology and Urodynamics* **21**, 167–178.

Ajzen I (1985) From intentions to actions: a theory of planned behaviour. In: Kuhl J, Beckmann J (eds) *Action Control: From Cognition to Behaviour*. Springer-Verlag, Berlin, chapter 2.

Barrett J (2002) Bladder and bowel problems after stroke. *Reviews in Clinical Gerontology* **12**, 253–267.

Booth J, Kumlien S, Zang Y, Gustafsson B, Tolson D (2009) Rehabilitation nurses practices in relation to urinary incontinence following stroke: a cross-cultural comparison. *Journal of Clinical Nursing* **18**, 1049–1058.

Booth J, Lawrence M, O'Neill K, McMillan L (2010) Exploring older peoples' experiences of nocturia: a poorly recognised urinary condition that limits participation. *Disability and Rehabilitation* **32**, 765–774.

Borrie MJ, Bawden M, Speechley M, Kloseck M (2002) Interventions led by nurse continence advisers in the management of urinary incontinence: a randomised controlled trial. *Canadian Medical Association Journal* **166**, 1267–1273.

Brittain K, Shaw C (2007) The social consequences of living with and dealing with incontinence: a carers perspective. *Social Science and Medicine* **65**, 1274–1283.

Brittain KR, Perry SI, Peet SM *et al.* (2000) Prevalence and impact of urinary symptoms among community-dwelling stroke survivors. *Stroke* **31**, 886–891.

Brown JS, Vittinghoff E, Wyman J *et al.* (2000) Urinary incontinence: does it increase risk for falls and fractures? *Journal of the American Geriatrics Society* **48**, 721–725.

Byles JE, Chiarelli P, Hicker AH, Bruin C, Cockburn J, Parkinson L (2005) An evaluation of three community based projects to improve care for incontinence. *International Urogynaecology* **16**, 29–33.

Carroll D, Dykes P, Hurley A (2009) Patients' perspectives of falling while in an acute care hospital and suggestions for prevention. *Applied Nursing Research* **23**, 238–241.

Cheater FM, Baker R, Gillies C *et al.* (2008) The nature and impact of urinary incontinence experienced by patients receiving community nursing services: a cross-sectional cohort study. *International Journal of Nursing Studies* **45**, 339–351.

Chiarelli P, Mackenzie L, Osmotherly P (2009) Urinary incontinence is associated with an increase in falls: a systematic review. *Australian Journal of Physiotherapy* **55**, 89–95.

Coll-Planus L, Denkinger M, Niklaus T (2008) Relationship of urinary incontinence and late-life disability: implications for clinical work and research in geriatrics. *Zeitschrift fur Gerontologie und Geriatrie* **41**, 283–290.

Crestodina LR (2007) Assessment and management of urinary incontinence in the elderly male. *Nurse Practitioner* **32**, 26–34.

Dingwall L, McLafferty E (2006) Do nurses promote urinary continence in hospitalised older people? An exploratory study. *Journal of Clinical Nursing* **15**, 1276–1286.

Dougherty MC, Dwyer JW, Pendergast JF *et al.* (2002) A randomized trial of behavioral management for continence with older rural women. *Research in Nursing and Health* **25**, 3–13.

DuBeau C, Simon S, Morris J (2006) The effect of urinary incontinence on quality of life in older nursing home residents. *Journal of the American Geriatrics Society* **54**, 1325–1333.

Eustice S, Roe B, Paterson J (2000) Prompted voiding for the management of urinary incontinence in adults. *Cochrane Database of Systematic Reviews* (2), CD002113.

Fonda D, DuBeau C, Harari D, Ouslander JG, Palmer M, Roe B (2005) Incontinence in the frail elderly. In: Abrams P, Cardozo L, Khoury S (eds) *Incontinence*, 3rd edn. Health Publications Ltd, Plymouth, UK, pp. 1163–1239.

French B, Thomas L, Leathley M *et al.* (2009) Preparing an intervention for incontinence after stroke: what might work? *International Journal of Stroke* **4** (Suppl. 2), 36.

Godfrey H (2008) Older people, continence care and catheters: dilemmas and resolutions. *British Journal of Nursing* **17**, 4–11.

Grimby A, Milsom I, Molander U, Wiklund I, Ekelund P (1993) The influence of urinary incontinence on the quality of life of elderly women. *Age and Ageing* **22**, 82–89.

Heckenberg G (2008) Improving and ensuring best practice continence management in residential aged care. *International Journal of Evidence Based Healthcare* **6**, 260–269.

Horrocks S, Somerset M, Stoddart H, Peters TJ (2004) What prevents older people from seeking treatment for urinary incontinence? A qualitative exploration of barriers to the use of community continence services. *Family Practice* **21**, 689–696.

Huang A, Brown J, Thom D, Fink H, Yaffe K (2007) Urinary incontinence in older community-dwelling women. *Obstetrics and Gynecology* **109**, 909–916.

Inouye S, Studenski S, Tinetti ME, Kuchel GA (2007) Geriatric syndromes: clinical, research, and policy implications of a core geriatric concept. *Journal of the American Geriatrics Society* **55**, 780–791.

Intercollegiate Stroke Working Party (2009) National Sentinel Stroke Audit Phase II (clinical audit) 2008 Report for England, Wales and Northern Ireland. Clinical Effectiveness and Evaluation Unit, Royal College of Physicians, London.

International Continence Society (2009) 4th International Consultation on Incontinence, Paris, 5–8 July 2008. Health Publication Ltd, Plymouth, UK.

Jenson J, Lundin-Olsson L, Nyberg L, Gustafson Y (2002) Falls among frail older people in residential care. *Scandinavian Journal of Public Health* **30**, 54–61.

Kincade JE, Dougherty MC, Carlson JR, Hunter GS, Busby-Whitehead J (2007) Randomized clinical trial of efficacy of self-monitoring techniques to treat urinary incontinence in women. *Neurourology and Urodynamics* **26**, 507–511.

Kirkevold M (1997) The role of nursing in the rehabilitation of acute stroke patients: toward a unified theoretical perspective. *Advances in Nursing Science* **19**, 55–56.

Kolominsky-Rabas PL, Hilz MJ, Neundoerfer B, Heuschmann PU (2003) Impact of urinary incontinence after stroke: results from a prospective population-based stroke register. *Neurourology and Urodynamics* **22**, 322–327.

Lekan-Rutledge D (2004) Urinary incontinence strategies for frail elderly women. *Urologic Nursing* **24**, 281–301.

Long A, Kneafsey R, Ryan J, Berry J (2002) The role of the nurse within the multiprofessional rehabilitation team. *Journal of Advanced Nursing* **37**, 70–78.

Martin JL, Williams KS, Abrams KS *et al.* (2006) Systematic review and evaluation of methods of assessing urinary incontinence. *Health Technology Assessment* **10** (6).

Mons B, Pons ME, Hampel C (2005) Patient reported impact of urinary incontinence: results from treatment-seeking women in 14 European countries. *Maturitas* **52** (Suppl.), 24–34.

Morris AR, Ho MT, Lapsley H, Walsh J, Gonski P, Moore KH (2004) Costs of managing urinary and faecal incontinence in a sub-acute facility: a bottom-up approach. *Neurourology and Urodynamics* **24**, 56–62.

Nicolson P, Kopp Z, Chapple CR, Kelleher C (2008) It's just the worry about not being able to control it! A qualitative study of living with overactive bladder. *British Journal of Health Psychology* **13**, 343–359.

Norton C (2006) Healthcare professionals, continence, stigma and taboos. Stigma conference papers available at www.labelmenot.org/index_files/Page476.htm

O'Connor S (1993) Nursing and rehabilitation: the interventions of nurses in stroke patient care. *Journal of Clinical Nursing* **2**, 29–34.

Oliver D, Daly F, Martin F, McMurdo M (2004) Risk factors and risk assessment tools for falls in hospital in-patients: a systematic review. *Age and Ageing* **33**, 122–130.

Ouslander JG, Schnelle JF, Uman G *et al.* (1995) Predictors of successful prompted voiding among incontinence nursing home residents. *Journal of the American Medical Association* **273**, 1366–1370.

Patient Safety Observatory (2007) *Slips, trips and falls in hospital*. National Patient Safety Agency, London.

Peterson JA (2008) Minimize urinary incontinence: maximise physical activity in women. *Urologic Nursing* **28**, 351–356.

Rodriguez N, Sackley C, Badger F (2007) Exploring the facets of continence care: a continence survey of care homes for older people in Birmingham. *Journal of Clinical Nursing* **16**, 954–962.

Roe B, Howell F, Riniotis K, Beech R, Crome P, Ong B (2008) Older people's experience of falls: understanding, interpretation and autonomy. *Journal of Advanced Nursing* **63**, 586–596.

Rowat A, Lawrence M, Horsburgh D, Legg L, Smith L and the Scottish Stroke Nurses Forum (2009) Stroke research questions: a nursing perspective. *British Journal of Nursing* **18**, 100–105.

Royal College of Physicians Healthcare of Older People Programme (2006) *Report of the National Audit of Continence Care for Older People (65 years and above) in England, Wales and N. Ireland*. Clinical Effectiveness and Evaluation Unit, Royal College of Physicians, London.

Royal College of Physicians Healthcare of Older People Programme (2010) *National Audit of Continence Care Report*. Clinical Standards Unit, Royal College of Physicians, London.

Schnelle J, Alessi C, Simmons S, Al-Samarrai N, Beck J, Ouslander J (2002) Translating clinical research into practice; a randomised controlled trial of exercise and incontinence care with nursing home residents. *Journal of the American Geriatrics Society* **50**, 1476–1483.

Shaw C, Tansey R, Jackson C, Hyde C, Allan R (2001) Barriers to help seeking in people with urinary symptoms. *Family Practice* **18**, 48–52.

Smith LN, Booth J, Cowey E *et al.* (2009) What factors influence the decision to insert an indwelling urinary catheter in newly diagnosed stroke patients? *International Journal of Stroke* **4** (Suppl. 2), 41.

Stewart R, Moore M, May F, Marks R, Hale W (1992) Nocturia: a risk factor for falls in the elderly. *Journal of the American Geriatrics Society* **40**, 1217–1220.

Swithinbank L, Hashim H, Abrams P (2005) The effect of fluid intake on urinary symptoms in women. *Journal of Urology* **174**, 187–189.

Thom D, Haan M, Van den Eden SK (1997) Medically recognised urinary incontinence and risks of hospitalisation, nursing home admission and mortality. *Age and Ageing* **26**, 367–374.

Thomas LH, Barrett J, Cross S *et al.* (2008) Prevention and treatment of urinary incontinence after stroke in adults. *Cochrane Database of Systematic Reviews* (1), CD004462.

Thomas L, Watkins C, French B *et al.* (2009) ICONS: Identifying Continence OptioNs after Stroke (poster presentation). Fourth UK Stroke Forum, Glasgow, 2 December 2009.

Tomlinson BU, Dougherty M, Pendergast JF, Boyington AR, Coffman M, Pickens S (1999) Dietary caffeine, fluid intake and urinary incontinence in older rural women. *International Urogynecology Journal* **10**, 22–28.

Tromp AM, Pluijm S, Smit J, Deeg D, Bouter L, Lips P (2001) Fall-risk screening test: a prospective study on predictors for falls in community dwelling elderly. *Journal of Clinical Epidemiology* **54**, 837–844.

Twigg J (2000) Carework as a form of bodywork. *Ageing and Society* **20**, 389–412.

Van Houten P, Achterberg W, Ribbe M (2007) Urinary incontinence in disabled elderly women: a randomised clinical trial on the effect of mobility and toileting skills to achieve independent toileting *Gerontology* **53**, 205–210.

Wagg A, Potter J, Peel P, Irwin P, Lowe D, Pearson M (2008) National audit of continence care for older people: management of urinary incontinence *Age and Ageing* **37**, 39–44.

Waters KA, Luker KA (1996) Staff perspectives on the role of the nurse in rehabilitation wards for elderly people. *Journal of Clinical Nursing* **5**, 105–114.

Williams KS, Assassa RP, Smith NK (2000) Development, implementation and evaluation of a new nurse-led continence service: a pilot study. *Journal of Clinical Nursing* **9**, 566–573.

Wyman JF, Fantl JA, McClish DK, Bump RC and the Continence Program for Women Research Group (1998) Comparative efficacy of behavioural interventions in the management of female urinary incontinence. *American Journal of Obstetrics and Gynecology* **179**, 999–1007.

Chapter 8

Promoting Physical Activity with Older People

Dawn Skelton, Marie McAloon and Lyle Gray

Introduction

For most body systems, the impact of ageing on everyday functional activities becomes noticeable from about the age of 30–40 years. Physical fitness, the ability to carry out daily tasks with vigour and alertness, without undue fatigue and with ample energy to enjoy our leisure time pursuits and to meet unforeseen emergencies is especially important as we all age. Often symptoms such as tiredness, breathlessness, falling and aches and pains are simply considered 'side effects' of ageing or disease, rather than signs of lack of fitness. The World Health Organization estimates that each year at least 1.9 million people die as a result of sedentary behaviour and the cost of inactivity is greater than the cost of smoking to health services (World Health Organization 2002). With an ever-increasing older population and longevity at its peak, we are now commonly dealing with people who have poor functional mobility and comorbidities associated with an inactive lifestyle. Indeed, significant mortality is associated with sedentary behaviour. But an active lifestyle is also important to ensure good quality of life. Evidence based guidelines and recommendations on amount and type of activity or exercise necessary to improve health, improve risk factors for disease, reduce symptoms of disease and maintain independence will be explored. Recognising that such guidance can only be effectively introduced in the context of an agreed values base, the case study will illustrate the importance of physical activity and the contributions of interdisciplinary working in a community of practice to promoting such activity among older people in hospital.

The added value of an active lifestyle

Active life expectancy, or the number of years an individual may expect to maintain the ability to perform the basic activities of daily living without significant disease or disability, is accepted as a key marker of physical, emotional and functional well-being and therefore of quality of life as we age (Katz & Branch 1983). Successful ageing is, in effect, the difference between active living and just being alive (Spirduso *et al.* 1996).

Evidence Informed Nursing with Older People, First Edition. Edited by Debbie Tolson, Joanne Booth and Irene Schofield.
© 2011 Blackwell Publishing Ltd. Published 2011 by Blackwell Publishing Ltd.

Active ageing, however, has many determinants, not all of which are easily changed (World Health Organization 2002). Regular exercise not only reduces risk for cardiovascular disease, osteoarthritis, osteoporosis, obesity, diabetes and insomnia but also significantly reduces risk for falls, depression and incontinence (US Department of Health and Human Services 1996; World Health Organization 1997, 2002; Dinan 2001; Young & Dinan 2005; Nelson *et al.* 2007). In the UK alone, it is estimated that the 'cost' of sedentary behaviour is £8.3 billion per year to the economy (Department of Health 2010).

Regular physical activity, more than any other intervention, has been shown to extend life, reduce disability and improve quality of life in older adults (Thompson *et al.* 1988; US Department of Health and Human Services 1996; Wagner 1997; World Health Organization 1997, 2002; Dinan 2001; Young & Dinan 2005; Nelson *et al.* 2007). At least 30 minutes of regular, moderate-intensity physical activity on 5 days per week reduces the risk of several common diseases and the impact of sedentary behaviour on an ever-broadening variety of health problems is clear (Thompson *et al.* 1988; World Health Organization 1997, 2002; Dinan 2001; Young & Dinan 2005). Because of the high prevalence of chronic conditions, frailer older people have the potential to gain most from regular physical activity and can potentially reverse loss of mobility (Thompson *et al.* 1988; US Department of Health and Human Services 1996; Dinan 2001; Young & Dinan 2005; Nelson *et al.* 2007). Regular, appropriate exercise training has been shown to improve the functional abilities and psychological well-being of both healthy older people (World Health Organization 1997; Young & Dinan 2005) and people with disabling symptoms common in old age (Thompson *et al.* 1988; Dinan 2001). The challenge to nurses working with older people is to understand the barriers and motivators to physical activity or exercise (Yardley *et al.* 2007).

Unfortunately, sedentary behaviour is common. For example, in the UK, 4 of 10 adults over the age of 50 are completely inactive and two-thirds of these believe they are doing enough activity to keep fit (Skelton *et al.* 1999; Department of Health 2010). Both older people, and professionals working with them, need to know how much activity is enough to maintain health, improve mobility and quality of life.

The impact of sedentary behaviour

Even healthy older people lose strength and power at some 1–3% per year (Skelton *et al.* 1995). The effect of sedentary behaviour exacerbates this loss and the resulting weakness and fatigue has important functional consequences for the performance of everyday life activities (Young & Dinan 2005). The contribution of sedentary behaviour to prevalence and cost of chronic illnesses exacts a significant burden in terms of morbidity and mortality and is a contributing factor for extended hospital stay and/or need for subsequent post-hospital care (Nichol *et al.* 1994; US Department of Health and Human Services 1996). It has been estimated that up to 37% of deaths from coronary heart disease could be attributed to inactivity (Britton & McPherson 2002).

It is known that a few weeks of immobilisation or disuse has a detrimental effect on muscle mass, muscle strength and power (Bloomfield 1997). The decrease in muscle strength is greatest, 3–4% per day, during the first week of immobilisation and up to a 40% decrease in isokinetic muscle strength has been seen after 3 weeks of immobilisation

(Bloomfield 1997). Bed rest causes an increase in calcium excretion and bone mineral loss in the weight-bearing bones such as the calcaneus, iliac crest and lumbar spine (Whedon 1984). High rates of inactivity in older people, especially those in residential or nursing accommodation, will lead to an increased loss of bone with increasing age. Nursing home residents spend up to 90% of their time either sitting or lying down (Tinetti 1994). This will mean that extremely sedentary people will see an 'active' loss of bone and muscle over and above the 'ageing' loss.

In particular, strength, balance and coordination appear to be key factors in maintaining upright posture. People with leg weakness have a threefold increased risk of recurrent falls compared to those with 'normal' strength for their age (Gillespie *et al.* 2009). Slow reaction time and decreased functional ability owing to lack of practice and/or physical pain, inadequate strength of the muscle–tendon complex, decreased joint flexibility, and lower limb asymmetry in strength and power are the main muscle factors involved in postural instability, falls and fractures (Skelton *et al.* 2005). This is illustrated by the changes in fracture site with increasing age: wrist fractures become more common in the forties and are prevalent up to the age of 65. Fractures of the hip become more prevalent after the age of 80, as slowing reaction times mean it is often no longer possible to get the hand out fast enough to prevent the body landing heavily on the hip and trunk.

Recommendations for physical activity and exercise in older people

Physical activity or exercise?

Physical activity is any activity which uses the muscular system in some exertion: gardening, walking and housework are all physical activities (World Health Organization 1997). For most older people increasing their physical activity will help improve their health without undue risk. Exercise is when the activity is structured and is aimed at improving one or more components of fitness (strength, endurance, balance, flexibility, etc.) with a purpose in mind (World Health Organization 1997). Supervised exercise ensures safe, up to date and evidence based exercise (no matter what the health or age of the person) but also provides strong motivational, social and psychosocial components.

The recommendation of regular moderate physical activity is based on the evidence necessary to prevent disease (such as heart disease or osteoporosis). It does not take into account those older people starting an exercise programme when they may already have extensive chronic disease. Nor does it take into account certain activities that are known to reduce the risk of falls, for example, but which would not be considered 'moderate' in intensity. This includes flexibility exercise to improve range of motion and strength training to maintain leg strength to use the stairs.

Tailored exercise programme at least twice a week

When the focus of the intervention is to improve or maintain quality of life or reduce symptoms of a disease, then the prescription gets more complicated. Improving and maintaining strength, balance and flexibility have been identified as key components of exercise programmes for older people (Skelton *et al.* 1995, 2005; Skelton & McLaughlin 1996; Dinan 2001; Nelson *et al.* 2007; Gillespie *et al.* 2009).

Research shows that in as little as 10–12 weeks, with regular strength or aerobic exercise training, newcomers to exercise can turn back the clock by up to 20 years in terms of their muscular and aerobic fitness (Skelton *et al.* 1995; Skelton & McLaughlin 1996; Malbut *et al.* 2002). For the over-75s, taking part in structured exercise and/or home exercise on three occasions a week helps maintain independence (Nelson *et al.* 2007). These older individuals may benefit more from improvements in muscle power (speed and strength of muscle) rather than strength alone (Skelton *et al.* 1995). Performing mobility-specific (power) exercises appears to produce greater improvements in functional outcomes than traditional resistance exercise (Skelton & McLaughlin 1996).

The forms of exercise shown to be beneficial for slowing or reversing age-related bone loss include brief bouts of weight-bearing exercise such as intermittent jogging (Kohrt *et al.* 2004), exercise classes (Welsh & Rutherford 1996) and also weight training using weights in excess of 80% of personal maximum (Nelson *et al.* 1994). Walking alone does not increase bone strength, only helps maintain it (Cavanagh & Cann 1988). However, regular exercise could delay the point at which osteopenia progresses to clinically significant osteoporosis (Nelson *et al.* 1994; Welsh & Rutherford 1996; Kohrt *et al.* 2004).

People with comorbidities and falls

Significant improvements in depression, mood, urinary urgency, postural hypotension, hypertension and vestibular function can be seen, at any age, with specific tailored exercise regimens three times a week (Biddle *et al.* 1994; World Health Organization 1997, 2002, 2007; Dinan 2001). Tailored exercise has a significant and large antidepressant effect in depressed older adults (O'Connor *et al.* 1993) and improves psychological function (Hill *et al.* 1993). For cardiac rehabilitation patients there is evidence of improved cognitive functioning and quality of life as well as improved aerobic capacity and reduced cardiac risk factors (Lavie & Milani 1995). Both aerobic exercise and combined aerobic and strength exercise are associated with improvements in cognitive function, with the combined aerobic and strength exercises being most effective (Nelson *et al.* 2007).

Individualised exercise interventions with balance training at the core of the programme are most effective for those at risk of falls (Robertson *et al.* 2001; Skelton *et al.* 2005). To prevent falls in younger older adults, physical activity is beneficial but t'ai chi stands alone as excellent prevention (Gillespie *et al.* 2009). Exercise to prevent another fall or reduce injury in frequent fallers must be individually tailored and concentrate on dynamic balance training, floor coping skills and resistance training (Skelton *et al.* 2005).

Frail older people with osteoporosis gain benefit from exercise. However, when working with these people, exercise must be low risk and low impact for safety. For example, those with a previous history of vertebral fractures should avoid unsupported spinal flexion, such as abdominal curls (Sinaki 1982). These people are likely to have weak back extensor muscle strength and must start with the lowest workload and progress slowly (Sinaki *et al.* 2002). Brisk walking in those with a history of falls and low bone density is not recommended as a single intervention as this can lead to an increased exposure to risk and greater chance of fractures (Ebrahim *et al.* 1997).

There are few major contraindications to exercise and most older people can exercise safely. Exercise referral schemes in primary care can result in sustainable improvements in physical activity (Biddle *et al.* 1994; Riddoch *et al.* 1998; Craig *et al.* 2000; Hillsdon *et al.* 2005; Dinan *et al.* 2006). Population based falls prevention programmes encouraging greater physical activity have been effective (Grahn-Kronhed *et al.* 2005; McClure *et al.* 2005).

A common concern when assessing older people for participation in a physical activity or exercise programme is whether or not a medical evaluation is needed (e.g. exercise treadmill testing to assess for the likelihood of adverse cardiac events) (Thomas *et al.* 1992; Jones & Rose 2005). For older people with no active cardiopulmonary symptoms embarking on a moderate intensity programme (as opposed to a vigorous one that causes the person to breathe hard and sweat profusely), formal testing is generally not necessary and is not supported by the current evidence (Jones & Rose 2005; Ory *et al.* 2005; Nelson *et al.* 2007). It can also deter participation by portraying exercise as potentially hazardous when the opposite message needs to be conveyed.

With all these caveats in mind, in order to see physiological change, the person must do more activity than they normally do, over a sustained period of time – increasing activity too gently will not cause an effective training effect! For the very deconditioned, suggesting they get off the bus one stop earlier, use the stairs rather than the escalators or lifts or go for a walk each morning is useful advice. For those with medical conditions requiring rehabilitative exercise, there are often outpatient-based programmes available but the challenge is to ensure the person continues the programme after discharge.

What makes older people take up or adhere to a referral or recommendation?

Those older people with the poorest health are most likely to receive a recommendation to become more physically active or be referred to an exercise programme, but may be most resistant to change (Dinan 2001; Skelton & Dinan 2008). This group, often with no previous positive experiences of activity, have perhaps the most to gain from undertaking an exercise programme, but present the greatest challenge in relation to motivation.

There are multiple barriers to improving physical activity levels in older people (Box 8.1). Poor vision and continence issues are also cited as reasons for avoiding activity in people concerned about falling (Yardley & Smith 2002) (see Box 8.2 for further information on barriers and eye conditions in older age). No single factor will predict whether or not an older person will start and sustain an exercise programme (Yardley *et al.* 2007). Participation is determined and regulated by a range of factors, unique to the individual, including their readiness to change and their exercise self-efficacy. Exercise self-efficacy, or confidence in one's ability to undertake regular exercise successfully (even when faced with difficulties), is a strong predictor of exercise adoption among older people (King *et al.* 1998; Marcus & Forsyth 2003; Yardley *et al.* 2007). Readiness to change may be significantly influenced by a referral from a health professional. This may best be done following the diagnosis of a chronic disease or following a significant life event such as a fall or heart attack. It may also be prompted when individuals recognise in themselves the tell-tale signs

Box 8.1 Revision notes: barriers for uptake and adherence to exercise and physical activity

Personal characteristics

Personal characteristics, often called intrinsic barriers, include individual perceptions and beliefs about exercise (often influenced by ageist stereotypes or negative images and myths about ageing); previous activity history and experiences (both positive and negative); current health status and fear of pain or discomfort; poor vision and continence issues. Exercise self-efficacy, or confidence in one's ability to undertake regular exercise successfully (even when faced with difficulties), is a strong predictor of exercise adoption among older people. Time (caring for others or other commitments perceived as more important) and cognitive impairment and dementia are also barriers to adherence to exercise.

Programme factors

Programme factors are associated with the design and delivery of the exercise programme, including mode (e.g. t'ai chi, dance, walking), intensity (where moderate exercise is more favoured by older participants), and the interpersonal skills of the instructor (e.g. providing individual attention and an empathetic teaching style). While social support from peers is frequently cited as a motivating factor among older people taking part in group activities, there is also evidence that large numbers of older people prefer activities that can be undertaken outside a formal class or group setting. Home exercise programming may be a good place to start or a good adjunct to group exercise to ensure benefits are reaped as early as possible.

Environmental (or extrinsic) factors

These also strongly influence participation and include the influence of significant others (e.g. positive support from peers, family, carer or health professional, particularly important among older women); ease of access (the provision of transport and timetabling, proximity of parks for walking and jogging); safe neighbourhoods (well-designed pavements and adequate street lighting) and perceptions of personal safety.

Source: Yardley *et al.* (2007) and Finch (1997).

Box 8.2 Revision notes: the eye and age-related changes

Dry eye is a common problem with increasing age. It can be caused by reduced tear production or poor tear quality. It is frequently associated with rheumatoid arthritis and is one of the triumvirate of signs in Sjögren's syndrome. Treatment is normally by the use of artificial tear solution, as necessary to resolve symptoms, although severe cases may need ophthalmological intervention. *Ectropion* (outward turning of the eyelid) or *entropion* (inward turning of the eyelid) are problems that occur due to age-related deterioration of the connective tissue in the eyelids and can cause exposure and mechanical damage to the ocular surface. Surgical intervention is indicated in severe cases of either ectropion or entropion.

Presbyopia, literally 'old eyes', is the most common age-related ocular condition. It arises through normal ageing changes in the crystalline lens that reduce the ability of the eye to focus at near distances. It is easily corrected by the prescription of reading glasses. *Cataract* is a common age-related change in the eye. In a cataract the lens material becomes opaque, preventing the formation of a clear image and causing blurred vision. Surgical removal is the only treatment option, but is straightforward and normally successful.

Ageing can also affect the neural components of the eye. Apoptosis of photoreceptor cells at the fovea, due to the action of free radicals, leads to *age-related macular degeneration* (AMD), and a reduction in detailed vision. This disease is progressive and currently untreatable, although lifestyle factors such as stopping smoking and dietary supplements are thought to slow the progression of the condition. A small number of patients may suffer from an acute form of the disease (wet AMD), which causes a rapid reduction of vision over a period of weeks and needs investigation and treatment by an ophthalmologist within 1–2 weeks of the onset of symptoms. *Primary open angle glaucoma* is an insidious disease causing damage to the optic nerve head, which is asymptomatic until significant visual loss has occurred. The disease becomes increasingly prevalent with age, but can be treated successfully with prostaglandin and/or beta-blocker eyedrops. Other changes with age include reduced *contrast sensitivity*, poor *dark–light adaptation* and reductions in *visual field*. These increase the risk of falls and may lead to inactivity through fear in older people.

that they are losing function (e.g. having difficulty using the stairs or crossing the road). Exploring the individual's readiness to change will reveal positive and negative attitudes towards participation and will determine the strategies to use when setting and agreeing realistic and meaningful goals (King *et al.* 1998; Chodzko-Zajko & Resnick 2004). It has been suggested that interventions might be more effectively aimed at semi-active older people who seem more positively disposed to participating but need help to get started or to stay involved (Marcus & Forsyth 2003; Chodzko-Zajko & Resnick 2004).

Recent research has showed that older people are more likely to take up and adhere to exercise if the benefits are explained in terms of positive effects on mobility, autonomy and social engagement. Greater commitment is found if the exercise programme is graded so that the benefits are felt quickly and people feel it is appropriate for them (Yardley *et al.* 2007). Motivators to exercise, particularly in frailer older people identified by Yardley *et al.* (2007), include:

- thinking that you are the kind of person who should do these activities;
- thinking other people think you should do these activities;
- believing that these activities will be enjoyable;
- thinking the exercise will benefit health conditions and help maintain independence;
- concern about avoidance of a future fall.

It is important that health professionals dispel some of the long-held myths and stereotypes associated with exercise (Box 8.3).

Box 8.3   Dispelling myths and stereotypes

There are five common myths and stereotypes about physical activity and ageing that need to be dispelled (Finch 1997; Jones & Rose 2005).

(1) *You have to be healthy to exercise*: find appropriate role models of people with chronic disease who have had improvements in their quality of life with exercise.
(2) *I'm too old to start exercising*: use appropriate images to show that age is not a barrier to physical activity.
(3) *You need special equipment and clothing*: apart from comfortable shoes and loose-fitting clothing, there is no special clothing or equipment. However, cultural and generational factors have to be taken into consideration.
(4) *No pain, no gain*: reinforce the notion that vigorous exercise is no longer recommended and that moderate physical activity can be easily incorporated into daily life.
(5) *I'm too busy to exercise*: help identify opportunities within their schedule.

How can we support a change to a more active lifestyle?

In the last decade, the growth in the literature on physical activity and exercise prescription in older people has led to the publication of a number of best practice guidelines and expert texts on the programming of exercise for relatively healthy older people wishing to engage in regular moderate to vigorous physical activity (British Heart Foundation 2009). Best practice guidelines for nursing staff working with frailer older adults on wards in hospital have also been published (NHS Quality Improvement Scotland 2005). An important point to understand is that sedentary behaviour is more risky than any physical activity and the role of the health professional in the promotion of active living amongst older adults is crucial. With the ever-increasing population of older adults the value of improved quality of life, reduced institutionalisation and increased productivity through active living should be a top priority.

There is an urgent need to appreciate the value of enthusiasm, positive images and sound advice about the benefits of physical activity and exercise for successful ageing. A great deal of disability associated with old age is a result of disuse not disease, symptoms could be ameliorated, and it is vital health professionals working with older people give positive information about the benefits of regular activity and exercise (British Heart Foundation 2009) (Case study 8.1).

In some instances there may be only one chance to encourage activity, but many health professionals will see older people over an irregular but long-term period. For these people, uptake of exercise or activity may be helped by support in the early stages (e.g. specific rehabilitation classes for some medical conditions) but often adherence stops when the professional support stops. The importance of involvement of peer mentors in the adoption and maintenance of exercise amongst other older adults and of professional support in adherence to a home exercise programme cannot be underestimated (Robertson *et al.* 2001;

Case study 8.1   Missed opportunities in promotion of physical activity

This case highlights the importance of promoting physical activity promotion at every opportunity throughout the older person's journey of care. Mrs Aitken, a 79-year-old lady, has been attending an outpatient clinic. She has chronic obstructive pulmonary disease and osteoporosis, poor vision and is extremely inactive. At these clinic appointments nothing was mentioned about the importance of regular physical activity to potentially improve the symptoms of her conditions. Mrs Aitken says she is too frightened to exercise as she feels that exercise will make her more breathless and increase her chances of falling. She feels exhausted with even the slightest exertion and it takes her a long time to recover. She feels her inactivity is made worse by her failing vision which she believes exposes her to hazards in her environment and again makes her feel frightened. So she is now almost housebound and increasingly immobile. In fact, regular exercise would reduce Mrs Aitken's breathlessness so she could do more activity without limitation. By avoiding activity her balance and strength also reduces so she is less able to correct a trip and more likely to fall.

Box 8.4   Peer mentors as a means of increasing uptake of exercise

In Kirklees, Yorkshire, 70 older peer activity mentors were trained. These volunteers work as 'buddies' and mentors. They meet and greet people at their first exercise referral meeting and in some instances accompany people to their sessions as encouragement. One mentor attracted 240 participants in 12 months to physical activity programmes.

Stewart *et al.* 2006). The project outlined in Box 8.4 highlights the importance of 'someone like me' in the motivation for an older person to become more active. Older people often perceive more empathy if the person encouraging them is of a similar age.

A recent trial of primary care exercise referral for older adults showed that, with structured support strategies including transport, it is possible to get high rates of uptake and adherence to exercise programmes even amongst frail older adults (Dinan *et al.* 2006). In people aged 75 and over, 89% took up the exercise programme; 73% completed stage I and 63% made the transition to the community stage II programme (Dinan *et al.* 2006).

Finally and importantly, designing and delivering exercise for older people with multiple medical conditions requires specialist skills and training. Shephard (1991) emphasised that programming physical activity for older people requires more care and more expertise than for any other age group, with only a fine line separating effective from dangerous procedures. The recognition of the importance of specialist skills culminated in the publication and current implementation of the International Curriculum Guidelines for Physical Activity Instructors of Older People (Ecclestone & Jones 2004). Within the UK, there is also the Register of Exercise Professionals (www.exerciseregister.org/) which has information on leisure-based instructors with appropriate qualifications to work with patients.

Teasing out some of the components for evidence informed nursing, key messages include:

- the importance of nurses recognising inactivity and sedentary behaviour in older people;
- nurses understanding the value of physical activity and mobility to older people, even those who are frail;
- interdisciplinary working towards promotion of healthy mobility and sustained physical activity in older people;
- user involvement at every stage and the value of negotiating activity programmes with older people based on informed choices;
- the importance of specific skills for nurses, essential to promoting movement and physical activity in the older person in different care settings.

A community of practice approach may be one way to ensure engagement of professionals and older people in implementing physical activity best practice guidelines. Case study 8.2 illustrates this.

Case study 8.2   Community of practice to increase physical activity

A practice development project was undertaken in a large university teaching hospital that aimed to create a community of practice (CoP) to accelerate the attainment of evidence based guidance relevant to promoting physical activity in the older person in hospital settings. This project was theoretically underpinned by the Caledonian Improvement Model (Tolson *et al.* 2005, 2006) in which the members of the CoP pooled their knowledge and resources to implement a best practice statement (NHS Quality Improvement Scotland 2005) and find practical solutions to the challenges associated with promoting physical activity in their particular area of practice. Learning, pooling of knowledge and knowledge translation were brought about in a virtual practice development college (Tolson *et al.* 2006), where the CoP met to plan, develop activities and support each other throughout the implementation project. The study recruited 44 practitioners, including nurses, physiotherapists and occupational therapists, from seven clinical sites across the health board area to form the CoP.

At the time of publication of the best practice statement (NHS Quality Improvement Scotland 2005) there was very little education and training provided in its use. Thus the project began with the CoP deciding to audit current practice in order to identify the areas where practice was aligned with the best practice statement and those areas where improvements were needed. Specific tools of evidence based review criteria derived from the best practice statement were used to conduct the audit. In total, 230 individual patient record audits and 25 clinical site audits were completed. The results highlighted a number of areas for development work but the CoP members wanted to prioritise involving older people, enabling choices and the development of active partnerships. The CoP members each developed an action plan for the duration of the project to address the main shortfalls identified in their individual audits and implement practice improvements in these areas.

A 'buddy' system was adopted to involve older people at every stage of the project. This system comprised CoP members asking patients their opinions on the relevant practice issues in the best practice statement. These views were fed back into the discussion forum in the virtual college for debate and subsequent changes to action planning and practice. This mechanism focused on enabling the patients to have a voice and as such promoted person-centred, respectful and dignified care. Other activities included disseminating posters in each of the clinical areas to heighten awareness of the project and enable patients and carers to see the positive work that was happening to improve their experiences of care. Additionally, community members embarked on disseminating the evidence based work of the CoP by presenting at both local and national conferences. Active members of the CoP used the cascade model of dissemination to ensure all clinical areas were provided with the information on the best practice statement. This involved cascading learning through teams and implementing revised local policies and practices. Educational resources based on the benchmarking audits were developed by CoP members and implemented across all clinical areas. These resources were banked in the virtual college for use by any member of the community. User statistics suggest approximately 50% of the community members actively contributed to changes in practice to produce the selected outcomes (see below). A number of key areas showed improvements on the outcome audits (Box 8.5) and in the expressed views of CoP members and older people (Box 8.6).

Box 8.5　Outcome audit results

(1) Evidence that the older person is involved in the decision-making and risk-taking process around physical activity (pre-CoP 50%, post-CoP 83%).
(2) Multidisciplinary documentation shows that therapeutic support has been offered or referrals made for specific disabilities affecting the person's ability to engage in physical activity (hearing, vision, cognitive, language) (pre-CoP 70%, post-CoP 81%).
(3) There is evidence that physical activity is offered to the older person on a regular basis (pre-CoP 80%, post-CoP 90%).
(4) Multidisciplinary documentation shows evidence that the older person exercises choice in participating in regular physical activity (pre-CoP 69%, post-CoP 83%).
(5) Multidisciplinary documentation shows evidence of structured activities, provided by multidisciplinary staff or others with appropriate training, which takes into account the older person's capabilities, preferences and interests (pre-CoP 46%, post-CoP 81%).

Box 8.6   Examples of participant views from a community of practice to improve physical activity among older people in hospital

'Working through the practice development process has helped me to change practice in other areas other than our chosen best practice statement and has assisted interdisciplinary working in our ward.' (Ward Manager)

'It is really useful speaking to other staff members across the directorate and it makes sure that we are providing standardised practice and most importantly involving our patients in their care.' (Ward Manager)

'It was the first time that anyone has included me in planning an exercise programme for my stay in hospital.' (Patient 4)

'Being involved has really motivated me and now I know the importance of exercise.' (Patient 1)

Summary

This chapter explores the positive influence of physical activity and exercise on the lives of older people. Improved fitness ensures a person has a better quality of life, even in the presence of disease, but a lack of knowledge among both older people and the health professionals coming into contact with them means the valuable contribution of self-management through exercise is missed. All professionals coming into contact with an older person in their journey of care should take the opportunity to discuss the person's current activity and discuss ways of increasing activity and engaging in the self-management of their conditions or symptoms. Best practice guidelines on physical activities that maintain health, reduce

Key messages

- Maintaining an active lifestyle is extremely important as we age and is even more important if we have medical conditions.
- It's never too late to take up exercise.
- Regular physical activity reduces the risk of many diseases and reduces many of the symptoms of disease.
- Self-management and reduction in morbidity can be enhanced by health professionals engaging older adults in a discussion about the value of exercise.
- Tailored supervised exercise can help in the management of disease and allows anyone, with any medical condition, to exercise safely and effectively.
- Developing a community of practice approach may be one means of ensuring effective dissemination of best practice guidance on encouraging and engaging older people in physical activity and exercise.

risk of falls, maintain independent living and quality of life do exist but their reach is negligible to older people if health professionals are not aware of them, do not promote active living or neglect to discuss the value of activity. Often avoidance of a discussion on exercise can lead to negative perceptions and further avoidance of activity. The role of a community of practice to ensure implementation of best practice statements has been shown to be successful and the Caledonian Model is one way to ensure that knowledge and skills are kept up to date, that users are involved in directing and disseminating information to ensure the greatest reach and the best chance of getting 'more people, moving more often'.

References

Biddle SJ, Fox K, Edmunds L (1994) *Physical Activity Promotion in Primary Health Care in England.* Health Education Authority, London.

Bloomfield SA (1997) Changes in musculoskeletal structure and function in prolonged bed rest. *Medicine and Science in Sports and Exercise* **29**, 197–206.

British Heart Foundation (2009) *Active for Later Life Resource.* Available at www.bhfactive.org.uk/older-adults/publications.html (accessed 1 May 2010).

Britton A, McPherson K (2002) *Monitoring the Progress of the 2010 Target for CHD Mortality: Estimated Consequences on CHD Incidence and Mortality from Changing Prevalence of Risk Factors.* National Heart Forum, London.

Cavanagh DJ, Cann CE (1988) Brisk walking does not stop bone loss in postmenopausal women. *Bone* **9**, 201–204.

Chodzko-Zajko WJ, Resnick B (2004) Beyond screening: the need for new pre-activity counseling protocols to assist older adults transition from sedentary living to physically active lifestyles. *Journal of Active Aging* **3**, 26–30.

Craig A, Dinan S, Smith A, Taylor A, Webborn N (2000) *NHS Exercise Referral Systems: A National Quality Assurance Framework.* The Stationery Office, London.

Department of Health (2010) *Chief Medical Officers Annual Report 2009.* The Stationery Office, London.

Dinan S (2001) Exercise for vulnerable older patients. In: Young A, Harries M (eds) *Exercise Prescription for Patients.* Royal College of Physicians, London, pp. 121–132.

Dinan SM, Lenihan P, Tenn T, Illiffe S (2006) Is the promotion of physical activity in vulnerable, older people feasible and effective in general practice? *British Journal of General Practice* **56**, 791–793.

Ebrahim S, Thompson PW, Baskaraon V, Evans K (1997) Randomized placebo-controlled trail of brisk walking in the prevention of postmenopausal osteoporosis. *Age and Ageing* **26**, 253–260.

Ecclestone NA, Jones CJ (2004) International curriculum guidelines for preparing physical activity instructors of older adults. *Journal of Aging and Physical Activity* **12**, 5–21.

Finch H (1997) *Physical Activity: At Our Age. Qualitative Research Among People Over the Age of 50.* Health Education Authority, London.

Gillespie LD, Robertson MC, Gillespie WJ *et al.* (2009) Interventions for preventing falls in older people living in the community. *Cochrane Database of Systematic Reviews* (2), CD007146.

Grahn-Kronhed AC, Blomberg C, Karlsson N (2005) Impact of a community-based osteoporosis and fall prevention program on fracture incidence. *Osteoporosis International* **16**, 700–706.

Hill RD, Storandt M, Malley M (1993) The impact of long-term exercise training on psychological function in older adults. *Journal of Gerontology* **48**, 12–17.

Hillsdon M, Foster C, Cavill N, Crombie H, Naidoo B (2005) *The Effectiveness of Public Health Interventions for Increasing Physical Activity Among Adults.* Health Development Agency, London.

Jones CJ, Rose DJ (2005) *Physical Activity Instruction of Older Adults.* Human Kinetics, Champaign, IL.

Katz DS, Branch LG (1983) Active life expectancy. *New England Journal of Medicine* **309**, 1213–1224.

King AC, Rejeski WJ, Buchner DM (1998) Physical activity interventions targeting older adults. A critical review and recommendations. *American Journal of Preventive Medicine* **15**, 316–333.

Kohrt WM, Bloomfield SA, Little KD, Nelson ME, Yingling VR (2004) Physical activity and bone health. American College of Sports Medicine Position Stand. *Medicine and Science in Sports and Exercise* **36**, 1985–1996.

Lavie CJ, Milani RV (1995) Effects of cardiac rehabilitation on exercise capacity, coronary risk factors, behavioural characteristics, and quality of life in a large elderly cohort. *American Journal of Cardiology* **76**, 177–179.

McClure RJ, Turner C, Peel N, Spinks A, Eakin E, Hughes K (2005) Population-based interventions for the prevention of fall-related injuries in older people. *Cochrane Database of Systematic Reviews* (1), CD004441.

Malbut KE, Dinan S, Young A (2002) Aerobic training in the 'oldest old': the effect of 24 weeks of training. *Age and Ageing* **31**, 255–260.

Marcus BH, Forsyth LH (2003) *Motivating People to be Physically Active.* Human Kinetics, Champaign. IL.

Nelson ME, Fiatarone MA, Morganti CM, Trice I, Greenberg RA, Evans WJ (1994) Effects of high-intensity strength training on multiple risk factors for osteoporotic fractures. A randomized controlled trial. *Journal of the American Medical Association* **272**, 1909–1914.

Nelson ME, Rejeski WJ, Blair SN *et al.* (2007) Physical activity and public health in older adults: recommendation from the American College of Sports Medicine and the American Heart Association. *Medicine and Science in Sports and Exercise* **39**, 1435–1445.

NHS Quality Improvement Scotland (2005) *Working with Dependant Older People towards Promoting Movement and Physical Activity.* NHS QIS, Edinburgh.

Nichol JP, Coleman P, Brazier JE (1994) Health and healthcare costs and benefits of exercise. *Pharmacoeconomics* **5**, 109–122.

O'Connor PJ, Aenchbacher LE, Dishman RK (1993) Physical activity and depression in the elderly. *Journal of Aging and Physical Activity* **1**, 34–58.

Ory MRB, Jordan PJ, Coday M *et al.* (2005) Screening, safety, and adverse events in physical activity interventions: collaborative experiences from behavior change consortium. *Annals of Behavioural Medicine* **29**, 20–28.

Riddoch C, Puig-Ribera A, Cooper A (1998) *Effectiveness of Physical Activity Promotion Schemes in Primary Care: A Review.* Health Education Authority, London.

Robertson MC, Devlin N, Scuffham P, Gardner MM, Buchner DM, Campbell A.J (2001) Economic evaluation of a community based exercise programme to prevent falls. *Journal of Epidemiology and Community Health* **55**, 600–606.

Shephard RJ (1991) Benefits of sport and physical activity for the disabled: implications for individuals and society. *Scandinavian Journal of Rehabilitation Medicine* **23**, 51–59.

Sinaki M (1982) Postmenopausal spinal osteoporosis: physical therapy and rehabilitation. *Mayo Clinic Proceedings* **57**, 699–703.

Sinaki M, Itoi E, Wahner HW *et al.* (2002) Stronger back muscles reduce the incidence of vertebral fractures: a prospective 10 year follow-up of postmenopausal women. *Bone* **30**, 836–841.

Skelton DA, Dinan SM (2008) Ageing and older people. In: Buckley JP (ed.) *Exercise Physiology in Special Populations. Advances in Sport and Exercise Science*. Elsevier Books, Edinburgh, pp. 161–224.

Skelton DA, McLaughlin A (1996) Training functional ability in old age. *Physiotherapy: Theory and Practice* **82**, 159–167.

Skelton DA, Young A, Greig CA, Malbut KE (1995) Effects of resistance training on strength, power and selected functional abilities of women aged 75 and over. *Journal of the American Geriatric Society* **43**, 1081–1087.

Skelton DA, Young A, Walker A, Hoinville E (1999) *Physical Activity in Later Life: Further Analysis of the Allied Dunbar National Fitness Survey and the Health Education Authority Survey of Activity and Health*. Health Education Authority, London.

Skelton DA, Dinan SM, Campbell MG, Rutherford OM (2005) Frequent fallers halve their risk of falls with 9 months of tailored group exercise (FaME): an RCT in community dwelling women aged 65 and over. *Age and Ageing* **34**, 636–639.

Spirduso WW, Francis KL, MacRae PG (1996) *Physical Dimensions of Aging*, 1st edn. Human Kinetics Books, Champaign, IL.

Stewart AL, Gillis D, Grossman M *et al.* (2006) Diffusing a research-based physical activity promotion program for seniors in diverse communities: CHAMPS III. *Prevention of Chronic Disease* **3**, 51–59.

Thomas S, Reading J, Shephard RJ (1992) Revision of the Physical Activity Readiness Questionnaire (PAR-Q). *Canadian Journal of Sports Science* **17**, 338–345.

Thompson RF, Crist DM, March M, Rosenthal M (1988) Physical effects of physical exercise for elderly patients with physical impairments. *Journal of the American Geriatrics Society* **36**, 130–135.

Tinetti ME (1994) Prevention of falls and falls injuries in elderly persons: a research agenda. *Prevention Medicine* **23**, 756–762.

Tolson D, McAloon M, Hotchkiss R, Schofield I (2005) Progressing evidence-based practice: an effective nursing model? *Journal of Advanced Nursing* **50**, 661–671.

Tolson D, Schofield I, Booth J, Kelly TB, James L (2006) Constructing a new approach to developing evidence-based practice with nurses and older people. *Worldviews on Evidence-Based Nursing* **3**, 1–11.

US Department of Health and Human Services (1996) *Physical Activity and Health: A Report of the Surgeon General. Executive Summary*. Centers for Disease Control and Prevention, National Center for Chronic Disease Prevention and Health Promotion, Atlanta.

Wagner EH (1997) Preventing decline in function: evidence from randomized trials around the world. *Western Journal of Medicine* **167**, 295–298.

Welsh L, Rutherford OM (1996) Hip bone mineral density is improved by high-impact aerobic exercise in postmenopausal women and men over 50 years. *European Journal of Applied Physiology and Occupational Physiology* **74**, 511–517.

Whedon GD (1984) Disuse osteoporosis. *Calcified Tissue International* **36**, S146–S150.

World Health Organization (1997) The Heidleberg guidelines for promoting physical activity among older persons. *Journal of Ageing and Physical Activity* **5**, 1–8.

World Health Organization (2002) *Reducing Risks. Promoting Healthy Life*. World Health Organization, Geneva.

World Health Organization (2007) A guide for population based approaches to increasing levels of physical activity Available at www.who.int/dietphysicalactivity/pa/en/index.html (accessed 24 November 2009).

Yardley L, Smith H (2002) A prospective study of the relationship between feared consequences of falling and avoidance of activity in community-living older people. *Gerontologist* **42**, 17–23.

Yardley L, Beyer N, Hauer K, McKee K, Ballinger C, Todd C (2007) Recommendations for promoting the engagement of older people in activities to prevent falls. *Quality and Safety in Health Care* **16**, 230–234.

Young A, Dinan S (2005) Active in later life. *British Medical Journal* **330**, 189–191.

Chapter 9

Age Related Hearing Problems

Debbie Tolson, Tracy Day and Joanne Booth

Introduction

Accumulating evidence shows that age related hearing disability is one of the most common impediments to communication in later life (Smeeth *et al.* 2002). Consequences of hearing loss for individuals and those close to them are many and can limit a person's participation in family and community life. Relational aspects of nursing care, and aspirations of working in partnership with older people are undermined when conversation is difficult or communication becomes one sided as a result of hearing difficulties. In Chapter 1 we included hearing problems in our list of geriatric syndromes (see Figure 1.2) which, in combination with other problems, contribute to poorer care outcomes. The association of hearing loss with other functional limitations is clearly demonstrated in the findings of a recent Spanish study (Lopez-Torres Hidalgo *et al.* 2009). Falls, another of the geriatric syndromes, has also been linked to hearing problems. For example, a Norwegian study of 332 older people admitted with hip fractures revealed that nearly 40% had hearing loss in isolation and a further 30% had combined visual and hearing loss (Grue *et al.* 2009). There is also evidence that hearing dysfunction may precede the onset of Alzheimer's disease, which raises the importance of early identification of problems due to their diagnostic implications given the development of medications that delay the advancement of early-stage disease (Gates *et al.* 2002). These research exemplars show that health risks associated with hearing loss need to be taken seriously and that our clinical and care interests should extend beyond a narrow concern of remediating communication problems. Despite the growing evidence base, management of hearing problems is rarely afforded the priority it deserves within gerontological practice and particularly within nursing.

The high numbers of older people living with hearing problems may explain why many people, including health professionals, accept hearing loss as a normal part of ageing. We will challenge this view, arguing that the negative impact of unmanaged hearing problems and associations with poorer outcomes make compelling reasons for intervention. To support older people and reduce hearing disability, nurses require an appreciation of how people hear and interpret sound including speech. Furthermore,

Evidence Informed Nursing with Older People, First Edition. Edited by Debbie Tolson, Joanne Booth and Irene Schofield.
© 2011 Blackwell Publishing Ltd. Published 2011 by Blackwell Publishing Ltd.

nurses need to make connections between the biological basis of problems, technological aspects of auditory rehabilitation, qualities of the listening environment and the interactions between emotional, cognitive and sensory processes within later life (Beck & Clark 2009).

We begin this chapter with a brief overview of how we hear and the influence of ageing, moving onto explore age related hearing problems and audiological rehabilitation options. In the second part of the chapter we examine nursing contributions to maximising communication with older people who have an age related hearing disability. Our best practice exemplar looks at implementation of evidence based care guidance drawing on previously unreported material from the Scottish Gerontological Demonstration Project (NHS Quality Improvement Scotland 2005; Tolson *et al.* 2006).

Hearing and ageing

The aetiology of sensorineural loss, the most common form of hearing loss in later life, is multifactorial and it is inappropriate to attribute this condition solely to age (Tolson & Swan 2006). Research suggests that sensorineural hearing pathology is most likely to be focused around changes in the outer hair cell functioning of the cochlea (Davis *et al.* 2007). Gates and Mills (2005) acknowledge that the evidence base to explain auditory ageing is incomplete and at times contradictory in part due to the difficulty in isolating ageing effects from the effects of noise trauma. In terms of healthcare interventions an important breakthrough is anticipated from biological studies of the stria vascularis in animals (more simply referred to as the 'battery' of the cochlea), which has given rise to the 'dead battery' theory of presbycusis. This biological theory has produced an engineering effort to create direct current hearing aids, which may lead to the next generation of treatments (Gates & Mills 2005, p. 1114). For decades hearing aid users, particularly older people, have voiced their dissatisfaction with hearing aids, many of which are discarded and left unused soon after issue. Research which examines user satisfaction as an outcome measure has shown progressive improvements in hearing aid use, user satisfaction and benefit, and a decrease in residual disability with each new generation of amplification devices, most recently the move from analogue aids to digital aids (Davis cited in Public Health Institute of Scotland 2003, p. 21). If investment in this area of research continues, then more effective solutions will in time become available. Nurses can do much to reassure older people that digital hearing aid technology is improving but the key to optimal benefit is early intervention (Carson 2005).

To orientate non-hearing specialists to the ear and hearing mechanisms, Box 9.1 provides revision notes on the ear and age related changes. For those wishing greater depth and an up to date account of the underlying pathophysiology we recommend Gates and Mills (2005). As noted in the description of changes within the inner ear (Box 9.1), sensorineural hearing impairment is usually more pronounced at high frequencies, which accounts for the common complaint among older people that they can hear people speaking but not understand what they are saying.

Box 9.1   Revision notes on the ear and age related changes

The human ear can be described in three main parts.

The external ear
Consists of the pinna (auricle) and the external auditory meatus. The shape of the pinna 'funnels' the sound into the ear, with both pinnae working together to locate the direction. The external auditory meatus channels the sound towards the tympanic membrane, which in turn transmits vibrations to the ossicles.

What can go wrong with the external ear in ageing?
Skin sagging can cause narrowing or collapse of the external auditory meatus, resulting in canal atresia and conductive deafness. Cerumen (wax) can collect and become impacted resulting in discomfort and hearing loss. The tympanic membrane can become scarred (tympanosclerosis) due to previous infection/healed perforation or noise damage.

The middle ear
The middle ear cavity is an air-filled space containing the ossicular chain, consisting of the stapes, incus and malleus bones. The flat 'footplate' of the stapes vibrates against the oval window of the cochlea transmitting the sound to the inner ear.

What can go wrong with the middle ear in ageing?
Ossicular discontinuity following trauma will result in a conductive hearing loss. Otitis media/suppurative otitis media can occur at any age, again resulting in a conductive or mixed loss. Cholesteatoma is a potentially life-threatening collection of dead skin cells and infection which can trigger meningitis if left untreated.

The inner ear
The inner ear consists of the semicircular canals (balance organ), vestibule (where all the structures join) and the cochlea. The cochlea is a fluid-filled snail-like structure that contains endolymph and perilymph separated by a thin membrane. The stapedial footplate causes waves in the perilymph, which in turn stimulates tiny hair cells that are arranged in order of pitch around the cochlear structure. These 'inner' and 'outer' hair cells are thought to contain nerve endings which convert kinetic energy into electrical energy that can be passed to the brain. The base of the cochlea corresponds to the high frequency (high pitch) sounds, while the apex registers the lower frequency (lower pitch) sounds.

What can go wrong with the inner ear in ageing?
General 'wear and tear' on the hair cells in the cochlea is the usual cause of hearing loss in the ageing population (presbycusis). The hair cells become damaged and worn and do not register the sound as effectively. The hair cells that receive high pitch sounds are usually first to be damaged as they lie at the beginning of the cochlea. High frequency loss is the hallmark of presbycusis.

Other factors to consider
Some hearing impaired individuals suffer from *recruitment*. This condition results in an abnormally rapid increase in perceived loudness of a sound caused by only a slight increase in intensity. The result may be difficulty in using any amplification device for that hearing loss.

Noise induced hearing loss is irreversible hearing loss attributed to exposure to high levels of noise. Noise induced hearing loss if often linked with recruitment (Heinz *et al.* 2005).

Tinnitus is defined as a noise heard without external stimulus. International studies suggest that 10% of adults have tinnitus, 5% describe it as moderately annoying, while 1% report tinnitus that severely affects their quality of life (Ferran & Phillips 2007).

In addition to the mechanisms within the ear, Gordon-Salant (2005) reminds us that changes in auditory temporal processing are equally important, hypothesising that for many older people the ability to process rapid acoustic information deteriorates with ageing. This problem becomes even more pronounced in noisy environments, with other distractions and if the speaker is heavily accented.

Successive studies have demonstrated that hearing difficulties reduce the quality of life of older people by interfering with communication, through social impacts and complex emotional responses linked to spoilt identity (Glavin 2003). Negative impacts have been consistently shown in studies of people who are independent and those who depend on others for care such as nursing home residents (Tsuruoka *et al.* 2001; Knussen *et al.* 2005).

The experience of hearing impairment has been equated to chronic long-term pain such as might be associated with a slipped disc (Davis *et al.* 2007). The onset of age related hearing problems is nearly always gradual so it is not seen as a health problem that requires urgent intervention. The insidious onset may explain why many people leave between 8 and 20 years before seeking help (Carson 2005).

Presbycusis

The term 'presbycusis' means age related hearing loss. Features of the presbycusis syndrome include:

- reduced hearing acuity
- high frequency hearing loss
- difficulties understanding speech in noise
- slowed processing of acoustic information
- impaired localisation of sound source.

The quotes shown in Box 9.2 illustrate older people's experience of presbycusis.

Box 9.2   Individual experiences of presbycusis

'When my hearing started to go I felt I missed out on so much. I missed the punch lines to jokes or I repeated what someone had said already. My family all have a good laugh at my expense. I can hear them speaking but can't make out the words.' (77-year-old lady with moderate presbycusis)

'The doctor came to see me in the ward but he just muttered something to himself. I had to ask the nurses later what he had said.' (80-year-old man with presbycusis)

'By the time I work out what someone has said, they've moved onto something else, or they say "never mind". I hate that!' (69-year-old man with mild presbycusis/noise induced hearing loss)

'I leave my front door unlocked so my home help can get in the house. I don't hear her at the door otherwise. My family say it's not safe but otherwise she'd have to knock on the window and that gives me a fright.' (85-year-old woman with severe presbycusis)

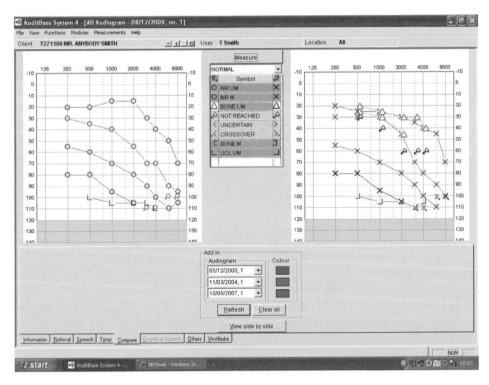

Figure 9.1 Audiograms showing progressing age related hearing impairment (presbycusis).

Risk factors associated with high frequency hearing loss include noise exposure, smoking, medication side effects and hypertension (Gates & Mills 2005, p. 1116). Some of these are shared risks associated with other geriatric syndromes (Inouye *et al.* 2007).

Problem assessment and diagnosis ideally includes physical examination following cerumen (ear wax) removal, evaluation of the impact of the problem on the person's life, and clinical screening such as spoken voice tests and the gold standard audiometric assessment. Figure 9.1 shows a typical audiogram of someone with presbycusis syndrome. The horizontal axis shows the frequency or pitch; the higher the number, the higher the pitch. The vertical axis is the volume required for the person to hear presented tones in decibels. Over a 7-year period repeated audiograms in both left and right ear demonstrate that progressively louder volumes are required at all frequencies with marked deterioration over time in the higher speech frequencies (4000, 8000 kHz).

In addition to the elevated pure-tone speech thresholds implicit in the prevalence figures, communication problems are for some compounded by executive function changes including attention span, memory and other cognitive changes. Beck and Clark (2009) argue for the integration of knowledge about cognition with that known about audition. They are critical of audiological rehabilitation approaches which fail to make these connections. The theoretical basis used by a number of leading studies which have integrated these elements are explained in an insightful commentary by Craik (2007). For readers interested in exploring this further Craik accessibly explains Trisman's levels of analysis model of selective attention within which interactions between 'bottom-up' auditory factors and 'top-down' cognitive factors may be understood. Several recent studies endorse the view that cognitive status and functioning needs to be considered alongside audiometric measures to explain the speech understanding abilities of older listeners (Humes 2005). Interpreting faster rates of speech is also particularly challenging for older listeners, a phenomenon attributed to slower information processing (Wingfield & Tun 2001). In general when a hearing loss occurs simultaneously with other age related declines, the person experiences a more severe disruption to communication. It has also, not unsurprisingly, been shown that hearing aid benefit and hearing use are lower in listeners with cognitive decline than those without (Lunner 2003; Gatehouse *et al.* 2006).

The size of the problem

Data derived from the UK National Study of Hearing estimates prevalence of hearing impairment in the better-hearing ear ≥ 25 dBHL at 37% in people aged 61–70 years, rising to 60% in people aged 71–80 years and escalating to 93% in people aged over 81 years. In the same age bands prevalence for hearing thresholds ≥ 45 dBHL (moderate impairment) were 7%, 18% and 64% respectively (Davis 1995). There are no reliable prevalence figures for institutionalised dependent older people, but extrapolations based on small samples suggest that hearing aid candidature may be higher than those of the community dwelling population (Tolson 1997).

The UK Medical Research Council (MRC) trial of the assessment and management of hearing problems among 32 656 community living older people found that provision of hearing aids fell short of need, and that for many people the performance of their hearing aid was considered inadequate (Smeeth *et al.* 2002). Many of the aids used by the participants were analogue. Of the subset of 14 877 who completed the whispered voice test, 3795 (26%) failed the test; 3028 (80%) of this hearing-impaired group had their ears examined by a nurse and 1148 of these people had ear wax. Interestingly, for the 710 people whose hearing was retested after wax removal, improved hearing was observed in just 3% as determined using the whispered voice test. This finding suggests that ear wax removal will help only a minority of older people with their ability to hear. Although the MRC trial is impressive in scale, the main weakness was a failure to use audiometric testing which is considered to be the gold standard measure. For hearing loss in the range 30–40 dBHL, the whispered voice test has a sensitivity of 90–100% and specificity of 70–87% (Pirozzo *et al.* 2003).

Arguably one of the most robust investigations of hearing problems and screening methods is that of Davis *et al.* (2007). This UK study concentrated on people aged between 55 and 74 years, and the multi-method design comprised a population study with a clinical effectiveness study followed by a case–control study. Over 34 000 people responded to a postal survey and 506 were interviewed. The clinical effectiveness study received 1461 replies from the first-stage questionnaire screen, with 306 people assessed in the clinic of whom 156 were fitted with hearing aids. The retrospective case–control study traced 116 previously fitted hearing aid users, who had been identified by a screen, and then conducted a case–control study using 50 participants.

Davis *et al.* (2007) found that 12% of people aged 55–74 years have a hearing problem that causes moderate or severe worry, annoyance or upset, but only 3% currently receive intervention through the use of hearing aids. Good amplification was shown to benefit about one in four of this 55–74-year-old population and the degree of hearing loss predicted benefit well.

Audiological rehabilitation pathways

The aim of audiological rehabilitation is to minimise the disability of hearing loss, enabling a person to maximise their communication abilities in day-to-day living. Since Goldstein and Stephens (1981) set out their preliminary model depicting an audiological procedural rehabilitation, a number of frameworks have been proposed. These include a model focused on the particular needs of dependent older adults (Tolson & Stephens 1997) and, more recently, a generic pathway outlining adult audiological assessment and management (Public Health Institute of Scotland 2003). The basic tenets involve problem evaluation, the setting of realistic goals, a phased management plan, hearing aid fitting, instruction and training. Findings from studies which have examined the benefits of training before or after hearing aid fitting are inconclusive, and recent investigations by Kelly *et al.* (in press) are critical of approaches that use didactic approaches and provide evidence that older people want support dealing with the emotional impact of hearing aid fitting as much as they want technical instruction. Research consistently shows that patient education can significantly improve health outcomes (Koelling *et al.* 2005) and hearing loss is no different. Older people can find explanations of what has changed in their hearing mechanism interesting and helpful. They often pass on this information to family members and this in itself can generate discussion within a family about the hearing loss and what can be done to help the hearing impaired person. It can also maintain realistic expectations when it comes to amplification.

In addition to hearing aid fitting and skill building, recommended care pathways include non-instrumental rehabilitation to support the person to relearn how to listen and develop new communication strategies (Public Health Institute of Scotland 2003). The American Academy of Audiology (AAA) have developed recommendations for improving the quality of life for people with hearing loss, including the use of screening procedures for identifying hearing loss and promoting funding for research in this area (American Academy of Audiology 2008, 2009). They also recommend a multifaceted approach towards aural rehabilitation where amplification should be used in partnership with effective instruction, good communication strategies, counselling and possibly group therapy. The AAA also advocate a non-auditory needs assessment including vision, manual dexterity, motivation, general health and cognitive ability. The success of hearing devices has been found to be closely related to experience, expectation, personality and attitude (Wong *et al.* 2003). These authors found expectation to be the greatest factor, not just with the individual, but with family and carers.

Readers who wish to further explore auditory rehabilitation for elderly people should refer to the excellent article by D'Wynter (2006). Practitioners working with older people anticipating hearing assessment and possible hearing aid fitting should familiarise themselves with current evidence based care guidance for ear care and in particular management of cerumen (ear wax) to ensure that they are equipped to provide safe and effective interventions (e.g. NHS Quality Improvement Scotland 2006).

As the above discussion indicates, there are many opportunities for nurses to work with older people who experience age related deterioration in their hearing abilities. What follows is a discussion of the findings from a community of practice tasked with developing and testing care guidance to optimise communication with presbycusic listeners as part of the demonstration project outlined in the first two chapters of this book.

Project Example: Delivering evidence informed practice: maximising communication with older people who have hearing disability

In 2004 NHS Quality Improvement Scotland commissioned the Gerontological Nursing Team at Glasgow Caledonian University to use participatory research methods to develop evidence based guidance to inform nursing with older people experiencing presbycusis. The theoretical framework that guided knowledge conversion processes used by the development community of practice was provided by the Caledonian Improvement Model, as described in Chapter 2 (Tolson *et al.* 2006; Booth *et al.* 2007). The impetus for the project was the conviction that effective communication is a prerequisite for quality relational-centred healthcare plus the known detrimental impact of presbycusis on a person's sense of well-being and independence.

Project aim

To collaboratively develop evidence informed best practice guidance for nurses to adopt in their contribution to the care of people with age related hearing loss.

Methods

Nurses working with older people in the NHS and independent sector in Scotland, and with a declared interest in communication, were recruited to form a community of practice to develop and demonstrate national care guidance in the area of age related hearing disability. An audiologist acted as an expert clinician to work with the community of practice and to lead the review of specialist research literature. The task of the group was to identify the nursing contribution and test the draft guidance for feasibility in two contrasting demonstration sites. The intention was to construct care guidance that would be applicable irrespective of the context of care.

A virtual collaborative workplace was established to act as an internet based place for discussions and online working, to act as an information repository using a similar design adopted throughout the Scottish Demonstration Project (Lowndes *et al.* 2007).

Constructing and testing the care guidance formed the bulk of the activities undertaken by the community of practice over the 12-month period. These included attending four face-to-face development days, two-weekly online synchronous learning sessions, one-to-one action planning and facilitated asynchronous themed discussion forums.

The procedural method of best practice statement development (Booth *et al.* 2007) was unchanged. It involved collaborative review by an expert advisor and members of the community of practice of the diverse evidence base relating to the topic. Alignment of the draft guidance with the community of practice's agreed value base for gerontological nursing was then undertaken with subsequent testing of the draft in two demonstration sites. Structured feedback from the demonstration sites and a national consultation were undertaken prior to the published best practice statement being distributed throughout the NHS and independent sector across Scotland.

Ethical issues

The longitudinal project received approval from the University Research Ethics Committee and as this study was focused solely on nurses' views and opinions and it commenced prior to the implementation of the Standard Operating Procedures for UK Research Ethics Committees (2004), it was not necessary to gain additional approval.

Participants

In forming the new community of practice 24 nurses were recruited through direct approaches to directors of nursing and through advertising using known national networks and the nursing press. A deliberate decision to over-recruit was made to allow for possible attrition. All participants were registered nurses practising with older people (Table 9.1) and all areas of practice were represented (Table 9.2).

Table 9.1 Membership of community of practice (CoP).

CoP members nursing roles	Number at outset	Number completing
Staff nurse	8	4
Charge nurse	8	4
Community specialist nurse	2	2
Lead nurse	1	1
Lecturer/practitioner	1	1
Practice development nurse	2	2
Nurse practitioner	1	1
Nursing director	1	1
Total	24	16

Table 9.2 Participants' areas of practice.

Practice area	N
Acute medicine for the elderly	4
Rehabilitation	6
Specialist mental health	2
Continuing care	6
Community	3
Independent sector	2
Higher education	1
Total	24

Statement	Reason for statement	How to demonstrate achievement in practice
Section 1 Extract: Promoting nurses' awareness of hearing disability in the older person		
Nurses and care staff are knowledgeable about: • age-related communication needs, and • the impact of hearing loss on older people's psychological and social well-being and overall quality of life	Age-related hearing disability can have a negative influence on a person's quality of life. The person may avoid social situations and is at increased risk of isolation Hearing loss may contribute to or exacerbate mental health problems such as depression or paranoid beliefs Family and other significant relationships may be affected by hearing loss There is evidence that age-related hearing loss is not recognised as a problem which is amenable to healthcare intervention	There are local guidelines on deaf awareness and communicating with older people with hearing disability Staff education and training programmes are in place. Staff training records provide evidence of education and training Access to local guidelines is made known to nursing and care staff at induction training
Section 2 Extract: Assessment and care planning		
The registered nurse undertakes screening for the presence of hearing disability on initial contact with the older person	Early identification of potential hearing deficits facilitates effective communication and enhances the well-being of older people with hearing disability, their spouses and other supporters	Self-reported hearing problems are documented in nursing records and lead to screening and in-depth assessment
A variety of screening approaches may be utilised according to the individual's presentation	Alternative means of screening, e.g. based on observation of body language, behaviour, voice and language use, are used to ensure all older people can be screened for age-related hearing disability	Screening is undertaken where a hearing disability is suspected, using an appropriate screening tool Findings from the initial screening are documented and inform subsequent assessment and collaborative care planning. Appendix 3 provides an example of a screening tool
Section 3 Extract: Maximising interaction opportunities for older people with hearing disability		
Nurses and care staff are aware that hearing aids do not restore full hearing ability and thus hearing disability may be reduced, but not eliminated	Age-related hearing loss commonly occurs at higher sound frequencies, which makes speech particularly difficult to understand, especially when there is background noise	Hearing devices other than hearing aids are used appropriately, e.g. visual alerting devices (including smoke detectors), communicators, loop induction systems
Where the older person has a hearing aid(s) nurses and care staff encourage them to wear it (them) and provide any support they require to insert, use and maintain it (them)	Devices to aid hearing only function correctly when properly used and maintained	Nursing and care staff are knowledgeable about different types of hearing aids, their proper usage, care and maintenance A range of equipment to maintain optimal hearing aid function is available to nursing and care staff, and hearing aid maintenance checks are routinely provided

Figure 9.2 Extracts from Sections 1–3 of the resultant care guidance. (Reproduced with permission from NHS Quality Improvement Scotland.)

Project outcomes

As indicated in Table 9.1, 24 nurses joined the community of practice but eight withdrew during the project leaving a group of 16. Lack of time was the reason given by four of the participants and family problems/sickness by a further three. One participant gave no reason for withdrawing. Nonetheless the care guidance was produced and field tested within 1 year, although during the early stages of development participation of the full group was limited.

The resultant best practice statement comprised four sections, focusing on raising staff awareness of the problem, assessment and care planning, strategies to maximise interaction opportunities and education and training. Extracts of the first three sections are shown in Figure 9.2. The original best practice statement displayed appropriate citations and the strength of the underlying evidence as determined by the evidence hierarchy adopted by the Scottish Intercollegiate Guideline Network (SIGN 2009). According to this evidence hierarchy, two-thirds of the evidence used to develop the best practice statement was graded as 'non-analytical studies (e.g. case reports, case series) or expert opinion', while only one-third of the evidence sources used were graded as strong in terms of the underlying research rigour. In other words a major challenge for the authors was that at the time of developing the care guidance the available evidence base was relatively weak and it was necessary to rely on what might be regarded as generally agreed good practice points.

Each section of the statement included a list of key points and list of challenges identified and subsequently resolved within the pilot demonstration sites, a remote rural community site and an inpatient hospital ward within a major city. Section 4 reflected that the nurses' contribution complemented that of hearing specialists and that major benefits could be accrued by nurses attending to interventions to improve the listening environment and enhancing self-care abilities of older people and regular communication partners.

This project was designed not only to produce care guidance but to evaluate its impact on practice and on the experiences of the members of the community of practice. Each demonstration site was successful in implementing a number of improvements to local practice guided by the draft best practice statement and each was able to provide regular feedback on the relevance, feasibility and achievability of the recommendations made to inform the final published guidance. The developments undertaken and achievements of the acute rehabilitation ward are presented in Table 9.3. This shows the alignment between the elements of the best practice statement and the specific plans made by the link nurses based on the results of their local audits. Some of the achievements relate to improvements in the facilities, such as designating an information site in the ward dedicated to hearing problems and negotiating new audiology referral guidelines. Other developments focused on improving direct patient care, including the introduction of the finger-rub screening test and of the presbycusis core care plan.

Analysis of the 'Thoughts about work' questionnaire showed a number of direct benefits that the members of the community of practice perceived and an overall positive response to the project approach. Following participation in this project the nurses reported increases in their sense of personal achievement, morale, job satisfaction, satisfaction with working conditions, communication with managers and feelings of being a valued employee. Significantly, the quality of care was perceived to have increased and stress levels decreased, despite the nurses reporting an increase in their responsibilities and their workload, together with decreased time for direct care (Table 9.4).

Table 9.3 Practice improvement activities and achievements in acute rehabilitation demonstration site.

Identified initial practice deficit	Planned actions	Reported achievements
There is lack of a training programme that includes all points required	Development of training materials to include: • Physiology of the ear • Impact of age related hearing loss • Types of hearing loss • Assessment and screening for hearing ability • Skills to aid communication with people who are deaf blind • Audiological rehabilitation strategies for patients who have other needs along with hearing loss • Type, use and care of hearing aids • Ear hygiene	Have met with in-service education department regarding need to develop division-wide education programme on hearing disability Have developed short PowerPoint training session on hearing loss in older people Current admission and assessment documentation due for review. Link nurse will take forward to include full assessment section for hearing All trained staff given information on assessing an older person for hearing disability and what is required for completion of this Have printed information on hearing aids for staff education purposes
No local guidelines available on communicating with older people with hearing loss	To provide local guidelines for use at ward level	Have implemented communication guidelines. All staff have been given a copy
There is no information available for patients and carers on communication strategies and how to access advice and services	To provide a range of information that patients and carers can access	Now have a designated information area in the ward foyer for hearing disability, for patients and carers to access, which includes information on different aspects of hearing disability, assistive devices, how to access services, communication guidelines and ear care
No formal screening programme available to assess for hearing loss and subsequent referral for audiology assessment	To provide a tool for screening for hearing loss To formalise referral system for audiology assessment	Have amended hearing disability assessment sheet originally devised by another link nurse for use in the ward to include the finger rub test Have visited and clarified with the Audiology Department their referral process and have devised a referral to audiology guideline for use in the ward
There is no formal recording of type of hearing aid used, its condition, usual usage or any other assistive devices used	Develop and implement a core care plan that can be individualised for use with people who have hearing loss	Have devised a core care plan exclusively relating to hearing disability Have printed information on hearing aids for staff education purposes
There is no care plan available which includes use of the hearing aid, help required with the hearing aid, other hearing devices used or required, named communication partners, ear wax management strategies, a record of ear irrigation, education about hearing loss and needs	Develop and implement a core care plan that can be individualised for use with people who have hearing loss	Have devised a core care plan exclusively relating to hearing disability Both link nurses are booked onto the ear irrigation course later this year Due to funds made available the ward has a new otoscope and electric ear irrigation machine for use

Table 9.4 Post-study 'Perception of workplace change' (*N* = 14).

Variable	Decreased	Stayed the same	Increased
Personal achievement	2	1	11*
Feeling valued	3	4	7*
Morale	2	2	8*
Quality of care	0	3	11*
Job satisfaction	1	4	9*
Satisfaction with working conditions	0	5	9*
Communication with managers	3	4	7*
Stress levels	7*	3	4
Responsibilities	0	3	11*
Workload	3	3	8*
Time for direct care	8*	2	4
Staffing levels	4	8*	1
Time to talk to patients	5*	5*	4*
Job security	3	7*	4
Resources	0	11*	3

*Asterisks indicate trends in data.

Discussion of best practice project

A number of challenges arose during this project that had not previously been encountered. A major challenge was the imposition of the task to be undertaken in the form of the best practice statement construction, testing and implementation within a time limit of 1 year and the particular subject area of communicating with older people with hearing disability. This contrasts with previous communities of practice where the subject of the guidance evolved through agreement among the members and emphasises the more technical approach adopted in this project where there was a central source of authority rather than supported autonomous decision-making within the group. While this approach created time and scope pressures, the community of practice was ultimately successful in achieving the project aims of developing evidence informed practice in maximising communication with older people with hearing disability, albeit with perhaps more limited enjoyment than experienced by other communities of practice.

Additionally, as these participants did not perceive themselves to be experts in the area of practice, a further challenge was their lack of confidence in identifying the specific needs and care for older people with presbycusis. So unlike the members of previous communities of practice who pooled expertise, these nurses were more reliant on the clinical expert and less able to appraise the evidence or suggest previously rehearsed implementation solutions.

I think the expert advisor is the major contribution and you listen to her and look up to her because she is the expert and I think that has been quite good specifically in this project because it's something we don't know a lot about is audiology and we've certainly learnt a lot from her. (Participant 110, para 109)

The group perceived their recognised knowledge deficits to be indicative of the low priority generally afforded to this area of care by nurses.

> *The nutrition's definitely the buzz at the moment and it has been for the last two or three years so there's a huge interest in that and I do find that hearing impairment does tend to go by the wayside and we're all kind of guilty of that you know.* (Participant 109, para 105)

> *Nurses ... see other things as a priority rather than hearing disability.* (Focus Group, p. 10, line 27)

The lack of hearing expertise among the nurses altered the dynamics of the relationship between the expert advisor and the community of practice and potentially affected the participants' sense of ownership of the completed best practice statement. In turn this may have impacted on their degree of motivation, which a number of authors (Breu & Hemingway 2002; McKenna & Green 2002) suggest is of greater importance to the success of virtual group working, than face to face.

Summary

There is compelling evidence that age related hearing loss is an important public health issue in terms of the large number of people affected and impact on their lives and well-being. Thankfully there are interventions that can make a difference, and recent advances in understanding the biological basis of hearing problems have influenced the technology of hearing aids. However, there is still a long way to go in terms of realising the potential of sound amplification devices in the new digital era. It is important that nurses work with older people and family carers to understand the benefits of early intervention, are enabled to make informed choices about auditory rehabilitation options and adopt appropriate self-care strategies to optimise communication and offset some of the negative consequences of presbycusis.

Key messages

- Age related hearing loss (presbycusis) is a prevalent condition that impacts on a person's ability to communicate and their well-being.
- The detrimental impact of unmanaged hearing problems include development of low mood and depression, social isolation, cognitive decline and self-imposed loss of independence; like other geriatric conditions, hearing impairment increases the risk of poor outcomes.
- Age related hearing pathology is thought to be mainly associated with changes in the outer hair cell functioning of the cochlea. There is currently no cure and much still to be discovered.
- Many older people are dissatisfied with the current generation of hearing aids and prematurely discard their hearing aids believing them useless. Nurses are well positioned to advocate with older people to ensure that they are fitted with the best possible aids and given appropriate information and counselling.
- There is much that nurses can contribute to maximising communication opportunities and promoting positive adjustments to life with a hearing aid.

References

American Academy of Audiology (2008) *Guidelines for the Audiologic Management of Adult Hearing Impaired*. Available at www.audiology.org/resources/documentlibrary/documents/haguidelines.pdf (accessed 9 March 2010).

American Academy of Audiology (2009) *Report of the Task Force on Hearing Impairment in Aged People*. Available at www.audiology.org/resources/documentlibrary/pages/hearingimpairmenti-nagedpeople.aspx (accessed 9 March 2010).

Beck DL, Clark JL (2009) Audition matters more as cognition declines. *Audiology Today* Mar/April, 48–59.

Booth J, Tolson D, Hotchkiss R, Schofield I (2007) Using action research to construct national evidence-based nursing care guidance for gerontological nursing. *Journal of Clinical Nursing* **16**, 945–953.

Breu K, Hemingway C (2002) Collaborative processes and knowledge creation in Communities of Practice. *Creativity and Innovation Management* **11**, 147–153.

Carson AJ (2005) What brings you here today? The role of self-assessment in help-seeking for age related hearing loss. *Journal of Ageing Studies* **19**, 185–200.

Craik FIM (2007) The role of cognition in age-related hearing loss. *Journal of American Academy of Audiologists* **18**, 539–547.

Davis AC (1995) *Hearing in Adults*. Whurr, London.

Davis A, Smith P, Ferguson M, Stephens D, Gianopoulos I (2007) Acceptability, benefit and costs of early screening for hearing disability: a study of potential screening tests and models. *Health Technology Assessment* **11** (42).

D'Wynter LC (2006) Keeping the conversation going: information and strategies for reducing the impact of sensory, motor and cognitive changes that affect the quality of communication in elderly patients in long term care. *Topics in Geriatric Rehabilitation* **22**, 256–267.

Ferran DJ, Phillips JS (2007) Tinnitus. *Journal of Laryngology and Otolaryngology* **121**, 201–208.

Gates GA, Mills JH (2005) Presbycusis. *Lancet* **366**, 1111–1120.

Gatehouse S, Naylor G, Elberling C (2006) Linear and nonlinear hearing aid fittings. Patterns of benefit. *International Journal of Audiology* **45**, 153–152.

Gates GA, Beisner A, Rees TS, D'Agostino RB, Wolfe PA (2002) Central auditory dysfunction may precede the onset of clinical dementia in people with probable Alzhiemer's disease. *Journal of the American Geriatrics Society* **50**, 482–488.

Glavin R (2003) The making of the disabled identity: a linguistic analysis of marginalisation. *Disability Studies Quarterly* **23**, 149–178.

Goldstein D, Stephens D (1981) Audiological rehabilitation: management model. *International Audiology* **20**, 432–452.

Gordon-Salant S (2005) Hearing loss and aging: new research findings and clinical implications. *Journal of Rehabilitation Research and Development* **42**, 9–24.

Grue EV, Kirkevold M, Ranhoff AH (2009) Prevalence of vision, hearing and combined vision hearing impairments in patients with hip fractures. *Journal of Clinical Nursing* **18**, 3037–3049.

Heinz MG, Issa JB, Young ED (2005) Auditory-nerve rate responses are inconsistent with common hypotheses for the neural correlates for loudness recruitment. *Journal of the Association of Research in Otolaryngology* **6**, 91–105.

Humes LE (2005) Do auditory processing tests measure auditory processing in the elderly? *Ear and Hearing* **26**, 109–118.

Inouye S, Studenski S, Tinetti ME, Kuchel GA (2007) Geriatric syndromes: clinical, research, and policy implications of a core geriatric concept. *Journal of the American Geriatrics Society* **55**, 780–791.

Kelly, T.B, Tolson, D. Smith, T.D, McColgan, G. (In press). Using the research process to develop group services for older persons with a hearing disability. In D. M. Steinberg (Ed.), *Orchestrating the Power of Groups: Overture, Movements, and Finale*. Whiting & Birch, London.

Knussen C, Tolson D, Swan IRC, Stott DJ, Brogan CA, Sullivan F (2005) The social and psychological impact of an older relative's hearing difficulties: factors associated with change. *Psychology, Health and Medicine* **10**, 57–63.

Koelling TM, Johnson ML, Cody RJ, Aaronson KD (2005) Discharge education improves clinical outcome in patients with chronic heart failure. *Circulation* **111**, 179–185.

Lopez-Torres Hidalgo J, Gras CB, Lapeira JT, Verdejo AL, del Campo del Campo JM, Rabadan FE (2009) Functional status of elderly people with hearing loss. *Archives of Gerontology and Geriatrics* **49**, 88–92.

Lowndes A, Smith J, Tolson D, Buggy T (2007) Evolution of a virtual Practice Development College for nurses (Stage 2). *ITIN. the Official Journal of the British Computer Society Nursing Specialist Group. Part of the British Journal of Computing* **18**, 8–13.

Lunner T (2003) Cognitive function in relation to hearing aid use. *International Journal of Audiology* **42**, 49–58.

McKenna K, Green A (2002) Virtual group dynamics. *Group Dynamics: Theory, Research and Practice* **6**, 116–127.

NHS Quality Improvement Scotland (2005) *Best Practice Statement: Maximising Communication with Older People who Have Hearing Disability*. NHSQIS, Edinburgh.

NHS Quality Improvement Scotland (2006) *Best Practice Statement: Ear Care*. NHSQIS, Edinburgh.

Pirozzo S, Papinczak T, Glasziou P (2003) Whispered voice test for hearing impairment in adults and children: systematic review. *British Medical Journal* **327**, 967–971.

Public Health Institute of Scotland (2003) *Needs Assessment Report on NHS Audiology Services in Scotland*. PHIS, Glasgow.

SIGN (2009) *Annex B: Key to evidence statements and grades of recommendations in SIGN 50: A guideline developers handbook*. Available at www.sign.ac.uk/guidelines/fulltext/50/annexb. html (accessed 25 March 2010).

Smeeth L, Fletcher AE, Ng ES *et al.* (2002) Reduced hearing, ownership and use of hearing aids in elderly people in the UK. The MRC Trial of the Assessment and Management of Older People in the Community: a cross-sectional survey. *Lancet* **359**, 1466–1470.

Tolson D (1997) Age-related hearing loss: a case for nursing intervention. *Journal of Advanced Nursing* **26**, 1150–1157.

Tolson D, Stephens D (1997) Age related hearing loss in the dependent elderly population: a model for nursing care. *International Journal of Nursing Practice* **3**, 224–230.

Tolson D, Swan IRC (2006) Hearing. In: Redfern S, Ross F (eds) *Nursing Older People*, 3rd edn. Churchill Livingstone, Elsevier, London, chapter 11.

Tolson D, Schofield I, Booth J, Kelly TB, James L (2006) Constructing a new approach to developing evidence based practice with nurses and older people. *World Views on Evidence Based Nursing* **3**, 62–72.

Tsuruoka H, Masuda S, Ukai K (2001) Hearing impairment and quality of life for the elderly in nursing homes. *Auris Nasus Larynx* **28**, 45–54.

Wingfield A, Tun P (2001) Spoken language comprehension in older adults: interactions between sensory and cognitive change in normal ageing. *Seminars in Hearing* **22**, 287–301.

Wong LLN, Hickson L, McPherson B (2003) Hearing aid satisfaction: what does research from the past 20 years say? *Trends in Amplification* **7**, 117–161.

Chapter 10

Low Mood and Depression

Andrew Lowndes, William McDonald
and Yvonne Awenat

Introduction

Depression and low mood are not normal aspects of growing older, but they have been identified as significant issues for some older people (Wilson *et al.* 2008). Furthermore, depressive disorders are more common in older people with physical illness than in those without (MacHale 2002). Holistic care models recognise that both physical and psychosocial care are essential to improving quality of life and care outcomes for older people (Jongenelis *et al.* 2004). In this chapter we examine the signs and symptoms of low mood and depression, focusing on their presentation and potential impact in older age. We explore some of the main factors that contribute to low mood and depression, highlighting their link with the risk of suicide. We examine recovery and relationship-centred approaches that are typical within Western and English-speaking healthcare systems (Department of Health 2001a,b, 2006; Scottish Executive 2006). Finally, we present a case study which shows how the care home nursing team demonstrated best practice in working with residents to prevent and detect depression.

The prevalence of low mood and depression in older age

In this section we identify the prevalence of low mood and depression in older people in the UK and describe some of the challenges in delivering relationship-centred care. In order that older people can continue to play a meaningful part in family and community life, good holistic health is essential (Department of Health 2006; Scottish Executive 2006; World Health Organization 2009). Although depression is not an inevitable or normal consequence of ageing, Baldwin (2008) identified that 10–15% of older people experience depressive symptoms at any point in time. It has been suggested that 3% will meet the criteria for clinical depression (American Psychiatric Association 2000; World Health Organization 2007).

Evidence Informed Nursing with Older People, First Edition. Edited by Debbie Tolson, Joanne Booth and Irene Schofield.
© 2011 Blackwell Publishing Ltd. Published 2011 by Blackwell Publishing Ltd.

> **Box 10.1**   Reflective activity: depression and ageing
>
> - Some professionals wrongly consider depression to be a normal part of ageing.
> - Reflect on your own practice and that of colleagues with whom you work.
> - Does this misconception seem evident in your own and your colleagues' attitudes and practice?

Worldwide, the under-diagnosis and under-treatment of depression in older people has been reported (Alexopoulos *et al.* 2002; Vanitallie 2005; Koritsas *et al.* 2006). Moreover, it is suggested that the prevalence of depression in older people will increase significantly in the next decade (Godfrey 2005a; Royal College of Psychiatrists 2005; Age Concern 2007). According to Craig and Mindell (2007) despite one in four older people in the UK having depressive symptoms severe enough to warrant intervention, only one-third of this group are likely to discuss this with their doctor. In a study carried out in China, 72% ($N = 178$) of physicians endorsed that 'becoming depressed was a natural part of being old' (Chen 2009).

Whilst the issue of poor mental health in older people, and depression in particular, has been described as an under-addressed area of public importance, it should be acknowledged that the majority of older people do not experience mental illness necessitating psychiatric care (Craig & Mindell 2007). The reflective activity in Box 10.1 will enable you to consider your own practice.

Dening and Milne (2009) have identified that depression in the UK doubles the risk of older people being admitted to a care home. Some nursing home residents, in addition to multiple physical health problems and associated loss of independence, experience high levels of depression; there is evidence that 30–40% of residents develop depression (Audit Commission 2000). Those people who do not suffer from depression on admission to long-term care often develop severe depression due to associated functional loss, chronic physical health problems, pain and social losses that lead to loneliness (Care Services Improvement Partnership 2006).

Causes of low mood and depression in older people

In this section we highlight biological, psychological and social causes of depression in older people, as well as other factors which influence an often complex picture of low mood and depression. Bostock & Millar (2003) identified the complex and interrelated nature of factors that are perceived by older people as being influential on mental well-being. They recognised retirement, the role of family and friends, keeping active and the loss of functional capacity as key aspects that impact on perceived mental well-being. These in turn were influenced by the attitudes of older people themselves, the attitudes of others, people's ability to adapt to life changes and experiences (for example bereavement), the importance of independence and choice, and access to appropriate resources. Specific to low mood and depression, there are several perspectives that offer possible explanations for their causes. Broadly these relate to biological, psychological and social factors (Box 10.2).

Box 10. 2 Causes of depression and low mood

Biological
- Disruption of chemicals in the brain, mainly thought to be serotonin and noradrenaline.
- Genetic predisposition.
- The influence of stress.
- May be worsened by alcohol, prescribed and recreational drugs.

Psychological
- Distorted perceptions in adulthood as a result of childhood experiences, in particular around loss and acceptance. This leads to feelings of low self-esteem, guilt and low mood.
- A lack of positive reinforcement leads to depressive behaviour.
- Individual thought processes. Rather than actual life events themselves, it is the individual's negative interpretation of these that lead to depression.

Social
- Thinking and behaviour are governed by social contexts and influences.
- Higher risk of bereavement in friends and families in older age.
- Social isolation.
- Adaptation to changing roles (e.g. following retirement or becoming dependant).
- Restrictions of physical health and illness.

However, the likelihood of an individual developing depressive symptoms in older age appears to be influenced by an often complex range of mental health protective and risk factors, as shown in Table 10.1.

Predisposing factors, for example biological aspects such as gender (the prevalence of depression is higher in women than men in all age groups), and past psychiatric history may all increase risk. There is a generally recognised link between physical illness and low mood, with common mental health problems occurring more frequently in patients with physical illness such as diabetes or cardiac problems, bowel problems, incontinence and chronic pain (Hitchcock Noël *et al.* 2004; Trivedi 2004; Alexopoulos 2005). Common health problems in older people, for example falls, incontinence, frailty, delirium and self-neglect, known as geriatric syndromes, are highly prevalent (Pavlou & Lachs 2006; Inouye *et al.* 2007). The effect of geriatric syndromes on quality of life, including mood, can be substantial, as they are mutually interactive and their multifaceted nature makes assessment and options about care planning complex and challenging.

As societies change, the opinions and beliefs of older members of those societies have also altered. Significantly, older people themselves may have to amend their expectations of later life and adapt to changes in their role. Transitions that result in a loss of status, independence and value in turn can lead to the lowering of mood. Beekman *et al.* (1997) found that older people's subjective views of health and perceived ability to function related more strongly to depression than the specific conditions or illnesses themselves. It is perhaps unsurprising that low mood is more

Table 10.1   Low mood and depression: protective and risk factors.

Resilience	Factors	Risk
Prepared, well adjusted to changing role	Retirement	Ill prepared, difficulty adapting to new role
Regular interaction, supportive, inclusive	Role of family and friends	Isolated, infrequent contact, lonely
Good physical health, opportunities to be active	Keeping active	Physically unwell, disability through ill health, no opportunities
Positive, optimistic, seeking opportunity	Attitude of individual	Negative, pessimistic, hopeless
Supportive, respectful, non-judgemental, see the individual	Attitude of others	Discriminatory, stigmatising, disrespectful
Appropriate response to new circumstances and experiences	Adaptable to life changes	Unable to adapt to changing circumstances and experiences
Meaningful participation in decision-making	Autonomy in choices	Unable or prevented from contributing to decision-making
Resources are available/ accessible in relation to proximity, cost, transport, etc.	Access to resources	Insufficient/inappropriate resources, inaccessible, prohibited by cost, location, etc.

Source: adapted from Bostock & Millar (2003).

likely in individuals who have developed low expectations of themselves and the societies in which they live.

The resilience and risk factors that influence depression in older people vary in significance for each individual and are the result of often complex personal and unique circumstances (Bowie 2001; Alexopoulos 2005; Godfrey 2005b). Much of this may be beyond individual control, for example for many people ageing is accompanied by diminishing physical ability that may be coupled with physical illness. Depending on the severity of their condition some individuals may have to move from their home to be supported in a care home. Changing roles in later life, for example through retirement, may lead an individual to experience feelings of reduced worth and importance in the way that they are able to contribute to their family or society. Reduced social networks, through population movement and bereavement, may also precipitate a loss of intimacy, and can result in isolation and feelings of loneliness. Many older people have a low income and poverty has also been recognised as a contributing factor in low mood and depression.

How does depression and low mood affect older people?

In this section we examine the presentation of depression and low mood in older people and suggest how low mood and depression differ from sadness as a typical response to unusual circumstances. The prevalence of depression in older people who are physically well is similar to that of the general adult population (Baldwin

> **Box 10.3**   Presentation of low mood and depression in older age
>
> Older people with depression may describe having the following:
>
> - Depressed or lowering of mood: most days and/or for most of the day.
> - Loss of interest, unable to feel enjoyment or pleasure (anhedonia).
> - Tired and lacking energy: results in decreased activity, fatigue following little effort.
> - Disturbed sleep pattern: difficulty getting to sleep or early morning wakening.
> - Poor concentration and ability to make decisions.
> - Disturbed appetite: possible weight loss or weight gain.
> - Poor self-esteem and self-confidence.
> - Persistent ideas of guilt, hopelessness and/or worthlessness.
> - Restlessness and agitation.
> - Recurrent thoughts of death: possible thoughts of suicide.
>
> Depending on the number and severity of the symptoms, a depressive episode may be specified as mild, moderate or severe.
>
> *Source*: adapted from World Health Organization (2007).

2008). Anyone can experience sadness as a part of their existence or in response to their life circumstances, so what is different in an older person experiencing such sadness and an individual who is low in mood or depressed? The difference lies in the severity, duration and impact of symptoms. In Box 10.3 we outline common symptoms and presentations of depression in older people. More detailed classifications can be accessed American Psychiatric Association (2000) and World Health Organization (2007).

Older people who are low in mood or depressed commonly describe feeling down and they may complain of feeling excessively tired and lacking in energy. They can also experience a loss of enjoyment, poor sleep patterns with early morning wakening, and loss of appetite with associated weight loss. Even with mild depression, individuals may express feelings of guilt, hopelessness or worthlessness, with poor self-esteem and a lack of confidence (Manthorpe & Iliffe 2007). Feelings of hopelessness can result in suicidal thoughts and behaviour and this important issue is discussed later in the chapter. Symptoms must be present for at least 2 weeks, and then depression is categorised as mild, through moderate to severe (World Health Organization 2007). Severity is measured by the number of symptoms and the degree of impact they have on the individual's ability to function in their daily life. So the more symptoms displayed and the greater the negative effect on the individual's capacity to cope, the more severe the depression.

The way that older people express their experience of depression is often different to that of younger adults. For example, they may place greater emphasis on somatic (physical bodily) symptoms (Hope 2003; Baldwin 2008; Snowden 2009) (see Box 10.3). Robert *et al.*

Box 10.4   Reflective point: symptoms of depression in older age

- Older people may present with the symptoms of depression and low mood as described in Box 10.3.
- These signs and symptoms of depression are the same in older age as in the general adult population.
- Baldwin (2008) also suggests that older people often present with somatic symptoms.
- Consider the symptoms in Box 10.3. Can you identify patients who have reported symptoms such as sleep or appetite disturbance?
- What additional signs or symptoms did they exhibit?

Box 10.5   Reflective point: suicide in older age

- Suicide is a risk for older people who are clinically depressed.
- What would make you suspect that someone may be contemplating suicide?
- What actions would you take in this event?
- You may wish to refer to the suicide intervention resources at www.livingworks.net.

(1997) suggest that it is the associated physical health issues and frailty that influence the mood of older people. Significant low mood and depression leads to significant morbidity, and lower quality of life (Goldney *et al.* 2000), functional impairment (Penninx *et al.* 1998) and increased healthcare utilisation (Huang *et al.* 2000). Major depressive disorder is associated with elevated mortality rates that increase with the severity of depression (St John & Montgomery 2009). The reflective point in Box 10.4 enables you to consider your own practice.

Care transitions, such as admission to hospital or transfer to a nursing home, can lead to anxiety and depression for some people who regard the transition as a loss of health, independence, role or status (Pot *et al.* 2005; Newson, 2008). O'Connell *et al.* (2004) identify that older people have a higher risk of completed suicide than any other age group worldwide. Baldwin (2001) identifies that whilst people in the UK aged over 65 make up 15% of the population, they disproportionally account for 20–25% of all completed suicides. Early recognition of low mood and depression in older people may therefore be life-saving. Depression is one of the main factors associated with suicide. Nurses who are knowledgeable about the symptoms of mild to severe depression and also of the predisposing factors for depression can provide timely and effective support for people experiencing suicidal thoughts and engaging in life-threatening behaviour. The activity in Box 10.5 enables you to consider your own practice with regard to suicide prevention.

Treatment for depression

There is an evidence base to support the use of a range of approaches that reduce risk factors and increase protective factors associated with depression in older people (National Institute of Mental Health 2007; National Institute for Clinical Excellence 2009a; Scottish Government 2009a). The evidence shows that older people benefit from specialist care that includes person-centred psychological and behavioural methods, the promotion of physical health and the prevention of discrimination and abuse. Despite this, antidepressant medication remains the main method of treatment for older people with depression (Department of Health 2006).

Nurses require an up to date understanding of the best evidence available relating to treatment approaches for older people who are low in mood or depressed. The prescribing of antidepressant medication remains the main treatment approach for those individuals identified with moderate to severe depression. Newer antidepressants such as the selective serotonin reuptake inhibitors (SSRIs) citalopram, fluoxetine and sertraline are advised as first choice by the National Institute for Clinical Excellence (2009a) as these tend to cause fewer side effects and are safer in the event of deliberate or accidental overdose. The older types of antidepressants, for example tricyclic antidpressants like amitriptyline, clomipramine and lofepramine, whilst still effective are less commonly prescribed due to their sedative effect. These tend to be reserved for people who have previously demonstrated benefit and tolerance to them. Monoamine oxidase inhibitors, for example moclobemide and phenelzine, require the avoidance of certain foods due to the risk of dangerous hypertension and are now rarely prescribed (Royal College of Psychiatrists 2009a).

When prescribing antidepressants for older people, the individual's age, physical health and other medications are taken into consideration. Generally it is advised to start with a lower dose and increase slowly, so 'start low, go slow' is a well-acknowledged prescribing rule. It is important that nurses discuss antidepressant medication with patients and remind them that they will usually be required to take these medications for longer periods, as benefits might not be expected until after 1–2 weeks, perhaps taking up to 6 weeks before the full effect is experienced (Royal College of Psychiatrists 2009a). Nurses are ideally placed to help individuals understand the ways that antidepressants differ from some other common medicines. Emphasis should be placed on the importance of continuing to take antidepressant medication even if the person feels better and, furthermore, that they always seek medical advice before stopping them. It is also important that nurses discuss the potential side effects of medication and that they carefully monitor people for unwanted side effects. For example, SSRIs can cause nausea and anxiety, and tricyclic antidepressants can cause dry mouth, tachycardia, confusion, hypotension and falls.

In more severe and enduring instances of depression, electroconvulsive therapy (ECT) continues to be used as a treatment option, although it is still regarded as controversial (Aveyard 2007). The treatment is given by passing an electric current through the front of the brain to induce a seizure intended to last between 20 and 50 seconds (Royal College of Psychiatrists 2009b). It is usually delivered in a specific ECT suite, following the administration of a

---

Box 10.6   Reflective point: use of ECT in older age

- ECT remains an emotive form of treatment and many nurses express negative attitudes towards it (Lutchman *et al.* 2001).
- For many people their understanding of ECT is based more on its representation in films and popular culture than more robust material.
- Consider your views and attitudes towards ECT. Are they based on contemporary clinical evidence? Would it be helpful to access more information?
- A useful starting point may be the Royal College of Psychiatrists (2009b) and the National Institute for Clinical Excellence (2009b).

---

general anaesthetic and a muscle relaxant. A course of six to eight treatments are usually prescribed, with ongoing assessment and review between sessions, with the possibility of up to 12 treatments being required. During the period following ECT some patients complain of headache, muscle aches and generally feeling 'muzzy'. Symptoms are usually treated successfully with support from nurses and analgesia. Most people do not appear to experience longer-term side effects, although some difficulties with memory and even personality changes have been reported. Whilst there is an important part for nurses to play in both the safe administration and monitoring of antidepressant medication, and in supporting people undergoing ECT, more detailed discussion of these goes beyond the scope of this chapter. However, it is useful to take time out to consider your understanding and views of this form of treatment for older people (Box 10.6).

Moving towards recovery-based approaches

In this section we explore recovery-based approaches to mental healthcare. Hitchcock Noël *et al.* (2004) suggest that recognition and treatment of low mood and depression have the potential to improve functioning and quality of life despite the presence of other medical comorbidities. However, only half of older people who are depressed are diagnosed as such, and antidepressant medication remains the main method of treatment for this group. According to Choi *et al.* (2009) health professionals reported feeling frustrated at the lack of referrals to specialist services and opportunities to engage in psychosocial treatments. They highlighted the use of antidepressant medication as first choice therapy. Choi *et al.* (2009) suggest that such medically driven approaches contribute to difficulties in maintaining the enthusiasm and motivation necessary for the provision of high-quality relationship-centred care.

Recovery-based models for mental healthcare have led to a shift from the dominant biomedical model. Recovery-based approaches were introduced following the writings of people who regarded themselves as 'survivors' within mental healthcare systems in the 1980s. These 'survivors' had themselves recovered from mental health challenges and wrote about their experiences of coping with symptoms, getting better, and regaining their sense of self (Anthony 1993). The concept of recovery, which has for some decades

> **Box 10.7**   Summary of definitions of mental health recovery (National Institute of Mental Health 2005)
>
> - A return to a state of wellness (e.g. following an episode of depression).
> - Achievement of a quality of life acceptable to the person (e.g. following an episode of psychosis).
> - A process or period of recovering (e.g. following trauma).
> - A process of gaining or restoring something (e.g. one's sobriety).
> - An act of obtaining usable resources from apparently unusable sources (e.g. in prolonged psychosis).
> - Recovering an optimum quality and satisfaction with life in disconnected circumstances (e.g. following a diagnosis of dementia).

been a central focus in the field of addictions, is now viewed in the Western world as the preferred approach model for mental health interventions (Department of Health 2006; Scottish Executive 2006; Ramon *et al.* 2007).

As a concept, recovery is seen as common and accepted in physical illness, trauma and care. Here recovery does not mean that symptoms are absent, suffering has disappeared and pre-morbid functioning has been restored, but that a person with a traumatic limb amputation following a road traffic accident can recover even though the limb has not regrown. Likewise despite criticism from writers such as Whitwell (1999), who denounced the idea of recovery as a return to prior functioning, there is evidence to support recovery approaches in mental healthcare. It has been identified that even patients with severe mental health problems may find a variety of ways to deal with difficult aspects of their illness and that rehabilitation and recovery is possible even though their illness is not cured (Hume & Pullen 1994). Recovery has developed a number of different meanings within mental healthcare and there is no one definition of the term acceptable to all stakeholders. The National Institute for Mental Health in England provides a number of definitions of recovery. These are summarised in Box 10.7.

Key to recovery approaches in mental health is that hope and restoration of a meaningful life are possible, despite serious illness (Deegan 1996; Buchanan-Barker 2009). Recovery is seen as an active experience for the client and is a deeply personal and individual experience. Through the supportive coaching of a committed mental health practitioner, recovery can lead to personal growth for the client who can discover new ways of coping, a sense of personal control and feelings of empowerment.

This change in thinking has resulted in a shift in approach from doing things to patients to working with them and doing things for them (Buchanan-Barker 2009), including patients in decision-making and fostering self-management in people to their best ability. In a relationship-centred approach people are viewed as unique individuals rather than clients or patients with generic needs and the focus is on understanding the person in the context of their relationships with others. It explores people's experience of ill health by listening to the meanings and values that individuals attach to it. This approach reflects government policy and professional guidance that extol the need for meaningful involvement of older people in decisions about the support that they receive whilst enabling responsibility for change to remain with the individual (Scottish Government 2007; NHS Education for Scotland 2008; Nursing and Midwifery Council 2009).

The value base

In this section we examine a developing value base for nursing older people and compare it with values accorded to contemporary mental healthcare (Table 10.2). The value base for gerontological nursing (Kelly *et al.* 2005) was described in Chapter 1. It was formulated by nurses from a range of practice settings working collaboratively, and involving older people, as part of the Scottish Gerontological Nursing Practice Project. This expression of core values resonates with similar value bases (Scottish Government 2009b; Department of Health 2010). These values are inherent in contemporary best practice guidelines and frameworks (Table 10.2). The move toward relationship-centred and recovery approaches has required nurses to re-evaluate many aspects of their care, but most particularly the values and beliefs which underpin care (Box 10.8).

Table 10.2   The underpinning values of gerontological and mental health nursing.

Gerontological nursing values (Kelly *et al.* 2005)	Mental health nursing values (Scottish Government 2009b)
Commitment to relationship-centred care	Relationship-centred care
Establishing equity of access	Promoting equality
Consistency of vision	Practising ethically
Promoting dignity and respect	Promoting dignity and respect
Maximising potential	Maximising independence
Commitment to an enabling environment	Promoting recovery
Commitment to negotiating care decisions	Working with service users
The value of reciprocity	Safeguarding rights
Commitment to developing innovative practice	Commitment to professional currency

Box 10.8   Reflective point: values in mental healthcare of older people

- The values which underpin mental health care and the care of older people are shown in Table 10.2.
- Consider the ways that you demonstrate each of these values in your practice with older people.

Promoting best practice in care homes

In 2003 the gerontological nursing research team at Glasgow Caledonian University, in collaboration with the Scottish Gerontological Link Nurse Network, NHS Quality Improvement Scotland and staff from a care home in Glasgow, collaborated to develop care guidance in the form of a best practice statement (NHS Quality Improvement Scotland 2004). The process for the development of evidence based care guidance has already been detailed in Chapter 2. One such best practice statement was *Working with Older People Towards Prevention and Early Detection of Depression*. We will now give an overview of the best practice statement with updated supporting references, which recognise the recovery-based approach to mental healthcare. The focus of the guidance was on the care of older people in transition, as in moving from hospital to continuing care or discharge from hospital to their own home. The guidance recognises that all nurses who work with older people have a role to play in promoting their mental healthcare. Furthermore, it acknowledges that it is important for nurses to be familiar with the roles of other mental health professionals, counsellors and referral systems.

The best practice statement is divided into four sections as follows.

Section 1: promoting nurses' awareness of depression in the older person

This section challenges nurses not to see low mood and depression as an inevitable consequence of ageing, but to recognise that prevention of depression is possible; furthermore, that early detection can lead to positive outcomes for the older person and their family. It recognises that despite the prevalence of symptoms of clinical depression amongst older people, symptoms frequently go undetected, misdiagnosed or untreated (Bagley *et al.* 2000; Age Concern 2007; Watson *et al.* 2009). It draws nurses' attention to the vulnerability of older people experiencing life and health challenges, such as separation from family, friends and pets, bereavement, chronic health problems, and care transition such as moving into a care home.

Section 2: promoting positive mental health and well-being

This section explores the type of support and care that older people need to help them make life, health or care transitions. The section emphasises the need to understand the older person as a unique individual with their own life history, hopes, fears and coping mechanisms. Recognising the individuality of the older person, their family carers and friends is the starting point for developing relationship-centred care. It highlights the importance of the older person playing an active and full part in decision-making about their care and future. Within recovery-based approaches the promotion of independence and individual choice is fostered by the nurses who seek to instil hope in their care. A supportive relationship is of central importance in order to empower the older person and encourage them to retain responsibility to change (Roberts & Wolfson 2004).

Section 3: assessment and care planning

It is important that nurses are able to identify not only the signs and symptoms of low mood and depression in older people through use of assessment and screening tools, but also potential risk factors, stressors and possible sources of support. Whilst it is recommended that older people have greater access to specialist care (Department of Health 2006), it is recognised that many people who experience feelings of low mood or depression will not come into contact with specialist mental health nurses (Age Concern 2007). It is therefore important that all nurses who care for older people come to view basic psychological assessment as an accepted part of their role. We recognise that nurses may lack experience and training in sensitive mental health issues such as self-neglect, self-harm or suicide; these issues are particularly challenging for most nurses to address. It is important therefore that when carrying out risk assessment all members of the multidisciplinary team are involved. The resources in Box 10.9 will help you to develop your skills in this area.

Carpenter (2002) found that older people with social support reported less depression, a more positive mood and a greater sense of happiness than those who lacked social support. Furthermore, half of older people experiencing depression have expressed a preference for psychological approaches over drugs, and effective communication is seen as key to a relationship-centred approach (Unützer *et al.* 2002). Possible psychosocial interventions that can be discussed with the older person are shown in Box 10.10.

Section 4: education and training

The final section of the best practice statement addresses aspects of education and training. It recognises that nurses working with older people experience difficulty in detecting depression and that symptoms of depression are often overlooked. Even brief training on depression can have an impact with demonstrable improvement (Eisses *et al.* 2005). Lyne *et al.* (2006) have studied the impact of brief training for care home nurses and identified that training care staff in systematic observation improves detection and treatment and slows the course of depressive symptoms. Furthermore, unnecessary treatment of non-clinically depressed residents can be avoided through improved detection and early intervention. The authors concluded that involving care staff in detecting mental health problems is feasible, and can lead to best practice.

Overview of study

This case study illustrates how demonstration of best practice in the prevention and early detection of depression contributed to the development of the best practice statement. The care home featured in the case study was an independent sector care home (nursing) with 61 residents and 50 staff. The skill mix ratio was one registered nurse to 11 unregistered staff. Staff turnover was slow and stable. Preliminary staff training covered general issues such as resident well-being at times of transition and values clarification on mental well-being. Specifically, training covered the definition of depression, main types of depression, causes of depression, treatment of depression and use of the Geriatric Depression Scale by registered nurses.

Training sessions on depression were held over a period of 2 days and all members of staff, including managers, attended except in cases of illness or absence. The aim of the sessions was to raise awareness of the staff in relation to low mood and depression. They were encouraged to explore their current practice in the home and to identify both positive and negative aspects of care. Many of the staff reported that they had been aware that residents were depressed but had not known what to do about it. Staff reported that the training gave them a better understanding of issues around depression and how to address them by carrying out preliminary screening, and where necessary referring to appropriate professionals. Staff were enabled to explore their own feelings and to recognise that they had an important role to play. It became clear that some staff members were unaware that their attitudes could affect others, including staff, residents and visitors:

> *It was a total shock to me to think that my behaviour while I was at work could affect my residents' moods. We were told that every contact we had with a resident should be a positive experience for that person. I really made up my mind to do the very best for my residents, and not take any of my personal life into work with me. I understood now that if I walked about with a gloomy face, this would affect my resident.* (Care assistant A)

The training reinforced that life transitions such as moving into a care home could be experienced as loss by residents. Of course at some level all staff realised how stressful this transition could be, but the training put it into perspective for many staff. For example:

> *Some come from home and some come from hospital. It must be awful to give up your home you might have stayed in for years, and you can't bring everything with you. That's just not possible.* (Care Assistant C)

Having addressed some of the underlying attitudes and issues, members of staff were able to see more clearly that they played an important role in relation to the implementation of the best practice statement and the overall well-being of their residents and colleagues.

The education programme included signs and symptoms of depression, and these were related to the documentation that registered nurses would complete when screening for depression. The Geriatric Depression Scale (Yesavage *et al.* 1983) was completed by registered nurses and incorporated into the documentation. The care assistants were able to see the link between paperwork and resident care as registered nurses took time to explain the findings to the care assistants thereby involving them in care delivery.

> *I like the questions on the form when it is completed. It lets you know if the resident is depressed.* (Care assistant B)

The impact of the training was felt immediately by staff:

> *When I went back to work after the training I felt as if I was on a mission to find out how many residents were depressed or sad and how I could help them.* (Care assistant A)

The care assistant began to look out for people who had depressive symptoms and to consider how she might help them. An example of her efforts is described in Box 10.11.

Box 10.9   Resources for mental health care
and assessment

- www.livingworks.net
- Depression in Older People (Expert Consensus Guideline Series): a guide for older people and their families (2001). www.psychguides.com/Geriatric%20Depression%20LP%20Guide.pdf
- Depression in Older Adults, Royal College of Psychiatrists (2009c). Information leaflet.
- Recognising and treating depression. A guide to helping nursing home residents with depression. American Geriatrics Society. www.healthinaging.org/public_education/rec_depression_booklet.php
- Analysis of a care planning intervention for reducing depression in older people in residential care. Lyne *et al.* (2006). www.well-beingandchoice.org.uk/ReducingDepression.htm

---

Box 10.10   Psychosocial interventions for depression

(1) Skills training interventions, e.g. health education interventions such as developing coping skills, relaxation training, anxiety management and assertiveness training (Manzoni *et al.* 2008).
(2) Physical exercise interventions, e.g. physical exercise programmes in groups (Strawbridge *et al.* 2002).
(3) Group support interventions, e.g. discussion groups (Cooper & Doherty 2000).
(4) Reminiscence interventions, i.e. life review or life storytelling (Bohlmeijer *et al.* 2003; Hsieh & Wang 2003).
(5) Social activities, e.g. visiting cultural sites, gardening, needlework (Greaves & Farbus 2006).

Box 10.11   Helping Mrs McPhee to prevent depression

Mrs McPhee had lived in the care home for 7 years. She moved into the home after a stroke which resulted in paralysis on her left side. She is mobile in an electric wheelchair. Mrs McPhee had been a very active person prior to her stroke. She has a supportive family and one son lives nearby and visits regularly and another son lives overseas, but is in frequent contact. Despite the family support she frequently said she was 'a bit down'.

Mrs McPhee's care assistant noticed a change in her mood after she returned from a holiday at another care home where she had the opportunity to go swimming.

She couldn't stop talking about the holiday and how much she enjoyed the swimming.
(Care assistant A)

Having attended the training in connection with implementing the best practice statement, the care assistant knew that physical activity and recreational activities increase a person's sense of well-being, and she could now relate this to Mrs McPhee. The care assistant took the initiative to arrange a swimming session for Mrs McPhee in the local community pool.

Finally, the big day arrived and Mrs McPhee went swimming. The care assistant describes the experience:

Mrs McPhee told us about her swimming when she came back. She was lowered into the water using a special chair. She said it was 'magic'. She felt a sense of freedom, even though her bad leg couldn't do much. Her son and grandchildren visited her that afternoon. She said to them, 'You'll never guess where I've been today. I went swimming.' Her grandchildren were giving their mum a hard time because they said they should have been there to swim with their gran. This experience had a very positive effect on how Mrs McPhee was feeling at the time. Her face still lights up when she talks about it.

The positive benefits of this were felt by the care staff as well as Mrs McPhee:

This is just one example of how the project has affected myself and the residents. All the staff really took on board what was discussed at the training. Residents have said that things are much better now and that staff seem to have more time to spend with them, and they are much happier at their work. (Care assistant)

Summary

The World Health Organization (2009) recommends that in relation to depression, there is no global single best practice model for the care of people with depression. Rather, it suggests that it is the local application of broad principles which is most likely to lead to success.

In this chapter we have provided an overview of low mood and depression in relation to older people. We have highlighted that low mood and depression are not a normal part of ageing. For older people who do experience low mood or develop depression, the causes are often complex and may be influenced by physical ill health, and social factors such as isolation, life changes or role transitions. Older people may focus on somatic or physical symptoms associated with depression so that identifying low mood can be more challenging. All older people have factors that increase risk or protect them against low mood and depression, and these are specific to each individual. It is important that nurses work closely with older people to identify their needs and strengths through collaborative relationships. The principles of partnership, respect for diversity and the instillation of hope are cornerstones of contemporary mental healthcare and underpin evidence informed care. The shift towards recovery-based and relationship-centred care acknowledges the importance of the individual's lived experience in making sense of their current difficulties and in directing the most appropriate interventions.

Key messages

- Low mood and depression are not inevitable consequences of ageing.
- Evidence supports the use of recovery-based approaches in the care and treatment of older people who develop low mood or depression.
- All nurses who work with older people have a role to play in the early detection of depression.

References

Age Concern (2007) Improving services and support for older people with mental health problems. Available at www.mhilli.org/documents/Inquiryfinalreport-FULLREPORT.pdf (accessed 21 September 2009).

Alexopoulos GS (2005) Depression in the elderly. *Lancet* **365**, 1961–1970.

Alexopoulos GS, Borson S, Cuthbert BN *et al.* (2002) Assessment of late life depression. *Biological Psychiatry* **52**, 164–174.

American Psychiatric Association (2000) *Diagnostic and Statistical Manual of Mental Disorders: DSM-IV Text Revision*, 4th edn American Psychiatric Press, Washington, DC.

Anthony WA (1993) Recovery from mental illness: the guiding vision of the mental health service system in the 1990's. *Psychosocial Rehabilitation Journal* **16**, 11–23.

Audit Commission (2000) *Forget Me Not: Developing Mental Health Services for Older People in England*. Audit Commission, London.

Aveyard B (2007) Enduring mental health issues. In: Neno R, Aveyard B, Heath H (eds) *Older People and Mental Health Nursing*. Blackwell Publishing, Oxford, pp. 182–194.

Bagley H, Cordingley L, Burns A (2000) Recognition of depression by staff in nursing and residential homes. *Journal of Clinical Nursing* **9**, 445–450.

Baldwin RC (2001) Suicide in older people: can it be prevented? *Reviews in Clinical Gerontology* **11**, 107–108.

Baldwin R (2008) Mood disorders: depressive disorders. In: Jacoby R, Oppenheimer C, Dening T, Thomas A (eds) *Oxford Textbook of Old Age Psychiatry*. Oxford University Press, Oxford, pp. 529–556.

Banazak DA, Mullan PB, Gardner JC, Rajagopalan S (1999) Practice guidelines and late-life depression assessment in long-term care. *Journal of General Internal Medicine* **14**, 438–440.

Bohlmeijer E, Smit F, Cuijpers P (2003) Effects of reminiscence and life review on late-life depression: a meta-analysis. *International Journal of Geriatric Psychiatry* **18**, 1088–1094.

Bostock Y, Millar C (2003) *Older People's Perceptions of the Factors that Affect Mental Well-Being in Later Life*. NHS Health Scotland, Edinburgh.

Bowie P (2001) The prognosis of depression in later life. In: Curran S, Wattis JP, Lynch S (eds) *Practical Management of Depression in Older People*. Arnold, London, pp. 27–43.

Buchanan-Barker P (2009) Reclamation: beyond recovery. In: Barker P (ed.) *Psychiatric and Mental Health Nursing. The Craft of Caring*, 2nd edn. Hodder Arnold, London.

Care Services Improvement Partnership (2006) *Long-term Conditions and Depression: Considerations for Best Practice in Practice Based Commissioning*. Care Services Improvement Partnership, University of Lancashire.

Carpenter B (2002) Family peer, and staff social support in nursing home patients. Contributions to psychological well-being. *Journal of Applied Gerontology* **21**, 275–293.

Chen S (2009) The prevalence of late-life depression and physicians' attitude toward it in primary care settings of China. *European Psychiatry* **24** (Suppl. 1), S626.

Choi NG, Wyllie RJ, Ransom S (2009) Risk factors and intervention programs for depression in nursing home residents: nursing home staff interview findings. *Journal of Gerontological Social Work* **52**, 668–685.

Cooper C, Doherty J (2000) Group work for older people with mental health problems. *Nursing Times* **96**(43), 42.

Craig R, Mindell J (2007) Health of older people. In: Craig R, Mindell J (eds) *Health Survey for England 2005*. The Information Centre, Leeds.

Deegan PE (1996) Recovery as a journey of the heart. *Psychiatric Rehabilitation Journal* **19**, 91–97.

Dening T, Milne A (2009) Depression and mental health in care homes. Special Issue: Depression, Suicide and Self-Harm in Older Adults. *Quality in Ageing* **10**, 40–46.

Department of Health (2001a) *National Service Framework for Older People*. Department of Health, London.

Department of Health (2001b) *The Journey to Recovery: the Government's Vision for Mental Health Care*. Department of Health, London.

Department of Health (2006) *From Values to Action: The Chief Nursing Officer's Review of Mental Health Nursing*. Department of Health, London.

Department of Health (2010) *New Horizons: Working Together for Better Mental Health*. Department of Health, London.

Eisses AMH, Kluiter H, Jongenelis K, Pot AM, Beekman ATF, Ormel J (2005) Care staff training in detection of depression in residential homes for the elderly. *British Journal of Psychiatry* **186**, 404–409.

Godfrey M (2005a) *Literature and policy review on prevention and services*. Completed for the UK Inquiry into Mental Health and Well-Being in Later Life. Age Concern and the Mental Health Foundation, London.

Godfrey M (2005b) Risk and resources for depression in later life. *Journal of Public Mental Health* **4**, 32–42.

Goldney RD, Fisher LJ, Wilson DH, Cheok F (2000) Major depression and its associated morbidity and quality of life in a random, representative Australian community sample. *Australian and New Zealand Journal of Psychiatry* **34**, 1022–1029.

Greaves CJ, Farbus L (2006) Effects of creative and social activity on the health and well-being of socially isolated older people: outcomes from a multi-method observational study. *Journal of the Royal Society for the Promotion of Health* **126**, 134–142.

Hitchcock Noël P, Williams JW, Unützer J *et al.* (2004) Depression and comorbid illness in elderly primary care patients: impact on multiple domains of health status and well-being. *Annals of Family Medicine* **2**, 555–562.

Hope K (2003) A hidden problem: identifying depression in older people. *British Journal of Community Nursing* **8**, 316–320.

Hsieh H-F, Wang J-J (2003) Effect of reminiscence therapy on depression in older adults: a systematic review. *International Journal of Nursing Studies* **40**, 335–345.

Huang BY, Cornoni-Huntley J, Hays JC, Huntley RR, Galanos AN, Blazer DG (2000) Impact of depressive symptoms on hospitalization risk in community-dwelling older persons. *Journal of the American Geriatrics Society* **48**, 1279–1284.

Hume C, Pullen I (1994) *Rehabilitation for Mental Health Problems*. Churchill Livingstone, Melbourne.

Inouye SK, Studenski S, Tinetti ME, Kuchel GA (2007) Geriatric syndromes: clinical research and policy implications of a geriatric concept. *Journal of the American Geriatrics Society* **55**, 780–791.

Jongenelis K, Pot AM, Eisses AMH, Beekman ATF, Kluiter H, Ribbe MW (2004) Prevalence and risk indicators of depression in elderly nursing home patients: the AGED study. *Journal of Affective Disorders* **83**, 135–142.

Kelly TB, Tolson D, Schofield I, Booth J (2005) Describing gerontological nursing: an academic exercise or prerequisite for progress? *International Journal of Older People Nursing* **14**, 1–11.

Koritsas S, Davidson S, Clarke D, O'Connor D (2006) Diagnosing and treating depressions in nursing home residents: challenges for GPs. *Australian Journal of Primary Health* **12**, 104–108.

Lutchman D, Stevens T, Bashir A, Orrell M (2001) Mental health professionals' attitudes towards and knowledge of electroconvulsive therapy. *Journal of Mental Health* **10**, 141–150.

Lyne KJ, Moxon S, Sinclair I, Young P, Kirk C, Ellison S (2006) Reducing depression among older people receiving care: an evidence-based approach. *Aging and Mental Health* **10**, 394–403.

MacHale S (2002) Managing depression in physical illness. *Advances in Psychiatric Treatment* **8**, 297–305.

Manthorpe J, Iliffe S (2007) Depression in later life. In: Neno R, Aveyard B, Heath H (eds) *Older People and Mental Health Nursing*. Blackwell Publishing, Oxford.

Manzoni GM, Pagnini F, Castelnuovo G, Molinari E (2008) Relaxation training for anxiety: a ten-years systematic review with meta-analysis. *BMC Psychiatry* **8**, 41.

National Institute for Health and Clinical Excellence (2009a) *Depression. The treatment and management of depression in adults*. Available at http://www.nice.org.uk/CG90 (accessed 20 September 2009).

National Institute for Health and Clinical Excellence (2009b) *Electroconvulsive therapy (ECT)*. Available at http://guidance.nice.org.uk/TA59/Guidance/pdf/English (accessed 29 September 2009).

National Institute of Mental Health in England (2005) *NIMHE Guiding Statement on Recovery*. Department of Health, London.

National Institute of Mental Health (2007) *Older Adults: Depression and Suicide Facts* (factsheet). Available at http://www.nimh.nih.gov/health/publications/older-adults-depression-and-suicide-facts-fact-sheet/index.shtml (accessed 10 May 2010).

Newson P (2008) Relocation to a care home, part one: exploring reactions. *Nursing and Residential Care* **10**, 321–324.

NHS Education for Scotland (2008) *Working with Older People in Scotland: A Framework for Mental Health Nurses*. NES, Edinburgh.

NHS Quality Improvement Scotland (2004) *Working with Older People Towards Prevention and Early Detection of Depression*. http://www.nhsqis.org/nhsqis/files/BPS%20Working%20 with%20Older%20.pdf (accessed 24 May 2010).

Nursing and Midwifery Council (2009) *Guidance for the Care of Older People*. NMC, London.

O'Connell H, Chin A-Y, Cunningham C, Lawlor BA (2004) Recent developments: suicide in older people. *British Medical Journal* **329**, 895–899.

Pavlou MP, Lachs MS (2006) Could self-neglect in older adults be a geriatric syndrome? *Journal of the American Geriatrics Society* **54**, 831–842.

Penninx BWJH, Guralnik JM, Ferrucci L, Simonsick EM, Deeg DJH, Wallace RB (1998) Depressive symptoms and physical decline in community-dwelling older persons. *Journal of the American Medical Association* **279**, 1720–1726.

Pot AM, Deeg JH, Twisk JWR, Beekman ATF, Zarit SH (2005) The longitudinal relationship between the use of long-term care and depressive symptoms in older adults. *Gerontologist* **45**, 359–369.

Ramon S, Healy B, Renouf N (2007) Recovery from mental illness as an emergent concept and practice in Australia and the UK. *International Journal of Social Psychiatry* **53**, 108–122.

Robert RE, Kaplan GA, Shema SJ, Strawbridge WA (1997) Does growing old increase the risk for depression? *American Journal of Psychiatry* **154**, 1384–1390.

Roberts G, Wolfson P (2004) The rediscovery of recovery: open to all. *Advances in Psychiatric Treatment* **10**, 37–49.

Royal College of Psychiatrists (2005) *Who Cares Wins: Guidelines for the Development of Liaison Mental Health Services for Older People.* Report of the Faculty of Old Age Psychiatry, Royal College of Psychiatrists, London.

Royal College of Psychiatrists (2009a) Antidepressants. Available at http://www.rcpsych.ac.uk/ mentalhealthinfo/problems/depression/antidepressants.aspx (accessed 12 March 2010).

Royal College of Psychiatrists (2009b) Electroconvulsive therapy (ECT). Available at http://www. rcpsych.ac.uk/mentalhealthinfoforall/treatments/ect.aspx (accessed 15 March 2010).

Royal College of Psychiatrists (2009c) Depression in older adults. Available at http://www.rcpsych. ac.uk/mentalhealthinformation/mentalhealthproblems/depression/depressioninolderadults.aspx (accessed 14 March 2010).

St John PD, Montgomery PR (2009) Do depressive symptoms predict mortality in older people? *Aging and Mental Health* **13**, 674–681.

Scottish Executive (2006) *Rights, Relationships and Recovery: The Report of the National Review of Mental Health Nursing in Scotland.* Scottish Executive, Edinburgh.

Scottish Government (2007) *All Our Futures: Planning for a Scotland with an Ageing Population.* Scottish Government, Edinburgh.

Scottish Government (2009a) *Towards a Mentally Flourishing Scotland: Policy and Action Plan 2009–2011.* Scottish Government, Edinburgh.

Scottish Government (2009b) *Rights, Relationships and Recovery: The National Review of Mental Health Nursing in Scotland. Charting Progress Two Years On.* Scottish Government, Edinburgh. Available at http://www.scotland.gov.uk/Resource/Doc/924/0065333.pdf (accessed 7 December 2009).

Snowden A (2009) Assessment and care planning. In: Kydd A, Duffy T, Duffy FJR (eds) *The Care and Wellbeing of Older People.* Reflect Press, Exeter.

Strawbridge WJ, Deleger S, Roberts RE, Kaplan GA (2002) Physical activity reduces the risk of subsequent depression for older adults. *American Journal of Epidemiology* **156**, 328–334.

Trivedi MH (2004) The link between depression and physical symptoms. *Journal of Clinical Psychiatry* **6** (Suppl. 1), 12–16.

Unützer J, Katon W, Callahan CM *et al.* (2002) Collaborative care management of late-life depression in the primary care setting. *Journal of the American Medical Association* **288**, 2836–2845.

Vanitallie TB (2005) Subsyndromal depression in the elderly: underdiagnosed and undertreated. *Metabolism: Clinical and Experimental* **54** (5 Suppl. 1), 39–44.

Watson LC, Zimmerman S, Cohen LW, Dominik R (2009) Practical depression screening in residential care/assisted living: five methods compared with gold standard diagnoses. *American Journal of Geriatric Psychiatry* **17**, 556–564.

Whitwell D (1999) The myth of recovery from mental illness. *Psychiatric Bulletin* **23**, 621–622.

Wilson K, Mottram PG, Vassilas C (2008) Psychotherapeutic treatments for older depressed people. *Cochrane Database of Systematic Reviews* CD004853.

World Health Organization (2007) *International Statistical Classification of Diseases and Related Health Problems*, 10th Revision. Available at http://apps.who.int/classifications/apps/icd/ icd10online/ (accessed 21 September 2009).

World Health Organization (2009) Ageing. Available at http://www.who.int/topics/ageing/en/ (accessed 21 September 2009).

Yesavage JA, Brink TL, Rose TL *et al.* (1983) Development and validation of a geriatric depression screening scale: a preliminary report. *Journal of Psychiatric Research* **17**, 37–49.

Chapter 11

Promoting Nutrition with Frail Older People

Jennie Jackson and Susan Polding-Clyde

Introduction

Good nutrition is essential throughout the life cycle to promote health and well-being. This is especially true in frail older people where nutrition can be the key to maintaining quality of life. The term 'malnutrition' has been defined as 'a state of nutrition in which a deficiency or excess (or imbalance) of energy, protein and other nutrients causes measurable adverse effects on tissues/body form (body shape, size and composition), bodily function and clinical outcome' (Elia 2000).

Malnutrition encompasses both over- and under-nutrition, and while the current obesity epidemic is impacting upon the health of younger adults, in frail older people under-nutrition is more common and of more significance. Indeed, the term 'malnutrition', in the context of older adults, generally refers to under-nutrition and this meaning will be used in the rest of this chapter. Older people have increased risk of malnutrition due to a variety of physiological, social, psychological and financial factors. Whatever the reasons, the result of poor nutrition may be devastating, resulting in immobility, poor health and increased risk of falls and pressure sores, and may lead to increased, and longer, hospital admissions.

This chapter discusses the role of nursing in addressing the problem of malnutrition in frail older people. The challenges for nurses are to identify those who are malnourished (or at risk of becoming so), understand the possible options for nutritional care, how and when to refer for further specialised intervention, and how to monitor nutritional status. Nutritional care means determining a person's individual preferences and cultural needs, defining his or her physical requirements and then providing the person with the food they need (Care Commission 2009). The best ways of providing nutritional care will depend on care setting and an individual person's needs, but care should ideally be evidence based and applied in the context of value-based gerontological nursing. This chapter highlights one such example of nursing care, i.e. the role of 'nutrition champions' in promoting nutrition in care homes.

Evidence Informed Nursing with Older People, First Edition. Edited by Debbie Tolson, Joanne Booth and Irene Schofield.
© 2011 Blackwell Publishing Ltd. Published 2011 by Blackwell Publishing Ltd.

Box 11.1   Effects of ageing which may affect food intake or nutrient absorption

- Decreased saliva production
- Diminished sense of smell and taste
- Tooth decay and edentulous mouths
- Receding gums
- Articulation of upper and lower jaw
- Decreased oesophageal peristalsis
- Decreased gastric secretions and atrophic gastritis
- Impaired vision
- Changes in gut microflora

Prevalence, causes and consequences of malnutrition in frail older people

Under-nutrition is common in older adults in the UK and worldwide. It is estimated that 10% of those aged 65 or over in the UK are malnourished (European Nutrition for Health Alliance 2006). Prevalence of malnutrition in older people who are unwell or require to be looked after is even higher. The British Association for Enteral and Parenteral Nutrition (2008) conducted a nutritional screening survey and audit of over 9000 people admitted to care homes, hospitals and mental health units and found that one-third of older people admitted to care homes or 'Care of older adults' hospital wards were classified as 'malnourished'. Investigations of the nutritional status of older people resident in nursing homes in Scotland found that food intakes were well below estimated requirements in spite of adequate food provision (Leslie *et al.* 2006) and about one in four older people in long-term residential care was malnourished (Clinical Research and Audit Group 2000). Community-living older people tend to be better nourished, but about 10% of older people living in sheltered housing in Wales were found to be at risk of malnutrition (Harris *et al.* 2008). The problem of malnutrition in older people is not restricted to the UK but is present in all developed countries and possibly many developing nations too (Shum *et al.* 2005; Suominen *et al.* 2005; Poojary *et al.* 2007; Aliabadi *et al.* 2008).

Older people are particularly at risk of malnutrition due to a variety of physical factors. Physical causes are partly attributable to body changes that occur with increasing age (Box 11.1).

For example, senses of taste and smell may be diminished, altering food choices and limiting food intake. Impaired vision and reduced mobility due to arthritis and other degenerative conditions may lead to difficulties in shopping and food preparation. There are also various changes in the gastrointestinal tract (especially associated with atrophic gastritis) which can lead to poor absorption of nutrients resulting in an increased prevalence of deficiencies of vitamin B_{12} and folate (Finch *et al.* 1998). Chronic illness and disability, particularly associated with neurological, respiratory or musculoskeletal conditions, can cause difficulty with eating, including swallowing disorders. Older people with few or no teeth eat a more restricted diet, e.g. they are less likely to choose apples, raw carrots, toast and oranges. This may lead to reduced intakes of iron, vitamin C, vitamin E and retinol (Finch *et al.* 1998).

Psychological factors, such as distress resulting from the loss of a loved one, can reduce the motivation to eat. Depression is common in this age group, and is probably under-diagnosed as symptoms may be attributed to physical problems. Low mood can lead to lack of interest in eating, poor intake and subsequent weight loss. Older people living alone often eat less well than those who eat with others, while practical issues such as access to shops and the cost of food also affect food choices. Money may be preferentially spent on heating or rent, and food is often treated as a flexible item and the first to be cut back.

The effects of medication can reduce appetite or sensory awareness and certain drugs interact with the absorption and metabolism of nutrients (Chan 2002).

All of the above may happen as part of normal ageing, and in addition it might be the person has a long-term condition, such as arthritis, which compounds the situation further. We can see how the older person might be further compromised if there are episodes of acute illness, and strong nursing assessment and leadership are needed to maximise good positive health and well-being.

Thus malnutrition is a key factor as both a consequence and a cause of ill health in frail older people and can result in the geriatric 'syndromes' or 'conditions' discussed in Chapter 1. Poor food intake may lead to increasing frailty and ill health. The resulting malnutrition can lead to poor recovery from illness, infections, immobility, increased risk of falls, poor cognition, the need for more medicines and general inability to cope with the activities of daily living. All this leads to a vicious circle where immobility and frailty reduce food intake, leading to worsening nutritional status, poor immunity and impaired recovery.

As well as the effect on health and well-being of individuals, there may be financial consequences for service providers. Malnutrition results in increased admissions to hospital, longer hospital stays and increased readmission rates, with an estimated £7.3 billion per year spent on malnutrition-related ill health and healthcare in the UK (most of this on older people) (European Nutrition for Health Alliance 2006).

The 'user perspective' of food provision and eating in older adults

Although there have been numerous studies on the causes and consequences of malnutrition, few have reported on the user perspective in terms of their thoughts on reasons for poor nutrition. However, a couple of studies have sought the views of older people about food provision in hospitals and long-term care. 'Hungry to be Heard' produced by the charity Age Concern UK (2006) consulted older people and their relatives and highlighted the problems experienced in terms of food provision in hospitals. Age Concern found examples of failure to provide assistance with eating, failure to check on whether food had been eaten, unsuitable foods provided (e.g. wrong texture), food left too long so cold and unpalatable, and food being left out of reach. Older people often lose weight after hospital admission and there appeared to be failure to react to this. People were experiencing these problems in hospitals that claimed to be meeting recommendations for good nutritional care proposed by the Department of Health (2004). Age Concern stress that the voices of older people, their relatives and carers must be heard. They should be consulted about the food available, their dietary needs and preferences and what type of help is required with eating.

A qualitative study of older people's perspectives of nutritional care in Denmark found that although satisfaction with meals was high, people lacked information about the meal service and person–staff communication about the food service was poor (Lassen *et al.* 2005). A similar qualitative study in two London teaching hospitals found that older people and those with physical disabilities experienced greatest difficult in accessing food. Half of the people reported feeling hungry during their stay. The difficulties in accessing food included organisational barriers (e.g. menus not providing information on best choices for their nutritional needs, unsuitable meal timing, inflexible ordering systems) and physical barriers (e.g. not being in a comfortable position, food out of reach, awkward utensils or difficult packaging). Environmental factors affecting food intake included staff interruptions, disruptive and noisy patients, repetitive sounds or nasty smells (Naithani *et al.* 2008). Using this information, Naithani *et al.* (2009) developed a tool to measure experience of food access in hospitals. Initial results using this tool in 29 wards in four hospitals in England revealed widespread problems of food access in hospitals.

Jones *et al.* (2005) explored the views of older people living on their own at home regarding provision of food. Eating alone was identified as one of the greatest factors limiting appetite, and older people also stressed variety, choice, presentation, smelling food cooking, activity and getting out the house as factors affecting their desire to eat.

How can under-nutrition be prevented?

In order to tackle the problem of malnutrition in frail older people, a multidisciplinary and holistic approach is necessary. Depending on the care system, this will require cooperative working by, for example, carers, relatives, nurses, medical staff, caterers, allied health professionals and social workers. The nurse has a key role in communicating with these partners and coordinating care to ensure that each person receives the best nutritional care. Such care should be based on best practice statements and guidelines, which should be evidence informed.

Systematic reviews are often used to identify best practice. There have been few undertaken focusing on older people and food, but Vanderkroft *et al.* (2007) conducted a systematic review to identify best practice in terms of preventing under-nutrition in hospitalised older people. Their comprehensive review identified 29 studies that included specific interventions to minimise malnutrition in people aged 65 years or older. Of these, 15 interventions involved giving oral nutritional supplements, six focused on tube feeding, four involved changes to the hospital food, one involved employing an extra staff member to promote nutrition and only three were concerned with the implementation of evidence based guidelines. They found evidence for the benefits of oral supplements in terms of improving weight and muscle mass, but the efficacy of the other interventions remained unclear, highlighting the need for further good-quality research. Other systematic reviews have also found some benefits in oral supplementation of older adults (Avenell & Handoll 2006; Milne *et al.* 2009). Otherwise, evidence in terms of systematic reviews and randomised controlled trials is scanty. Most 'best practice' guidelines are based on less robust evidence and expert opinion, highlighting the need for more good-quality research to inform best practice in ensuring good nutrition for older people. The values of both health carers and older people should also be considered in deciding on optimum delivery of nutritional care.

Nurses' role in alleviating malnutrition

Food and fluid play an essential role in all our lives in terms of our physical, philosophical, spiritual, cultural and social well-being, and therefore sit easily with the nursing philosophy of holistic practice. Nutritional needs vary over time, depending on age and physical activity. Illness may result in changes to an individual's requirements, and may alter the appetite, the ability to eat and to communicate needs.

Nurses have a key role in providing help and advice on food and fluid intake in an appropriate manner for the person, if necessary by obtaining help with shopping and cooking and in providing food in formal care settings. It is important that food is tasty, attractive and of good nutritional value. To enjoy meals people should feel clean and comfortable; they should also have been offered the opportunity to use the toilet and/or wash their hands. Care settings should provide a pleasant environment that is quiet and calm, and offer as many sensory clues as possible, such as cooking smells, to stimulate the appetite. Some people might benefit from specially designed cutlery and other eating utensils.

Nutrition is essential to life and as vital as medication or any other type of intervention to support older people, not only through the actions of the individual nurse but also as a member of a team working together to promote the well-being of older people. Nurses are responsible for assessing, planning and evaluating the nutritional and hydration needs of older people in their care, working in partnership with other members of the multidisciplinary team, including caterers, doctors, dietitians, and speech and language therapists, who also have an important role to play in the provision of effective nutrition and hydration for individuals. It is only through a multidisciplinary approach that good nutritional care can be achieved.

The particular role of nurses within the multidisciplinary team in relation to nutritional care has been discussed by Savage and Scott (2005) who identified several key responsibilities (Box 11.2).

Box 11.2   Key responsibilities for nurses in relation to nutritional care

- Initial nutritional assessment, monitoring and referral to specialist staff, where appropriate.
- Screening for dysphagia.

- Implementing the advice of dietitians and speech and language therapists.
- Helping patients to complete menu cards.
- Ensuring that patients receive their chosen meal, including special diets.
- Providing snacks (such as toast and tea) for patients who cannot eat a full meal.
- Helping any patients who need it to eat and drink.
- Organising nursing work around protected patient mealtimes.

Nutrition screening and assessment

Malnutrition is rife, but nurses may still have difficulty in recognising undernourished older people (Suominen *et al.* 2009). The benefits of nutrition screening are well established, with potential to reduce length of stay, reduce hospital costs and improve people's health. Screening all older people for risk of malnutrition on admission to a hospital or care home is recommended by many guidelines (NHS Quality Improvement Scotland 2002, 2003; National Institute for Health and Clinical Excellence 2006) but is not always implemented (Elia 2000). There are various validated screening tools available for use with older people, reviewed by Green and Watson (2006). These include the Malnutrition Universal Screening Tool (MUST) (British Association for Enteral and Parenteral Nutrition 2009) and the Mini-Nutritional Assessment (Guigoz 2006). MUST was developed by the British Association for Enteral and Parenteral Nutrition for use by nurses, other health professionals and carers. It is quick and easy and can be used in most settings. MUST is a five-step screening tool that calculates the overall risk of malnutrition score based on body mass index, unplanned weight loss and effect of acute disease. Depending on the score, guidelines are given to help devise a care plan. The MUST score has been shown to predict mortality and length of hospital stay in acutely ill older people (Stratton *et al.* 2006).

As well as initial screening to identify people at immediate risk who require referral or intensive nutritional support, nurses have a role in a more detailed assessment to develop a nutritional care plan (National Institute for Health and Clinical Excellence 2006). Nurses should carry out a complete and holistic nursing assessment of the older person's needs, regardless of the reason for the intervention. Usually, an assessment framework, based on a nursing model, is used. The purpose of this stage is to identify the person's nursing needs and to maximise their independence; these needs are expressed as either actual or potential. For example, an older person who has fractured their arm after a fall may be assessed as having difficulty carrying out their shopping or preparing a meal. The nurse's role is to consider all the person's immediate needs, then to recognise the actions required to ensure long-term independence for that person.

Capturing a nursing history and communicating with the person prior to any physical examination allows a nurse to establish a rapport with the older person and family. Elements of the history will include:

- health status
- course of present condition including symptoms

- current management of illness
- past medical history including family's medical history
- social history
- perception of the condition.

The purpose of this assessment is to devise a personal care plan that will optimise the nutritional status and well-being of the person. A nurse's assessment may include a physical examination and the recording of observations (e.g. height and weight, pulse or blood pressure) identified as relevant. There are many assessment tools that focus on specific aspects of care, for example the Waterlow score which deals with a person's risk of developing a pressure sore, and there are various pain scales available to support assessment.

Key to any assessment process would be to ensure that the person understands why they have been involved in this discussion and are being assessed, what they would hope to gain during this time and what they would like to achieve. Documenting the assessment is necessary to share information with others; this recording may be on paper or as part of an electronic record which can be accessed by all members of the care team. Documentation is identified as a crucial part of the process to ensure that the person is not asked the same questions again.

The importance of communicating and acting on the information gathered during assessment and care planning cannot be underestimated. Documentation alone is not enough. It is the implementation of the care plan by those directly involved in the care of the older person that is essential to make changes and improve nutritional care.

Care planning to provide optimal nutrition

In terms of nutrients, dietary recommendations generally do not differ much between younger and older adults (although a supplement of vitamin D may be needed in those over 65 years) (Department of Health 1991). However, since energy intakes of older people are generally less and absorption of some nutrients may be poor, the diet must be of high nutritional value in order to meet requirements for all vitamins and minerals. In practice, the nutritional requirements of most can be met by three nutritious meals per day, plus snacks to maximise energy density and increase eating opportunities. Plenty of variety increases the likelihood of all nutrient requirements being met (Bernstein *et al.* 2002; Caroline Walker Trust 2004).

The challenge is in making sure that all older people have access to such a diet. Nurses are pivotal in ensuring that care plans are implemented and appropriate actions are taken to improve the nutritional status for all older people across all care settings. The nurse is the key to identifying the need for the involvement of other professionals, for example the dietitian for intensive nutritional support, speech and language therapist for swallowing assessment, occupational therapist for adapted utensils, physiotherapist to optimise eating position, and doctor for provision of medical support. Liaison with the catering staff to ensure that the appropriate therapeutic diet is delivered is a critical aspect of improving a person's nutritional status.

In recent years there has been a focus on improving hospital food (Scottish Government 2008). This national programme to improve nutritional care in hospitals has introduced a

Box 11.3   Themes related to patient safety affecting nutritional care

- Dehydration: patients transferred to hospitals dehydrated.
- Choking: patients choking whilst eating a meal.
- Inappropriate diet: patients receiving normal food when requiring textured modified diet.
- Incorrect artificial feeding: potential for incorrect dose of enteral feed given or wrong total parenteral nutrition given.
- Nil by mouth (prolonged): impact of fasting for days.
- Nil by mouth (patient fed): patient given breakfast and theatre then having to be cancelled.
- Missed meals: patient declined breakfast and not given lunch.
- Transfer of care: poor communication between different care settings, both verbal and written.
- Pressure sores: nutritional status identified as a contributing factor to pressure sore development.
- Catering services: unable to supply appropriate meals.

partnership approach to the provision of meals and introduced 'nutrition champions' to support the process. There have been various strands to this programme (e.g. standardising recipes, provision of educational tools to support learning and the development of a website) to improve nutrition in hospitals. The introduction of protected mealtimes can be identified as one of the developing areas. Protected mealtimes have been described as 'protected uninterrupted time to focus on providing an environment conducive to eating', when there should be no clinical interventions and all staff focus on people's nutritional needs. The ambition is to ensure a relaxed and leisurely mealtime in order to maximise well-being and nutritional intake. Ensuring that the intake of food is a priority in the care of older people is a significant move in recognising that good nutrition and adequate intake of fluid are both key to the physical and emotional well-being of individuals.

Protected mealtimes have been introduced in many hospitals and care homes, but a review of hospitals across England and Wales found that implementation remained variable between hospitals and between wards within hospitals. There were inconsistencies around which mealtime services and which clinical areas were protected (National Patient Safety Agency 2007). Being able to access food 24 hours a day to give to people who are hungry or who have missed meals due to investigations is essential for nurses to be able to supply nutritional care.

The nurse, as clinical leader, has a vital role in looking after and protecting older people around the issue of nutrition and its relationship to safety, particularly in our hospitals. The NHS National Patient Safety Agency (www.nrls.npsa.nhs.uk) recognises that poor nutritional care can threaten safety of patients and identifies a number of key themes to consider (Box 11.3).

Nurses need to ensure activities at mealtimes are focused on the meal and the person, ensuring that the person is ready to eat and making sure that the environment encourages eating. Nurses should be recognising and providing assistance to older people who cannot manage to eat their meal without support, observing the person and monitoring the difficulties

---

Box 11.4　Key messages for nurses on improving safety

- Observing and monitoring the appropriate diet and fluids
- Assessing for swallowing problems
- Ensuring adequate diet and fluid intake

---

to make sure they are eating and drinking fluids. Crucially, this information should be recorded on the care plan and other documentation to ensure information is communicated to other colleagues.

By following the checklist in Box 11.4, patient safety and the risk of malnutrition and dehydration can be minimised. In order to provide good nutritional care nurses are responsible for ensuring that their care is focused on the following.

- Providing person-centred care that is evidence based. This means ensuring that all aspects of nutrition are taken into account and acted upon in the context of the person's individual needs.
- Keeping up to date though accessing and using quality information and evidence about nutrition and hydration through continuous professional development.
- Challenging poor practice in relation to nutrition and hydration.
- Assessing the environment and ensuring it supports good nutritional care.
- Evaluating the impact of nutrition and hydration care plans and making necessary changes.
- Contributing to multidisciplinary and multi-agency working that achieves seamless nutritional care.
- Dedicating time to prioritise the nutritional needs of individuals with protected mealtimes.

All nurses, in their leadership role, are responsible for enabling others to provide good nutritional care.

Hand in hand with good nutrition is the need to encourage adequate hydration and prevent dehydration in older people. There is an increased risk of dehydration in older people due to reduced fluid intake and increased fluid loss. Intakes may be reduced because older people may not feel thirsty until dehydration is apparent. Issues such as swallowing problems, incontinence, dementia and use of diuretics all exacerbate the problem. Fluid losses are greater because the kidney becomes less adept at concentrating urine and more urine is excreted. There is strong evidence to suggest that good hydration assists in the management of diabetes and helps prevent pressure ulcers, constipation, urinary infections and incontinence, kidney stones, heart disease, cognitive impairment, falls, poor oral health, skin conditions and many other illnesses. Encouraging the drinking of fluids will help reduce incidence of common ailments and better hydration improves well-being.

Older people have similar fluid requirements to those of younger adults. Although there is currently no agreed recommended daily intake in the UK, estimates range from approximately 1.2 to 3.1 L/day. A conservative estimate for older adults is that the daily intake of fluids should not be less than 1.5 L/day (World Health Organization 2002). Unfortunately, many older people do not drink adequate amounts; a recent survey of water provision in UK care homes for older people found that most residents consumed only two to four glasses of fluid per day (480–960 mL) (www.water.org.uk/home/water-for-health/older-people/rsph-survey). The principles of assessment, care planning and putting the actions in place to support nutrition are equally as important for hydration of older people.

Case study 11.1   Improving Nutrition in Care Homes for Older People programme: the introduction of nutrition champions to improve nutritional care in care homes

Improving nutritional care for older people across all care sectors continues to be one of the Scottish Government's objectives. In 2007, the Government funded a programme to support improving nutritional care in 100 of Scotland's care homes (Care Commission 2009). The partners were the Scottish Government, the Care Commission and the Care Homes for Older People Dietitians Network. Making sure residents in care homes have nutritious food and drinks is essential to good care. Food is fundamental to quality of life and, for older people in particular, can be critical to their health and well-being. Unplanned or unexplained weight loss can make older people vulnerable to disease and may be fatal. People's appetites also reduce with age, so keeping older people interested in food is a challenge. Malnutrition and dehydration are serious and common problems among older people in care homes (Copeman 2000).

There is extensive research showing that many older people in care homes are malnourished and there is much guidance on best practice to deliver nutritional care (Scottish Executive 2001; NHS Quality Improvement Scotland 2002; Caroline Walker Trust 2004). However, the challenge is to implement the guidelines and put them into practice on a day-to day basis. The Clinical Research and Audit Group (2000) report sought changes to culture and practice rather than more legislation. The Improving Nutrition in Care Homes programme aimed to do just that, by introducing nutrition champions.

The programme partners invited staff from care homes across Scotland to become nutrition champions in developing practice in their own care homes by planning and implementing and evaluating their own projects. The programme reflected the complexity of delivering nutritional care at mealtimes. This complexity reflects organisational commitment to change and skills such as practical know-how, problem solving, interpersonal skills and flexibility. The nutrition champions needed to be able to explore the emotional, social, practical and physical factors that support and hinder good nutrition and eating well.

The nutrition champions planned and implemented a project in their care home that would enrich the quality of care delivered to older people around nutritional issues and more widely enhance mealtimes. The projects were focused around the following categories.

- Improving the dining room experience, including protected mealtimes when all non-urgent activity stops.
- Introduction of the MUST.
- Improving menus, according to nutritional value, likes and dislikes.
- Sharing knowledge with other staff in the care home.
- Making food more accessible and attractive.
- Developing recording systems to support audit.
- Improving levels of intake of fluid and other drinks.

It is hoped that the Scottish Government will consider funding and support to extend the nutrition champions programme across all care homes in Scotland.

For one care home, the project chosen by the nutrition champion aimed to make mealtimes an enjoyable part of the day by introducing protected mealtimes. This care home was a privately run 35-bed care home with nursing care provision. The residents were frail and many had cognitive impairment. Most required intensive support for activities of daily living and were dependent on carers to support their needs. By introducing protected mealtimes, even the care home group manager was not allowed to go into the dining room at mealtimes unless invited!

To some this change might seem a task that was easy to achieve, but a great deal of discussion took place and agreement had to be reached both within and outwith the care home. Within the care home consideration had to be given to individual preferences about when mealtimes should take place, ensuring staffing schedules were planned to meet the individual needs of people requiring support. This agreement had to be achieved before starting to consider the nutritional components and requirements.

The nutrition champion then had to liaise and consult with all the visitors to the care home, including general practitioners, podiatrists, district nurses, physiotherapists, as well as family and friends of the people who lived in the care home. The intention was that everyone would know when mealtimes occurred and would understand that mealtimes would not be interrupted for anyone or anything. Family and friends of people in the care home were always welcomed at mealtimes, and the introduction of protected mealtimes was viewed positively by them and offered them the opportunity to continue to be involved with, and participate in, the care of their loved ones.

Ultimately, the professionals viewed this change positively, as they were dissatisfied interrupting the person at their meal, particularly if they were enjoying their food. The care home manager now feels more empowered in protecting the people in the care home and their needs at mealtimes. Any unexpected visitors are advised politely that they will need to come back at a convenient time.

The nutrition champion also introduced a communication tool to help record people's needs. This tool was used in discussion with the person and their families to ensure individual preferences and wishes were known. This, together with increased knowledge about nutrition for staff, has led to people in the care home gaining weight. The improved communication between carers and chefs has had a huge impact in identifying an individual's needs and sharing this with all those involved in their care. The nutrition champion has learnt the value of involving people in the process of change to move forward.

Some quotes from nutrition champions who took part in the programme are shown in Box 11.5.

Box 11.5   Views of nutrition champions

'One change leads to the next. You have to find a way of keeping the momentum going.'

'The key to success is to include others in the decision-making process. It's important to know your people and anticipate the resistance to your suggestions and have your answers prepared.'

Challenges and ethical issues

Unfortunately, malnutrition is only too common in frail older people and there are many challenges facing nurses in addressing the problem. Providing nutritional care to older people who live in their own home has its own challenges. Nurses need to work in health and social care partnership (often in community teams) taking account of many issues: the public health agenda; providing support to carers and those who support older people at home; the issue of poverty and access to benefit maximisation; as well as the role of nursing for the wider population. Advice for older people at home needs to be clear, accessible and understandable and take into account individual needs, for example people with dementia will have specific issues. The role of the nurse must remain pivotal in the prevention and early detection of malnutrition in older people, the coordination of others involved in delivery of support and care, and identifying the need for specialist support. Nurses must also provide appropriate educational opportunities to ensure that good nutrition and the identification of malnutrition is a component of student training.

A further challenge is the need to maintain the individual's autonomy and dignity, which are integral parts of value-based nursing. Being able to choose one's own food is vital in maintaining autonomy. It is difficult to choose food for another person since an individual's preferences are strongly influenced by beliefs about appropriate food behaviour, which are formed by life course events and even childhood experiences. When making food choices, older people consider social context, sensory factors, financial considerations, convenience and physical well-being (Falk *et al.* 1996). As far as is possible nurses should seek to do the same when working with, or on behalf of, an older person.

Maintaining dignity is core to providing nursing care and must be taken into account in the provision of nutritional care. Older people may be embarrassed by needing help, by the time taken to eat a meal, and the implications of tying a baby bib around the neck of an older person in place of a napkin should not be underestimated (Age Concern 2006). Negotiating care decisions and maintaining dignity and autonomy may be difficult in certain cases where older people may not be able to choose, for example in older people with dementia. Malnutrition is common in older people with dementia, even in the early stages of the disease (Kagansky *et al.* 2005; Orsitto *et al.* 2009). Older people with dementia may forget to eat, fail to recognise food, may not feel the normal drive to eat or may have difficulties chewing and swallowing. In the later stages, as the disease progresses, choking is common and alternative means of feeding are often considered. Enteral tube feeding involves the administration of artificial food and fluids via a nasogastric or PEG (percutaneous endoscopic gastrostomy) tube, commonly referred to as 'tube feeding'. A survey in the USA found that one in three nursing home residents with advanced cognitive impairment were tube fed. The decision to insert a tube and start feeding is difficult and ethically challenging. There may be pressure from relatives who find it painful to watch an older person refusing to eat or drink or being incapable of doing so. Medical and nursing staff may fear legal consequences if they do not intervene and they may feel that in order to provide reliable nutrition, hydration and medication tube feeding is essential (Bryon *et al.* 2008). However, a systematic review by Sampson *et al.* (2009) found no evidence that tube feeding in this client group improved quality of life, prolonged life, decreased infections or led to improved nutritional status. They found no literature on the possible adverse effects of tube feeding older people with advanced dementia. Alternative options to tube feeding include assisted feeding. A systematic review of interventions to promote eating in older people with dementia reported on studies involving changes to meal service systems, staff assignment, nutritional screening, altered food texture, behavioural interventions and introducing music in the dining room (Watson & Green 2006). They concluded that further research was needed into how nurses could best help older people with dementia to eat. However, current guidelines for feeding older people with dementia give many practical suggestions and highlight issues that should be considered, for example timing and presentation of meals, offering finger foods, high energy snacks and ensuring food is of suitable texture (Caroline Walker Trust 1998; Alzheimer's Society 2009).

Recognising the end of life is a further challenge in older people's nutrition. There is likely to be a point at which nutritional intervention (be it food or 'tubes') is of no benefit in terms of improving nutritional status, quality of life or the well-being of the older person. Great sensitivity and expertise is needed when approaching and negotiating any decisions once this point has been reached. A partnership approach is crucial, which should have included the older person and their family, to ensure that everyone involved is in agreement with the focus on the best interests of the older person.

Summary

People aged 80 years and over are the most rapidly growing population group. It will become ever more important to ensure good nutrition in later life to maintain good health and well-being, and there is potential for increased demand on services. For nurses, and other healthcare professionals, it is necessary to recognise the importance of optimal nutrition and hydration in preventing ill health and maintaining good health in older people.

Health professionals have a role in helping older people and their families to understand the importance of good nutrition, and what that really means, and discussing how this has an impact on overall health and well-being. Nurses must also encourage conversation with older people about future wishes and wants within an anticipatory care planning process, which might include 'tube feeding' or what they might wish to happen, and which will inform their future care needs.

Although there is a need for more good-quality research to inform best practice in improving nutritional status in frail older people, there is much scope for improving nutritional care by enabling the implementation of existing guidelines. It should be noted that there is a plethora of guidelines, best practice statements and policies relating to nutrition and improving nutrition. Therefore, the future focus of any activity must be to ensure that existing guidelines and policies are put into practice to make change happen, i.e. to recognise and treat malnutrition in older people as early as possible.

Finally, sharing positive messages as part of the wider public health agenda for children and adults with regard to nutrition offers an opportunity to share information with the population that supports good nutrition in later years. The ambition is that the individual will take ownership of their own nutritional needs and solutions and make good choices.

Key messages

- Under-nutrition is common in frail older people and is the cause and consequence of ill health.
- It is only through a multidisciplinary approach that good nutrition can be achieved.
- Nutritional care and food provision in many hospitals and care homes fails to meet the needs of nutritionally vulnerable older adults.
- Nurses have a major role in screening, assessment and care planning to ensure that older people receive appropriate food and drinks and get help to eat when they need it.
- The introduction of nutrition champions to promote good practice within nursing homes can help to improve nutritional care.

References

Age Concern (2006) *Hungry to be Heard. The Scandal of Malnourished Older People in Hospital.* Available at www.ageconcern.org.uk

Aliabadi M, Kimiagar M, Ghayour-Mobarhan M, Shakeri M, Nematy M, Ilaty A (2008) Prevalence of malnutrition in free living elderly people in Iran: a cross-sectional study. *Asian Pacific Journal of Clinical Nutrition* **17**, 285–289.

Alzheimer's Society (2009) *Food for Thought: Eating and Nutrition.* Available at www.alzheimers. org.uk

Avenell A, Handoll HG (2006) Nutritional supplementation for hip fracture aftercare in older people. *Cochrane Database of Systematic Reviews* (4), CD001880.

Bernstein MA, Tucker KL, Ryan ND, O'Neill EF, Clements K, Nelson ME (2002) Higher dietary variety is associated with better nutritional status in frail elderly people. *Journal of the American Dietetic Association* **102**, 1096–1104.

British Association for Enteral and Parenteral Nutrition (2008) *Nutrition Screening Survey in the UK in 2007: a Report by BAPEN.* Available at www.bapen.org.uk/pdfs/nsw/nsw07_report.pdf

British Association for Enteral and Parenteral Nutrition (2009) *MUST Malnutrition Universal Screening Tool* Available at www.bapen.org.uk/must_tool.html

Bryon E, Dierckx de Casterlé B, Gastmans C (2008) Nurses' attitudes towards artificial food or fluid administration in patients with dementia and in terminally ill patients: a review of the literature. *Journal of Medical Ethics* **34**, 431–436.

Care Commission (2009) *Promoting Nutrition in Care Homes for Older People.* Available at www. carecommission.com/images/stories/documents/publications/reviewsofqualitycare/promoting_ nutrition_in_care_homes_-_january_09.pdf

Caroline Walker Trust (1998) *Eating well for older people with dementia. A good practice guide for residential and nursing homes and others involved in caring for older people with dementia. Report of an expert working group.* Available at www.cwt.org.uk/pdfs/Dementia%20Report.pdf

Caroline Walker Trust (2004) *Eating well for older people.* Caroline Walker Trust, London.

Chan L-N (2002) Drug–nutrient interaction in clinical nutrition. *Current Opinion in Clinical Nutrition and Metabolic Care* **5**, 327–332.

Clinical Research and Audit Group (2000) *National Nutritional Audit of Elderly Individuals in Long Term Care, Scotland.* Clinical Research and Audit Group, Edinburgh.

Copeman J (2000) Promoting nutrition in older people in nursing and residential care homes. *British Journal of Community Nursing* **5**, 227–284.

Department of Health (1991) *Dietary Reference Values for Food Energy and Nutrients for the United Kingdom. Report of the Panel on Dietary Reference Values of the Committee on Medical Aspects of Food Policy.* Report on Health and Social Subjects 41. HMSO, London.

Department of Health (2004) *Standards for Better Health.* Available at www.dh.gov.uk

Elia M (ed.) (2000) *Guidelines for Detection and Management of Malnutrition. A Report by the Malnutrition Advisory Group.* British Association for Enteral and Parenteral Nutrition, Maidenhead.

European Nutrition for Health Alliance (2006) *Malnutrition Among Older People in the Community: Policy Recommendations for Change.* Available at www.european-nutrition.org/

Falk LW, Bisogni CA, Sobal J (1996) Food choice processes of older adults: a qualitative investigation. *Journal of Nutrition Education and Behavior* **28**, 257–265.

Finch S, Doyle W, Lowe C (1998) *National Diet and Nutrition Survey: People aged 65 years and over. Vol. 1 Report of the diet and nutrition survey.* The Stationery Office, London.

Green SM, Watson R (2006) Nutritional screening and assessment tools for older adults: literature review. *Journal of Advanced Nursing* **54**, 477–490.

Guigoz Y (2006) The Mini Nutritional Assessment (MNA) review of the literature. What does it tell us? *Journal of Nutrition Health and Aging* **10**, 466–485.

Harris DG, Davies C, Ward H, Haboubi NY (2008) An observational study of screening for malnutrition in elderly people living in sheltered accommodation. *Journal of Human Nutrition and Dietetics* **21**, 3–9.

Jones C, Dewar B, Donaldson C (2005) *Recipe for Life: Helping Older People to Eat Well.* Available at www.qmu.ac.uk/copa/publications/documents/Recipe%20for%20Liife%20 research%20report2.pdf

Kagansky N, Berner Y, Koren-Morag N, Perelman L, Knobler H, Levy S (2005) Poor nutritional habits are predictors of poor outcome in very old hospitalized patients. *American Journal of Clinical Nutrition* **82**, 784–791.

Lassen KO, Kruse F, Bjerrum M (2005) Nutritional care of Danish medical inpatients: patients' perspectives. *Scandinavian Journal of Caring Science* **19**, 259–267.

Leslie WS, Lean ME, Woodward M, Wallace F, Hankey CR (2006) Unidentified under-nutrition: dietary intake and anthropometric indices in a residential care home population. *Journal of Human Nutrition and Dietetics* **19**, 343–347.

Milne AC, Potter J, Vivanti A, Avenell A (2009) Protein and energy supplementation in elderly people at risk from malnutrition. *Cochrane Database of Systematic Reviews* (2), CD003288.

Naithani S, Whelan K, Thomas J, Gulliford MC, Morgan M (2008) Hospital inpatients' experiences of access to food: a qualitative interview and observational study. *Health Expectations* **11**, 294–303.

Naithani S, Thomas JE, Whelan K, Morgan M, Gulliford MC (2009) Experiences of food access in hospital. A new questionnaire measure. *Clinical Nutrition* **28**, 625–630.

National Institute for Health and Clinical Excellence (2006) *Nutrition Support in Adults: Oral Nutrition Support, Enteral Tube Feeding and Parenteral Nutrition.* NICE, London. Available at http://guidance.nice.org.uk/CG32/?c=91500

National Patient Safety Agency (2007) *Protected Mealtimes Review.* Available at www.npsa.nhs. uk/EasySiteWeb/GatewayLink.aspx?alId=2654

NHS Quality Improvement Scotland (2002) *Best Practice Statement on Nutrition for Physically Frail Older People.* Available at www.nhsqis.org/nhsqis/2074.html

NHS Quality Improvement Scotland (2003) *Food, Fluid and Nutritional Care in Hospitals.* Available at www.nhshealthquality.org/nhsqis/files/Food,%20Fluid%20Nutrition.pdf

Orsitto G, Fulvio F, Tria D, Turi V, Venezia A, Manca C (2009) Nutritional status in hospitalized elderly patients with mild cognitive impairment. *Clinical Nutrition* **28**, 100–102.

Poojary S, Lemke R, Hunter P (2007) Screening for malnutrition in the elderly. *Internal Medicine Journal* **37** (Suppl. 3), A63-A88.

Sampson EL, Candy B, Jones L (2009) Enteral tube feeding for older people with advanced dementia. *Cochrane Database of Systematic Reviews* (2), CD007209.

Savage J, Scott C (2005) *Patients' Nutritional Care in Hospital: an Ethnographic Study of Nurses' Role and Patients' Experience*. Royal College of Nursing, commissioned by NHS Estates. Available at www.rcn.org.uk/development/practice/clinical_governance/patient_focus/rcn_publications

Scottish Executive (2001) *Care Homes for Older People. National Care Standards*. Available at www.scotland.gov.uk/publications/2001/11/10336

Scottish Government (2008) *Food in Hospitals: National Catering and Nutrition Specification for Food and Fluid Provision in Hospitals in Scotland*. Available at www.scotland.gov.uk/Publications/2008/06/24145312/0

Shum NC, Hui WW, Chu F, Chai J, Chow T (2005) Prevalence of malnutrition and risk factors in geriatric patients of a convalescent and rehabilitation hospital. *Hong Kong Medical Journal* **11**, 234–242.

Stratton R, King CL, Stroud M, Jackson AA, Elia M (2006) Malnutrition Universal Screening Tool predicts mortality and length of hospital stay in acutely ill elderly. *British Journal of Nutrition* **95**, 325–330.

Suominen M, Muurinen S, Routasalo P, Soini H, Suur-Uski I, Peiponen A (2005) Malnutrition and associated factors among aged residents in all nursing homes in Helsinki. *European Journal of Clinical Nutrition* **59**, 578–583.

Suominen M, Sandelin E, Soini H, Pitkala KH (2009) How well do nurses recognize malnutrition in elderly patients? *European Journal of Clinical Nutrition* **63**, 292–296.

Vanderkroft D, Collins C, Fitzgerald M, Lewis S, Neve M, Capra S (2007) Minimising under nutrition in the older inpatient. *Joanna Briggs Institute Library of Systematic Reviews* **5**, 134–229.

Watson R, Green SM (2006) Feeding and dementia: a systematic review. *Journal of Advanced Nursing* **54**, 86–93.

World Health Organization (2002) *Keep Fit for Life. Meeting the Nutritional Needs of Older Persons*. Geneva. Available at www.who.int/nutrition/publications/olderpersons/en/index.html

Chapter 12

Pain and Older People

Derek Jones and Pat Schofield
(with acknowledgement to Ron Marsh)

Introduction

In order to draw attention to the limited consideration given to pain in older people, the journal *Pain* published an editorial entitled 'Is there such a thing as geriatric pain?' (Melding 1991). Since then, the International Association for the Study of Pain has designated 2006–2007 an International Year Against Pain in Older Persons, and in a critical review Gagliese (2009) has reinforced the argument that pain and ageing is a sub-field in its own right, drawing attention to research demonstrating important differences between older people and younger people clinically and at the level of biological mechanisms.

The experience of pain at whatever stage of life has far-reaching consequences for the individual (in terms of general health and function), their friends and family (in terms of maintaining social networks) and society at large (in terms of the costs of poorly managed pain and hidden costs of carers). There is increasing recognition that access to pain management is a fundamental human right (Brennan *et al.* 2007) and that (in addition to pulse, respiration, blood pressure and temperature) pain should be treated as the '5th Vital Sign' (Jackson 2002) requiring assessment and monitoring.

Despite the continuing increase in numbers of older people as a proportion of the population, the assessment and management of pain in older people remains to be adequately addressed and presents particular challenges in terms of the complications and comorbidities associated with ageing, limited research into the applicability of existing interventions developed for younger populations, and attitudinal barriers.

Although there are many similarities between acute pain, chronic pain, cancer pain and non-cancer pain in terms of neural mechanisms and management, there are also important differences. For these reasons, and because chronic pain is increasingly recognised as a condition in its own right (Niv & Devor 2007), the focus of this chapter is on non-cancer pain (in particular chronic pain). This chapter addresses the key issues identified in the early chapters of this book in the context of pain, as illustrated in Figure 12.1.

We begin this chapter by looking at the scope of the problem of pain in older people through epidemiological studies and we address issues around the definition of pain and

Evidence Informed Nursing with Older People, First Edition. Edited by Debbie Tolson, Joanne Booth and Irene Schofield.
© 2011 Blackwell Publishing Ltd. Published 2011 by Blackwell Publishing Ltd.

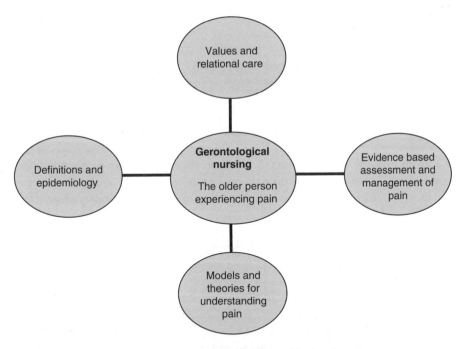

Figure 12.1 Evidence informed nursing of older people with chronic pain.

chronic pain in particular. This information is then put in the context of the theory base that informs best practice in the assessment and management of pain. An essential requirement of professional practice is that it is informed by the best available research and we highlight some of the evidence supporting current interventions for chronic pain in older people. Of course evidence based practice is not just about the research; it should be remembered that it is about the use of the best available evidence in combination with clinical reasoning and knowledge of the values and preferences of the client. To this end we consider the application of the principles and evidence of pain management in the context of caring values and relational care.

Pain and ageing: definitions and epidemiology

The first issue to clarify relates to who we are talking about when we refer to older people. There is no objective definition and the point at which a person becomes defined as an older person is influenced by politics (the point at which people begin to experience discrimination on the basis of age), organisational pragmatism (what are the age limits for using a service), and epidemiology (at what point do most people begin to experience noticeable declines in biological systems and/or functional capacity). Participants in research into pain in older people have ranged from mid-50s to over 80 (Gagliese 2009). We take a pragmatic approach in this chapter, using the definition of older people as it appears in the literature referred to.

Pain and chronic pain

Pain is often thought of as a sensation but is more accurately conceived of as a perception (like vision, or hearing, smell or touch) and as such is subject to the same kind of influences (memory, mood, context, culture, etc.). It is more than simply the stimulation of receptors (called nociceptors) in the peripheral nervous system that are sensitive to actual or potential tissue damage. For reasons that will be explained later it is preferable to refer to these structures as damage receptors rather than pain receptors. It is well known that people can experience pain (and display all the physiological responses associated with pain) in the absence of tissue damage and have evident major tissue damage and yet report no pain. These features of the pain experience are reflected in the definition provided by the International Association for the Study of Pain in their widely accepted definition of pain (Mersky & Bogduk 1994, p. 210):

> *An unpleasant sensory and emotional experience associated with actual or potential tissue damage, or described in terms of such damage.*

The picture becomes more complicated when we consider the often made distinction between acute and chronic pain. Acute pain is commonly described in terms of tissue damage resulting from trauma (accidental or surgical) and some diseases that lead to the activation of nociceptors; it is considered to be relatively short-lived (Loeser & Melzack 1999). Bonica (1990), one of the central figures in the development of pain medicine, drew attention to the fact that acute pain serves the function of alerting the individual to the fact that something is wrong and acts as a stimulus to seek help or engage in some behaviour that promotes healing or prevents further injury. By contrast, he noted, chronic pain serves no such simple biological function but does have severe emotional, physical, social and economic consequences for the individual and society.

Although such definitions emphasise biological events, Carr and Goudas (1999) have noted that patients' attitudes, beliefs and context influence the experience of acute pain and that the division of pain into acute and chronic are problematic. Of course the attitudes, beliefs and behaviours of health professionals also contribute to that experience.

Epidemiology

Difficulties in distinguishing between acute and chronic pain complicate the efforts of epidemiologists to quantify the incidence (number of new cases of a disease appearing per year) and prevalence (number of people with the disease at a point in time) of chronic pain. Nevertheless, it is clear that pain is a common problem amongst older people. Although methods to measure pain prevalence in the older age group vary between studies, there is clear evidence that the prevalence of a number of pain conditions (e.g. hip, knee, shoulder and widespread body pain) increases with age (Macfarlane *et al.* 2005). Further, a recent study of persons initially free of pain demonstrated that, over a 3-year period, the onset of 'pain that interferes with life' increased from 16% in persons aged 50–59 years to 35% in those aged over 80 years (Thomas *et al.* 2004). Thus, older people are more susceptible to the experience of pain than any other age group in society

(Pickering *et al.* 2006). This increase in pain can be explained in part by a number of known risk factors that increase with older age, for example reduced physical activity (Evenson *et al.* 2002) and increased morbidities. At a social level Peat *et al.* (2004) demonstrated that being widowed and the absence of close friends and relatives were significantly associated with functionally disabling pain.

In addition to the increase in risk factors for chronic pain in older people, the impact of pain becomes more noticeable with greater negative consequences for independence and well-being (Thomas *et al.* 2004). These consequences include helplessness, depression, isolation, family breakdown and functional impairment (Cornell Institute for Translational Research on Aging 2006). Chronic pain affects not only the individual but also those around them, as can be seen in terms of personal costs to carers facing increased responsibilities and, more generally, economic costs to the healthcare system (Smith *et al.* 2001; Picker Institute 2007).

The effective assessment and management of pain requires an understanding of the neural mechanisms of pain and an appropriate model to assist the clinician in framing intervention.

Models and theories for understanding pain

Different models and theories for understanding pain have been evident throughout history. As Hanson and Gerber (1990) have noted, patients and professionals hold a conceptual model of pain that will determine treatments that are both offered and considered acceptable. Professionals not specialised in this area do not necessarily share this broader picture and their inappropriate biases and assumptions can lead to a breakdown in client–professional relationships and confusion on the part of the patient (Nielson 2001).

The biomedical model of pain

A conceptual model of pain commonly held by patients and clinicians can be labelled the biomedical model. Box 12.1 outlines key features of a biomedical model of pain (Bendelow & Williams 1995; Main & Spanswick 2000).

Box 12.1   Key features of a biomedical model of pain

- Pain = harm (if it hurts there must be damage occurring and you should stop what you are doing).
- A simple 1 : 1 relationship between tissue damage and pain (more pain means more damage).
- A focus on sensation and a separation between mind and body (pain is physical and if no physical cause is evident or the response is disproportionate to the amount of tissue damage, then it must be psychological).

This model leads to curative and symptom-focused approaches that attempt to resolve or correct underlying pathology or relieve specific symptoms (Hanson & Gerber 1990). Whilst this approach has some value in dealing with acute pain, practitioners who base their understanding of chronic pain within this model can become frustrated with individuals who still report pain after healing time has thought to have occurred, or in the absence of ongoing tissue damage. In the absence of pain relief from increasing doses of stronger and stronger drugs, they may infer that patient reports of pain are motivated by psychological problems or that they are 'malingering' (Nielson 2001). People with chronic pain themselves may begin to doubt their own experience and as a result are faced with challenges to self and identity (Bury 1991; Kelly & Field 1996).

It is now well recognised that tissue healing does not always stop pain, that neurobiological changes can long outlast tissue damage and that pain is not *either* biological *or* psychological. An alternative to the biomedical perspective is a biopsychosocial model (associated with the work of Engel 1977) and when applied to pain and its management this model views pain as a multidimensional experience that incorporates sensory, emotional, affective, cognitive, behavioural and interactional (people and the environment) elements. The next section reviews key features of biopsychosocial models of pain.

Biopsychosocial pain models

Multidimensional (biopsychosocial) models of pain have been proposed by a number of pain experts (Loeser 1982; Hanson & Gerber 1990; Waddell & Main 1998). Such models shift the emphasis from biomedical attempts to 'cure' chronic pain to the involvement of patients in 'managing' their pain. The following statement by Hanson and Gerber (1990, p. 57) makes a distinction between the classical biomedical model and a broader biopsychosocial model regarding the management of pain:

> *The foundation for self-management is the biopsychosocial model of pain. We suggest that more effective control over chronic pain requires a thorough and accurate understanding of the nature of pain. Dualistic notions that consider pain as either entirely physical or psychological must be abandoned. All pain involves a combination of biological or physiological factors, psychological factors (mental, emotional and behavioural) and social-environmental factors.*

Since the effect of pain on the life of the sufferer is multidimensional, involving a combination of biological, psychological and social–environmental factors, current best practice in pain assessment and management reflects the importance of these components of the pain experience. An understanding of the neural mechanisms of pain provides a scientific basis for the validity of this model.

Neural mechanisms of pain

There are whole books and chapters in books dedicated to explaining the neural mechanisms of pain and it is beyond the scope of this chapter to go into great detail on this topic. For more in-depth information an excellent resource is the book by Butler and Moseley

---

Box 12.2   Pain mechanisms: key messages

- Tissue damage is neither necessary nor sufficient for the experience of pain (Butler & Moseley 2008).
- Because pain is a perception constructed in the brain, it is best to avoid talking about pain receptors or (use the technical term 'nociceptor' or 'danger/damage detectors' if using lay language).
- Events in the peripheral nervous system and spinal cord are important, but the experience of pain is crucially determined by complex interactions within and between higher centres in the brain.

(2008) that provides a user-friendly introduction to pain written with professionals and their patients in mind. The following summary of mechanisms is influenced by this text and the key messages are summarised in Box 12.2.

Damage detection

Pain specialists make a distinction between 'nociception', the activation of nerve endings sensitive to noxious stimulus, and 'pain', a perception occurring in the brain (Johnson 1997; Jones 1997; Butler & Moseley 2008). Nociceptors are nerve endings found in skin and deep tissues (such as muscles and joints and viscera) and are activated by stimuli associated with actual or *potential* tissue damage (Mannion & Woolf 2000). There are different classes of nociceptive afferent fibres. Aδ (delta) fibres are high-threshold mechanoreceptors; they are small myelinated fibres with distinctive receptive fields that respond to intense (high-threshold) mechanical stimuli (Galea 2002). These fibres transmit nerve impulses at up to 30 metres per second and are associated with the initial 'sharp' sensation when we injure ourselves. C fibres are smaller still and unmyelinated. They therefore carry signals at a much slower rate than Aδ fibres (up to 2 metres per second). These fibres are responsible for the 'dull', 'aching' experience. Because they respond to mechanical, thermal and chemical (including the body's own chemicals) stimuli, they are known as polymodal nociceptors (Sukiennik & Wittink 2002).

From nociception to pain perception

Figure 12.2 provides a simplified overview of the process of pain perception. Under normal circumstances, actual or potential tissue damage causes particular types of nerve fibre to fire off signals. This process is called transduction: the conversion of one type of stimulus into an electrical signal. However, this is only the start of a process that includes transmission and interpretation (perception) of the signal. There is also another element that is considered in this section called modulation (modifications to the transmission of the signal through the system).

Before pain can be perceived the nociceptive signal must travel along the primary afferent nerve to the spinal cord. In the spinal cord this nerve fibre may synapse with many neurones, each of which also receives inputs from other afferent fibres or from systems descending

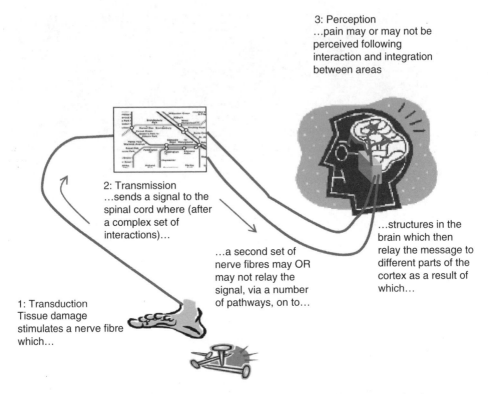

Figure 12.2   Simplified illustration of the stages in the process of perception of pain.

from higher brain centres. As a result of these interactions the modulated nociceptive signal may or may not begin the second stage of its journey on to the brain. On the second stage of the journey the noxious information is transmitted along multiple parallel pathways (Hunt & Mantyh 2002). Nociceptive information arriving in the brain via this route is projected to multiple areas of the brain. These areas include the hypothalamus (with links to the autonomic, endocrine and immune systems), the limbic system (which influences mood and emotional response) and the frontal lobe, which is involved in the cognitive evaluation of pain (meaning, and subsequent motor planning in order to escape from the stimulus) (Johnson 1997; Treede *et al.* 1999). The existence of these different pathways and their onward projections highlights the important role of thoughts and feelings about pain and provides the theoretical basis for psychological interventions in pain management and emphasises the importance of seeing pain as a holistic experience rather than a simple sensation.

The preceding information has considered the major pathways for transmission of nociceptive messages. However, at various stages of its journey the nociceptive signal can be altered or blocked and this process is called modulation.

Pain modulation

The transmission of the nociceptive signal can be modulated (altered) at all levels, including the peripheral nerve endings, spinal cord, brainstem and cortex. The interaction of incoming information from the peripheral nervous system with information from structures within the cortex concerned with emotion, memory and cognition determines the perception of pain. Pain perception is affected by cognitive processes related to attention and distraction, independent of the scale of tissue damage (Peyron *et al.* 2003). Other cognitive processes that may negatively influence the endogenous opioid system (the body's own analgesic system) include anxiety, depression, past pain experiences, and attitudes and beliefs (Watson 1982; Benedetti *et al.* 2003). Understanding of the complex interactions taking place within the cortex reinforces the importance of a biopsychosocial model of pain and its use.

The neuromatrix

The concept of the neuromatrix represents a development of the highly influential gate control theory and takes into account genetic influences and neural–hormonal mechanisms of stress (Melzack 1999). The neuromatrix is the entire nervous system as influenced by genetic factors and the environment through sensory input. Melzack (1999) proposed that the neuromatrix is profoundly influenced by the effect of the stress hormone cortisol. The impact of stress on the neuromatrix highlights the important role of psychosocial interventions.

Neuropathic pain

The material discussed up to this point has been concerned with pain arising from the stimulation of nociceptors by tissue damage and inflammation (as in the case of rheumatoid arthritis for example), typically referred to as nociceptive pain. Neuropathic (or pathological) pain is pain resulting from nerves that have altered their functioning and in this situation there may or may not be clear evidence of damage (Koltzenburg 2002). The nerves affected can be in the peripheral or central nervous system and examples include phantom limb pain, post-herpetic neuralgia and complex regional pain syndrome (Basbaum & Bushnell 2002).

Pain mechanisms and ageing

A number of changes have been identified that have important implications for the assessment and management of pain in older people. These are summarised in Box 12.3 (Gibson 2005; Fine 2009).

Box 12.3   Pain mechanisms and ageing

- The increase in pain perception threshold and the widespread change in the structure and function of peripheral and central nociceptive pathways may place the older person at greater risk of injury (actual or potential damage is less easily recognised).
- Reduced efficacy of endogenous analgesic systems, a decreased tolerance of pain and the slower resolution of post-injury hyperalgesia (increased sensitivity to stimuli that may result in pain) may make it more difficult for the older adult to cope, once injury has occurred.

Ageing also leads to degenerative changes within all structures of the spine which may lead to pain. Furthermore, the influence of lifestyle, genetics and the environment over the lifespan leads to greater variability in physiology amongst older people; as a result, in the management of pain the importance of focusing on the individual is heightened.

Evidence based assessment and management

Issues around the selection and use of measurement tools for pain research purposes are complicated by debates about validity and reliability and sensitivity to change. These issues are important given that good assessment forms the basis of pain management and it is important that tools that are easy to use and interpret are available for use in the clini-cal setting. Fortunately, 2007 saw the publication of guidelines (jointly produced by the British Pain Society and British Geriatric Society) that point the busy clinician in the right direction, with examples of suitable measures and a step-by-step procedure (algorithm) to follow. The guideline directs all healthcare professionals to 'think about the possibility of pain in all contacts with older people, enquire about it routinely, be aware of behaviours that indicate underlying pain and have pathways for management' (British Pain Society and British Geriatrics Society 2007, p. 4).

Because pain is a perception and tissue damage is neither necessary nor sufficient for the experience of pain, self-report measures are the gold standard. There is no objective measure of pain and McCaffery back in 1968 proposed the influential definition of pain as 'whatever the person experiencing the pain says it is' (McCaffery & Ferrell 1996).

This next section deals with general issues around pain assessment in older people. The more complex task of assessing pain in cognitively and/or sensory impaired older people is outwith the scope of this chapter.

Pain assessment

The first step in pain assessment is to simply ask as part of routine assessment if an older person is sore, aching or hurting anywhere. These terms may well produce different responses to asking outright if a person is in pain. Depending on the response to this ques-tion further enquiries should attempt to identify the nature of the sensation being com-municated (stabbing, throbbing, like an electric shock, etc.), its location (outlines of the human figure that can be drawn on are helpful here) and the intensity of the sensation.

Research into the measurement and assessment of pain has identified that numeric rat-ing scales and verbal descriptor scales are useful in assessing pain intensity, while the McGill Pain Questionnaire is good for assessing the qualities and location of pain. Questions have been raised about the ability of visual analogue scales to capture pain intensity adequately in older people (Gibson 2006; Gagliese 2009).

As the biopsychosocial model suggests, it is important that we capture not only the bio-logical aspects of the pain experience (intensity, quality and location) but also the psychologi-cal and functional aspects. Depression is a common comorbidity for pain and psychological distress in general is an important factor to assess given its ability to exacerbate the pain experience (as understanding of neural mechanisms and the role of emotional centres in the brain demonstrates). Many tools for assessing mood and functional assessments are readily available and suitable for use with older people who do not have cognitive impairments. However, in a busy clinical environment the Brief Pain Inventory has much to offer (Keller *et al.* 2004). The Brief Pain Inventory is a freely available 15-item scale assessing pain severity, impact on daily living, and impact on mood and enjoyment of life; it is quick and easy to administer and score, and is recommended by the British Pain Society and British Geriatrics Society (2007). For a detailed review of the assessment of pain in older adults, an interdisciplinary expert consensus statement on assessment of pain in older persons is available (Hadjistavropoulos *et al.* 2007).

Of course assessment of pain is of little value if findings are not acted upon using evidence based interventions.

Evidence based pain management

The biopsychosocial model underpins the assessment and management of pain. It follows that if pain assessment should be multidimensional, it is also important that pain management takes into account all aspects of the pain experience. Pharmacological and other physical interventionist modalities (e.g. spinal cord stimulation) can play an important role in modulating activity within the CNS; however, the psychological response to pain also needs to be addressed and strategies provided to manage the functional consequences of pain. Of course all these aspects are connected, so addressing one on its own may have some impact but not as great as addressing all.

One limitation of the research into the treatment of pain in older people is that much of the existing evaluations do not include older people within the sample; thus whilst there is good evidence from systematic reviews and randomised controlled trials into the effectiveness of certain interventions, we cannot be sure if these findings apply to older people. Indeed Gibson (2006) has highlighted that until relatively recently older people in the USA were actually excluded from pharmacotherapy trials. Similarly, the evidence supporting multidisciplinary pain management programmes is compromised by the fact that older people are under-represented in referral to this kind of service (which is often limited in availability to begin with). The next section focuses on those approaches to pain management that nurses may find themselves involved with.

Pharmacology

Nurses have a key role to play in the pharmacological management of pain, both in the administration and monitoring of drugs but also (following the 2000 NHS Plan) increasing authority for suitably qualified nurses to independently prescribe non-controlled drugs.

As highlighted in the section on neural mechanisms, research suggests age-related changes in a number of important body systems; this in turn has important implications for the pharmacological management of pain in older people. Freedman (2002) and Fine (2009) highlighted anatomical and physiological changes in the heart, liver, kidneys and other body systems that all have the potential to impact upon drug concentrations and metabolism and as a result there may be increased side effects and risk of toxicity.

American Geriatric Society (2009) guidelines on the management of pain in older people paid particular attention to pharmacology. Original guidelines recommended older people use over-the-counter or prescription non-steroidal anti-inflammatory drugs (NSAIDs) or cyclooxygenase (COX)-2 inhibitors such as aspirin or ibuprofen before being prescribed an opioid drug. The updated guidelines pointed to newer information suggesting that this is a risky strategy in older persons (because of increased cardiovascular risk and gastrointestinal toxicity). These risks were judged to outweigh the benefits and, as a result, the guidelines were revised to reflect newer clinical trials and clinical observation findings. The result was a recommendation that NSAIDs and COX-2 inhibitors be used only in highly specific individuals. The guidelines recommend that all patients with moderate to severe pain or diminished quality of life due to pain should be considered for opioid therapy.

Guidelines such as those produced by the American Geriatric Society are important because in older people with pain pharmaceutical management predominates. Hanlon *et al.* (2005) reported that over half of community-dwelling older persons report analgesic use, most commonly NSAIDs, paracetamol or opioids. Denneboom *et al.* (2006) demonstrated that in around one-third of community-dwelling older persons, improvements to their medication could be identified which were considered to be of direct clinical relevance, indicating that these individuals may be getting insufficient pain relief and/or suboptimal other medication. Others have found that older adults living both in the community and in institutional settings receive less potent analgesia (Zyczkowska *et al.* 2007), but that adverse effects of analgesics are more common in this age group (Ruoff 1998). This suggests that additional non-pharmaceutical pain management strategies need to be developed alongside the use of medication in order to deliver the best possible pain management in older people (Gibson 2006). A cognitive behavioural approach is seen as key to the management of chronic pain and a range of interventions has demonstrated varying degrees of efficacy when delivered using the principles of cognitive behavioural therapy (Gibson 2006; Lunde *et al.* 2009). Box 12.4 details the central assumptions of this approach (Turk & Meichenbaum 1994).

Box 12.4   Principles of cognitive behavioural therapy applied to pain management

- People actively process (interpret) information from the senses.
- What people think influences how they feel both emotionally and in terms of physiological responses (sympathetic nervous system responses).
- Thoughts act as a driver for behaviour.
- Behaviour is influenced by individual and environmental factors.
- People can learn positive ways of thinking which in turn influences feeling and behaviour.
- Individuals should be active collaborators with health professionals in bringing about change.

> **Box 12.5**   Key components of multidisciplinary pain management programmes
>
> - Education about pain mechanisms, the psychology of pain (links between fear of pain and avoidance of activity; stress, and depression) and effective use of medication.
> - Exercise to improve physical conditioning.
> - Advantages and disadvantages of assistive devices.
> - Setting goals and pacing activity levels.
> - Relaxation.

Multidisciplinary pain management programmes often involve nurse pain specialists and use a cognitive behavioural therapy approach to deliver a number of interventions (key components of pain management programmes are detailed in Box 12.5; British Pain Society 2007).

There is good evidence from systematic reviews and meta-analysis to support the effectiveness of pain management programmes in the adult population (Morley *et al.* 1999; Guzmán *et al.* 2002; Hoffman *et al.* 2007) and there is some evidence to support the use of this type of programme with older people (Gibson 2006). However, it has been shown that older adults are rarely referred to pain management programmes (Kee *et al.* 1998; Spiers 2006).

A meta-analytic review of the effectiveness of cognitive behavioural therapy based approaches for older people (outwith formal multidisciplinary pain management programmes) covering 16 separate interventions found evidence for effectiveness on self-reported pain experience but limited impact on symptoms of depression, physical functioning and medication usage (Lunde *et al.* 2009). These findings support the importance of multidimensional approaches to pain management.

Pain management programmes are not the only services designed to focus on helping participants to play an active part in the management of their healthcare. A focus on self-management (as envisaged in the UK within the NHS Expert Patient Programme; see www.nhs.uk/conditions/Expert-patients-programme-/Pages/Introduction.aspx) is increasingly a feature of health policy and this approach shares many principles with pain management programmes.

Self-management

Self-management is a term that is widely used but can be difficult to pin down: it can be used to refer to treatments or self-designed protocols autonomously accessed and controlled by individuals (e.g. use of over-the-counter medications or alternative and complementary therapies) or to approaches based on the Chronic Disease Self Management Programme originally designed by Kate Lorig in the USA (Lorig 1996) (see Box 12.6 for key features of this approach).

Box 12.6   Key assumptions of the Chronic Disease Self Management Programme (Lorig 1996)

- A belief that people with chronic diseases are faced with common problems in managing the consequences of their illnesses.
- People can learn to manage their own health on a day-to-day basis.
- Success in self-management improves health status and reduces use of services.

A narrative review of chronic disease self-management programmes by Jonker *et al.* (2009) found good evidence for an increase in physical exercise, decrease in health distress, improvement in self-care and beneficial effects on self-efficacy. Although chronic disease self-management programmes typically involve trained laypersons delivering at least part of the programme, the evidence for this as a requirement for positive outcomes is equivocal (Bury *et al.* 2005).

Assistive devices

Although traditionally associated with occupational therapists, the prescription of assistive devices is also a role that can be undertaken by community-based nurses in particular. Assistive devices are prescribed to prevent further impairment, compensate for range of motion restrictions, promote safety, and manage pain during self-care and other activities of daily living (Klinger & Spaulding 2001).

Mann *et al.* (1999) conducted a high-quality randomised controlled trial in the USA of an assistive devices/environmental adaptations service designed to maintain independence and reduce home care costs for the frail elderly. The service, led by an occupational therapist (assisted by a nurse and technician), provided a comprehensive functional assessment, provision of devices and home modifications as required, training in their use and continued follow-up and additional assessment and provision as required. Although over an 18-month period there was a significant decrease in function for the intervention group, there was significantly *greater* decline for the control group. Pain also increased significantly more for the control group.

The potential of specialist equipment to have a positive impact on the quality of life of older people with chronic pain is illustrated by the following quote from a nursing home resident as reported in a study by the Picker Institute (2007, p. 20):

> *I mean this bed has made a big difference ... it's really marvellous because I mean you can adjust it to what you want ... but this mattress has made a heck of a difference, otherwise I should think I would be ... I'd probably have a lot more aches than what I have.* (Woman aged 79 years)

The same report also drew attention to the potential of equipment to cause pain rather than alleviate it:

They tried to use the hoist but I don't want it, with my shoulders being painful it hurts me ... (Man aged 95 years)

Applying the biopsychosocial model of pain within gerontological practice

The biopsychosocial model of pain has been crucial in informing the development of pain assessment and management. It has emphasised that pain has a biological basis and that evokes an interpretation and response at a psychological level and that this response is influenced by the social environment in which this takes place. The biopsychosocial model has also drawn attention to the influence of social variables such as age, gender, culture and socioeconomic status on the pain experience. However, within the pain literature there has been less attention to how social context shapes care, how care is conceptualised or how 'patient'–professional relationships are understood.

Pain and caring values

Caring remains a core (if complex) value of nursing practice and what it means to be cared for may vary according to each patient or situation. For example the older person who is experiencing pain may have different requirements than the person who is experiencing loss or who is dying. An essential element of caring does appear to be the personal nature of the relationship. The following quote is from a participant in a seminar series involving the authors of this chapter and illustrates the importance of the personal aspect of care:

> *I'm admitted to hospital, I'm unwell, in pain, out of my comfort zone and confused in an unusual environment. I need care and the one I turn to is the nurse ... the fundamental [behaviours] are those that reassure me and help my progress on the hospital journey, the more 'personal' actions. That belief is confirmed by my memory of past events. I clearly remember and am convinced that these 'personal' behaviours of nurses helped me benefit from treatment.* (An older man with chronic pain)

Other chapters in this book have highlighted that many healthcare settings have value statements and philosophies that are designed to demonstrate organisational commitment to promoting good-quality care. This is all irrelevant if the staff delivering that care do not have the caring attributes (attitudes, beliefs and behaviour) to deliver such philosophies. Fox (1995) drew attention to sociological analyses of care that have distinguished between 'care for' a person and 'care about' a person. He highlighted a tension between care delivered within the confines of rational/scientific procedures of a professional discipline (disciplinary care, or 'care for') and care delivered with a focus on respectful relationships (care as 'gift', or 'care about'). This type of conceptualisation of care and those highlighted in this book are increasingly influencing policy (and hopefully) practice.

> ### Box 12.7   The New Pain Manifesto
>
> - Education: so that pain is an integral part of all professional training.
> - Empowerment: to support people to make decisions about their condition.
> - Collaboration: so that all stakeholders share in a joined-up patient strategy.
> - Early access: to prevent acute pain becoming chronic pain.
> - Measurement: of pain as the fifth vital sign.

A recent initiative bringing together patients, carers, politicians and professionals is the Chronic Pain Policy Coalition (www.paincoalition.org.uk/cppc), whose New Pain Manifesto is detailed in Box 12.7 (Chronic Pain Policy Coalition 2007).

Helping to manage pain is an essential attribute of caring that appreciates the impact of persistent pain on an individual and their quality of life, and so regardless of the situation, relief of pain is a fundamental human right (Brennan *et al.* 2007) and failure to attempt to relieve pain constitutes neglect of care and so breaches that concept of care promoted by this book.

Despite the increasing recognition of the destructive impact of poorly managed pain (across the lifespan), deficiencies in service provision and the attitudes and behaviours of some professionals persist. It is widely believed that with increasing age comes the potential for increased pain and that this is wrongly believed to be an inevitable consequence of normal ageing (Cowan *et al.* 2003). One of the consequences of this belief was highlighted by the Picker Institute (2007) who found that more than 39% of carers said that healthcare professionals 'never' or 'only occasionally' reviewed patients' pain levels.

Older patients themselves often have a strong desire to be a 'good patient', one who does not complain, who accepts pain and the lack of treatment as normal (Sofaer-Bennett *et al.* 2007). A report on older people and pain commissioned by Help the Aged (now Age UK) reported reflections and experiences of pain from an older person's perspective and highlighted similar themes, in particular the loss of dignity and ability to engage in meaningful activities (Kumar & Allcock 2008).

Misconceptions around pain in later life lead to barriers amongst patients and healthcare workers which, ultimately, may result in poor pain management for this population. A range of strategies are usually delivered by pain services, although provision varies across the UK and they are not likely to be as easily available and accessible to older adults (Spiers 2006).

Two reports of note highlight the experiences of older people with pain and the inadequate response of healthcare professionals in terms of clinical management but also, more importantly, the lack of care demonstrated in some cases. Qualitative research commissioned by the Patients Association into pain and older people in residential care (Picker Institute 2007) reflected many of the findings already highlighted in this chapter, noting problems around the review of medication (and limited effort to support concordance with recommended protocols), people suffering in silence as a result of a combination of stoicism on the part of the older person and failure to enquire about pain by care home staff, and lack of support for residents' own efforts to relieve pain.

This last point is illustrated by a quote from one woman interviewed for the report:

> *The only one that I had any help from was a TENS machine, but I had to stop using that because I couldn't put it on for myself. That was for my back when the vertebrae collapsed... and I don't think they want to be bothered here.* (Woman aged 82 years)

Whilst it is clear that limited resources, poor management and other organisational barriers have some responsibility for poor pain management, the following quotes from the report highlight the responsibility of individuals and the importance of the concept of care held by staff. These quotes illustrate variation in staff attitudes and behaviour, sometimes within the same care home:

> *Some are better than others and that's it... there's a certain few that are really very, very good and you can tell that they're... you know they're different from the rest, so I mean you have to be thankful for those people.* (Woman aged 79 years)

> *They're excellent staff, I mean I know as I say I've worked in places like this and half the time the staff never took any notice of you at all but these do, they're always there if you need them and the night staff as well.* (Woman aged 83 years)

The second publication (Kumar & Allcock 2008) reported reflections and experiences of pain from an older person's perspective and highlighted similar themes, in particular the loss of dignity and ability to engage in meaningful activities.

Summary

Pain is a complex biopsychosocial phenomenon that is a significant problem for older people and which is often poorly assessed and managed. Organisational barriers (low levels of staff, inadequate resources, poor integration of services across agencies, lack of services and waiting lists for non-pharmacological treatments such as pain management programmes) inevitably make the provision of care difficult. Also the attitudes of older people (acceptance of pain as inevitable, dislike of medication, not wanting to make a fuss, expectation that professionals know best) can also be a challenge to nurses who want to do the right thing and engage patients with their own management. However, what has been said emphasises that there are steps that individuals can take to improve quality of life and these are grounded in the quality of relationship staff have with their patients. This does not require material resources, rather the development of attitudes and beliefs that build on the key messages delivered by this chapter.

Key messages

- Pain is not inevitable.
- Pain is what the person says it is.
- Pain is multidimensional and requires attention to the emotional and psychosocial impact.
- Older people may be more not less susceptible to pain than younger populations.
- Older people may be reluctant to report pain out of stoicism or reluctance to make a fuss, therefore suitable assessment strategies need to be in place that give the opportunity (and permission) to report pain.
- Multidimensional approaches that recognise the importance of relationships are required to manage pain.

References

American Geriatric Society (2009) Pharmacological management of persistent pain in older persons. *Journal of the American Geriatric Society* **57**, 1331–1346.

Basbaum A, Bushnell MC (2002) Pain: basic mechanisms. In: Giambardino MA (ed.) *Pain 2002: an Updated Review*. IASP Press, Seattle, pp. 3–10.

Bendelow GA, Williams SJ (1995) Transcending the dualisms: towards a sociology of pain. *Sociology of Health and Illness* **17**, 140–165.

Benedetti F, Pollo A, Maggie G, Vighetti S, Rainero I (2003) Placebo analgesia: from physiological mechanisms to clinical implications. In: Dostrovsky JO, Carr DB, Koltzenburg M (eds) *Proceedings of the 10th World Congress on Pain*. Progress in Pain Research and Management 24. IASP Press, Seattle, pp. 315–323.

Bonica JJ (1990) Definitions and taxonomy of pain. In: Bonica JJ (ed.) *The Management of Pain*. Lea and Febiger, Philadelphia.

Brennan F, Carr DB, Cousins M (2007) Pain management: a fundamental human right. *Anesthesia and Analgesia* **105**, 205–221.

British Pain Society (2007) *Recommended Guidelines for Pain Management Programmes for Adults*. British Pain Society, London.

British Pain Society and British Geriatrics Society (2007) *Guidance on the Assessment of Pain in Older People*. British Pain Society and British Geriatrics Society, London.

Bury M (1991) The sociology of chronic illness: a review of research and prospects. *Sociology of Health and Illness* **13**, 451–468.

Bury M, Newbould J, Taylor D (2005) *A Rapid Review of the Current State of Knowledge Regarding Lay Led Self Management of Chronic Illness*. National Institute for Health and Clinical Excellence, London.

Butler DS, Moseley L (2008) *Explain Pain*. Noigroup Publications, Adelaide.

Carr DB, Goudas LC (1999) Acute pain. *Lancet* **353**, 2051–2058.

Chronic Pain Policy Coalition (2007) *Our Campaign*. Available at www.paincoalition.org.uk/cppc/our-campaign (accessed 14 May 2010).

Cornell Institute for Translational Research on Aging (2006) *Taking Community Action Against Pain: Translating Research on Chronic Pain Among Older Adults*. Available at www.citra.org/Assets/documents/pain%20conference%20summary.pdf (accessed 12 May 2010).

Cowan DT, Fitzpatrick JM, Roberts JD, While AE, Baldwin J (2003) The assessment and management of pain among older people in care homes current status and future directions. *International Journal of Nursing Studies* **40**, 291–298.

Denneboom W, Dautzenberg MG, Grol R, De Smet PA (2006) Analysis of polypharmacy in older patients in primary care using a multidisciplinary expert panel. *British Journal of General Practice* **56**, 504–510.

Engel GL (1977) The need for a new medical model: a challenge for biomedicine. *Science* **196**, 129–136.

Evenson KR, Rosamond WD, Cai J, Diez-Roux AV, Brancati FL (2002) Influence of retirement on leisure-time physical activity: the Atherosclerosis Risk in Communities Study. *American Journal of Epidemiology* **155**, 692–699.

Fine PG (2009) Chronic pain management in older adults: special considerations. *Journal of Pain and Symptom Management* **38**, S4–S14.

Fox N (1995) Postmodern perspectives on care: the vigil and the gift. *Critical Social Policy* **15**, 107–123.

Freedman GM (2002) Clinical management of common causes of geriatric pain. *Geriatrics* **57**, 36–41.

Gagliese L (2009) Pain and aging: the emergence of a new subfield of pain research. *Journal of Pain* **10**, 343–353.

Galea MP (2002) Neuroanatomy of the nociceptive system. In: Strong J, Unruh AM, Wright A, Baxter GD (eds) *Pain: a Textbook for Therapists*. Churchill Livingstone, Edinburgh.

Gibson SJ (2005) Age differences in psychosocial aspects of pain. In: Gibson SJ, Weiner DK (eds) *Pain in Older Persons*. Progress in Pain Research and Management 35. IASP Press, Seattle, pp. 87–107.

Gibson SJ (2006) Older people's pain. *Pain Clinical Updates XIV* (3). IASP, Seattle.

Guzmán J, Esmail R, Karjalainen K, Malmivaara A, Irvin E, Bombardier C (2002) Multidisciplinary bio-psycho-social rehabilitation for chronic low back pain. *Cochrane Database of Systematic Reviews* (1), CD000963. Update *Cochrane Database of Systematic Reviews* 2006 (2), CD000963

Hadjistavropoulos T, Herr K, Turk DC *et al.* (2007) Interdisciplinary expert consensus statement on assessment of pain in older persons. *Clinical Journal of Pain* 23, S1–S43.

Hanlon JT, Guary DR, Ives TJ (2005) Oral analgesics: efficacy, mechanism of action, pharmacokinetics, adverse effects, drug interactions, and practical recommendations for use in older adults. In: Gibson SJ, Weiner DK (eds) *Pain in Older Persons*. Progress in Pain Research and Management 35. IASP Press, Seattle, pp. 111–134.

Hanson RW, Gerber KE (1990) *Coping with Chronic Pain: a Guide to Self-management*. Guilford Press, New York.

Hoffman BM, Papas RK, Chatkoff DK, Kerns RD (2007) Meta-analysis of psychological interventions for chronic low back pain. *Health Psychology* **26**, 1–9.

Hunt SP, Mantyh PW (2002) Understanding the neurobiology of chronic pain: molecular and cellular biology. In: Giambardino MA (ed.) *Pain 2002: an Updated Review*. IASP Press, Seattle.

Jackson M (2002) *Pain, the 5th Vital Sign*. Random House, Canada.

Johnson MI (1997) The physiology of the sensory dimensions of clinical pain. *Physiotherapy* **83**, 526–536.

Jones AKP (1997) Pain, its perception and imaging. *IASP Newsletter* May/June, 3–5.

Jonker AAGC, Comijs HC, Knipscheer KCPM, Deeg DJH (2009) Promotion of self management in vulnerable older people: a narrative literature review of outcomes of the Chronic Disease Self Management Program. *European Journal of Aging* **6**, 303–314.

Kee WG, Middaugh SJ, Redpath S, Hargadon R (1998) Age as a factor in admission to chronic pain rehabilitation. *Clinical Journal of Pain* **14**, 121–128.

Keller S, Bann CM, Dodd SL, Schein J, Mendoza TR (2004) Validity of the Brief Pain Inventory for use in documenting the outcomes of patients with non cancer pain. *Clinical Journal of Pain* **20**, 309–318.

Kelly MP, Field D (1996) Medical sociology, chronic illness and the body. *Sociology of Health and Illness* **18**, 241–257.

Klinger L, Spaulding SJ (2001) Occupational therapy treatment of chronic pain and use of assistive devices in older adults. *Topics in Geriatric Rehabilitation* **16**, 34–44.

Koltzenburg M (2002) Classification of neuropathic pain. In: Giambardino MA (ed.) *Pain 2002: an Updated Review.* IASP Press, Seattle.

Kumar A, Allcock N (2008) *Pain in Older People: Reflections and Experiences from an Older Person's Perspective.* Help the Aged, London.

Loeser (1982) Concepts of pain. In: Stanton-Hicks M, Boas R (eds) *Chronic Low Back Pain.* Raven Press, New York.

Loeser JD, Melzack R (1999) Pain: an overview. *Lancet* **353**, 1607–1609.

Lorig K (1996) Chronic disease self management: a model for tertiary prevention. *American Behavioral Scientist* **39**, 767–783.

Lunde LH, Nordhus IH, Pallesen S (2009) The effectiveness of cognitive and behavioural treatment of chronic pain in the elderly: a quantitative review. *Journal of Clinical Psychology in Medical Settings* **16**, 254–262.

McCaffery M, Ferrell BR (1996) Correcting misconceptions about pain assessment and use of opioid analgesics: educational strategies aimed at public concerns. *Nursing Outlook* **44**, 184–190.

Macfarlane GJ, Jones GT, McBeth J (2005) Epidemiology of pain. In: McMahon S, Koltzenburg M (eds) *Wall and Melzack's Textbook of Pain.* Churchill Livingstone, Edinburgh.

Main CJ, Spanswick CC (2000) Models of pain. In: Main CJ, Spanswick CC (eds) *Pain Management: An Interdisciplinary Approach.* Churchill Livingstone, Edinburgh.

Mann WC, Ottenbacher KJ, Fraas L, Tomita M, Granger CV (1999) Effectiveness of assistive technology and environmental interventions in maintaining independence and reducing home care costs for the frail elderly. *Archives of Family Medicine* **8**, 210–217.

Mannion RJ, Woolf CJ (2000) Pain mechanisms and management: a central perspective. *Clinical Journal of Pain* **16**, S144–S156.

Melding PS (1991) Is there such a thing as geriatric pain? *Pain* **46**, 119–121.

Melzack R (1999) From the gate to the neuromatrix. *Pain Supplement* **6**, S121–S126.

Mersky H, Bogduk N (1994) Classification of chronic pain. In: Mersky H, Bogduk N (eds) *Definitions of Chronic Pain Syndromes and Definition of Pain Terms*, 2nd edn. IASP, Seattle.

Morley S, Eccleston C, Williams A (1999) Systematic review and meta-analysis of RCT trials of cognitive behaviour therapy and behaviour therapy for chronic pain. *Pain* **80**, 1–13.

Nielson WR (2001) The concept of pain. *Clinical Journal of Pain* **17**, S5–S7.

Niv D, Devor M (2007) Position paper of the European Federation of IASP Chapters (EFIC) on the subject of pain management. *European Journal of Pain* **11**, 487–489.

Peat G, Thomas E, Handy J, Croft P (2004) Social networks and pain interference with daily activities in middle and old age *Pain* **112**, 397–405.

Peyron R, Rainville P, Predrag P, Garcia-Larrea (2003) Cognitive modulation of cortical responses to pain. In: Dostrovsky JO, Carr DB, Koltzenburg M (eds) *Proceedings of the 10th World Congress on Pain.* Progress in Pain Research and Management 24. IASP Press, Seattle, pp. 277–293.

Pickering G, Jourdan D, Dubray C (2006) Acute versus chronic pain in Alzheimer's disease. *European Journal of Pain* **10**, 379–384.

Picker Institute (2007) *Pain in Older People: a Hidden Problem.* The Patients Association, London.

Ruoff G (1998) Management of pain in patients with multiple health problems: a guide for the practising physician. *American Journal of Medicine* **105**, 53S–60S.

Smith BH, Elliott AM, Chambers WA, Cairns Smith W, Hannaford PC, Penny K (2001) The impact of chronic pain in the community. *Family Practice* **18**, 292–299.

Sofaer-Bennett B, Walker J, Moore AP, Lamberty J, Thorp T, O'Dwyer J (2007) Perseverance by older people in the management of chronic pain: a qualitative study. *Pain Medicine* **8**, 263–280.

Spiers JA (2006) Expressing and responding to pain and stoicism in home-care nurse–patient interactions. *Scandinavian Journal of Caring Sciences* **20**, 1–9.

Sukiennik A, Wittink H (2002) Pathophysiology of pain: a primer. In: Wittink H, Hoskins Michel T (eds) *Chronic Pain Management for Physical Therapists*, 2nd edn. Butterworth Heineman, Boston.

Thomas E, Peat G, Harris L, Wilkie R, Croft PR (2004) The prevalence of pain and pain interference in a general population of older adults. *Pain* **110**, 361–368.

Treede R-D, Kenshalo DR, Gracely RH, Jones AKP (1999) The cortical representation of pain. *Pain* **79**, 105–111.

Turk DC, Meichenbaum D (1994) A cognitive-behavioral approach to pain management. In: Wall PD, Melzack R (eds) *Textbook of Pain*. Churchill Livingstone, Edinburgh, pp. 1337–1348.

Waddell G, Main CJ (1998) A new clinical model of low back pain and disability. In: Waddell G (ed.) *The Back Pain Revolution*. Churchill Livingstone, Edinburgh.

Watson J (1982) Endogenous pain control mechanisms. *Australian Journal of Physiotherapy* **28**, 38–45.

Zyczkowska J, Szczerbin'ska K, Jantzi MR, Hirdes JP (2007) Pain among the oldest old in community and institutional settings. *Pain* **129**, 167–176.

Chapter 13

Protecting Older People from Healthcare Associated Infections

Kay Currie and Jacqui Reilly

Defining the nursing practice issue

Infection prevention and control is a key component of providing safe and effective care for all patients, yet advancing age poses an increased risk of infection and greater associated morbidity and mortality. This chapter discusses the nature, prevention and management of healthcare associated infections (HCAI) across the range of care settings that older people may experience, such as general or specialist acute care hospital facilities, community hospital settings, care homes, or indeed the person's own home. The discussion identifies the challenges posed by the most common infections faced at various points on a potential patient journey.

In the following sections, the significance of infection for the older person will be identified through international prevalence data, with evidence of specific risk factors highlighting links to the key clinical features and syndromes of older age identified in Chapter 1. Each section applies evidence drawn from international research and guidelines to common practice issues related to screening for infectious organisms, management of colonisation or infection, and prevention of transmission. Furthermore, the core principles and values of gerontological practice, such as truth-telling, involving patients and their carers in decision-making, and optimising health outcomes, will be explored.

When thinking about the implications of HCAI for older people, it is useful to have an understanding of the terminology often used in relation to research in this area. Box 13.1 gives a brief description of key terms.

Box 13.1   Revision notes: defining infection prevention and control terminology

Healthcare associated infection

HCAI are not present when healthcare begins for a patient, but arise thereafter as an unintended consequence of that healthcare. The simplest definition is: an infection which was not present or was incubating on admission. An arbitrary cut-off time of 48 hours after admission is frequently used to make this judgement (Centers for Disease Control 2008).

Evidence Informed Nursing with Older People, First Edition. Edited by Debbie Tolson, Joanne Booth and Irene Schofield.
© 2011 Blackwell Publishing Ltd. Published 2011 by Blackwell Publishing Ltd.

Colonisation

Colonisation occurs when a patient has an organism, such as meticillin-resistant *Staphylococcus aureus* (MRSA), in or on a body site but has no clinical signs or symptoms of disease. A person colonised with MRSA may be a temporary or a longer-term carrier of MRSA. Certain carriers may shed MRSA into the environment (e.g. patients with dermatitis or burns). Those who carry MRSA are at greater risk of self-infection and cross-transmission of colonisation to others whilst in healthcare environments. The distinction between colonisation and infection is a clinical one. Such a distinction should be determined by signs and symptoms of the infection, not by culture results alone.

Infection

Infection occurs when an organism enters a body site and multiplies in body tissue causing clinical manifestations of disease. This is usually evident by symptoms such as fever, a rise in the white blood cell count, or purulent drainage from a wound or body cavity. Infection is distinct from colonisation, but both play a part in the transmission of HCAI in healthcare settings.

HCAI are monitored and reported in research studies using two main approaches: incidence and prevalence.

Incidence

In an incidence survey, information on a healthcare associated infection in a selected population (e.g. a specialty in a hospital) is gathered by regular observation of that population *over a period of time*. An example of this is patients who have surgery for hip fracture being followed up after the surgery to see if surgical site infection occurs. The follow-up would be to 30 days after operation as the infection would be considered to be related to the surgery up until that point. Therefore, surgical site infection may actually be detected following discharge into other care settings, such as the community, nursing home or rehabilitation unit. Incidence data are helpful in assessing trends in infection rates over time.

Prevalence

In prevalence surveys the number of specified events is counted in a specified population at a point in time (point prevalence) or over a short period (period prevalence). Large well-conducted surveys are helpful in establishing a snap-shot baseline value for a healthcare associated infection and in estimating the burden at a given point or period in time. Repeated, well-designed surveys can also provide useful data on infection trends, whether the number of infections are reducing or increasing, and therefore the efficacy of infection prevention and control measures. However, the results are usually of more limited value than those obtained from incidence studies, which determine the rate of new cases of infection. Prevalence studies are therefore a useful adjunct to other surveillance methods. Most of the information relating to HCAI which has informed policy over the last 25 years has been derived from prevalence surveys.

Having grasped the key terminology, the next section highlights the significance of the problem of HCAI for older people in hospital in terms of prevalence and known risk factors.

The scale of the HCAI problem for older people

Infection prevention and control is a priority in healthcare. HCAI are an important public health threat; they are damaging and distressing, and can cause disability and death. Like many other public health problems, HCAI are substantially preventable, and although governments have called for zero tolerance, the 'irreducible minimum' (or the amount of HCAI that cannot be prevented) remains unknown (National Audit Office 2004). Unlike other infectious diseases, less than 10% of HCAI occur in the context of outbreaks (European Centre for Disease Prevention and Control 2008).

Hundreds of millions of people worldwide every year suffer from HCAI. Estimates of the European burden of HCAI suggest that approximately 4 million people acquire a healthcare associated infection in the EU every year. The consequences of these infections in terms of additional length of stay and associated opportunity costs amount to billions of Euros within the EU each year, and the number of deaths occurring as the direct consequence of these infections is estimated to be at least 37 000 (European Centre for Disease Prevention and Control 2008). The burden of HCAI has been described in individual country point prevalence surveys in the literature in recent years and indicates a prevalence of 3.5–10.5% (European Centre for Disease Prevention and Control 2008). In all these prevalence surveys, advancing age is demonstrated as an independent risk factor for infection. Table 13.1 summarises significant intrinsic and extrinsic risk factors for HCAI in older people.

Table 13.1   Intrinsic and extrinsic risk factors for healthcare associated infections.

Intrinsic risk factors Increasing age Underlying comorbidities, such as diabetes, renal impairment, cancer, immunocompromise, presence of pressure ulcers, exfoliating skin conditions (eczema) depression Nutritional status/body mass index (BMI): very low BMI or very high BMI adds risk Immobility Previous infection
Extrinsic risk factors Extended length of hospital stay Invasive device use (risk increases with increasing time *in situ*), e.g. urinary catheters, central venous lines, peripheral infusions, ventilators Surgery Prior treatment with antibiotics

Increasing age means increasing risk of infection

The increasing number of people over 65 years of age forms a special population at risk for HCAI. A large prospective study of all HCAI in Scotland identified increasing age as an independent risk factor for infection (Reilly *et al.* 2007). Those who were older than 65 years were at risk and there was a linear trend in risk with increasing age thereafter. Alongside increasing age, other important predictors of HCAI in acute hospitals include (i) surgical, medical and care of the elderly specialties due to the underlying comorbidities of these patients; (ii) the winter months, because more respiratory tract infections are imported into, and transmitted within, healthcare settings during this time of the year; and (iii) the subsequent secondary infections, such as *Clostridium difficile*, arising due to antibiotic use. The vulnerability of the older age group is related to impairment of immune responses and to life circumstances, such as residence in care homes and nutritional status. Morbidity and case fatality associated with HCAI is higher in older people as a result of age related frailty arising from multiple comorbidities and the vulnerabilities described previously. This 'domino effect' in older people makes them a special risk group with respect to HCAI and prevention should therefore be the focus for nursing care. Alongside infection prevention strategies, early detection of these infections when they do occur, with early intervention, is critical in their management and control. However, identifying infection in older people presents particular challenges, as presentation of infection is often atypical, with delirium frequently being the first indicator that infection may be present. Gerontological nurses are in a prime position to recognise the often subtle changes in a patient's condition or behaviour that may herald the onset of serious infection. It is therefore essential that careful observation, monitoring and reporting of the patient's general condition takes account of the potential for infection to be incubating.

Common infections in older people: microorganisms and clinical context

When thinking about the most common types of infections experienced by older people, nurses should consider both the common organisms causing infection and the clinical situations where infection is most likely to occur.

The microorganisms responsible for causing the majority of these infections are predominantly S*taphylococcus aureus*, in particular MRSA, and *C. difficile*. These are organisms of concern in older patient populations with particular reference to the resistance mechanisms within them, i.e. the ability of the organism to withstand the effects of antibiotics and the subsequent potential inability to treat patients in some circumstances.

MRSA has been a predominantly hospital-related pathogen for many years, but is now seen in non-hospital settings as a result of patient movement from hospital to care home, readmissions from the community reservoir to hospital, antibiotic selection and cross-transmission in all settings. Thus, MRSA infection poses a threat to older people in a variety of care settings, including their own home.

Risk factors for colonisation with MRSA include known previous MRSA-positive status, previous admissions or transfers from other hospitals or care homes, and presence of skin lesions such as venous ulcers or exfoliating conditions (e.g. eczema). Nurses should be aware of these particular risk factors and take them into account during the admission and management of patients in any care setting. Many hospitals now routinely screen for MRSA colonisation on admission. A recent study (Health Protection Scotland 2008) of universal screening of patients being admitted to acute hospitals found that the prevalence of colonisation was higher in those over 65 years when compared to those under 65 years and three times higher still in those being admitted from care homes. Duration of colonisation and the factors affecting this are not fully known. For MRSA infection, risk factors include recent antibiotic treatment, advanced age, invasive procedures such as surgery, invasive devices such as urinary catheters or intravenous infusion lines, prolonged hospital stay, the care environment (i.e. poorer staffing ratios) and low compliance with infection control practices.

Other healthcare threats to older people in terms of antimicrobial resistance include vancomycin-resistant *Staphylococcus aureus*, vancomycin-resistant enterococci and extended-spectrum β-lactamase-producing Enterobacteriaceae. Infection prevention and control measures must therefore take account of the complexities of the HCAI agenda, including the reservoir of infection imported from the community to hospital and back again, emerging infections and antibiotic resistance mechanisms.

The emergence of *C. difficile* has affected predominantly older people in healthcare. More than 80% of all reported cases in the UK are in those aged 65 and over (Health Protection Scotland 2008). In addition to advancing age, prior antimicrobial treatment is an important risk factor. It is not surprising therefore that many of the recent outbreaks of *C. difficile* in the UK have occurred in older people and the case fatality rate has been estimated to be around 10% in the UK (Health Protection Scotland 2008).

Clostridium difficile and MRSA may be the focus currently in healthcare, but other organisms are becoming increasingly important. A European review of data from several national prevalence surveys (European Centre for Disease Prevention and Control 2008) also found *Pseudomonas aeruginosa*, *Enterococcus*, coagulase-negative staphylococci, *Candida*, and other Enterobacteriaceae such as *Klebsiella* and *Enterobacter* to be the most prevalent. Emerging strains of microorganisms and resistance mechanisms cause a ubiquitous threat to infection prevention, control and management.

The majority (80%) of HCAI described in published national studies of hospital prevalence (European Centre for Disease Prevention and Control 2008) are urinary tract infections, lower respiratory tract infections (including pneumonia) and surgical site infections. The remaining infection sites include bloodstream infections, gastrointestinal infections (mainly *C. difficile* recently), skin and soft tissue infections, and central nervous system infections. In long-term care hospital settings, where there is a higher average age and different speciality distribution, the types of HCAI are different to that in acute care (Reilly *et al.* 2007). The most common types of HCAI in older patients in long-term care settings noted in this first UK national study were urinary catheter associated infections, skin and soft tissue infections such as pressure ulcers, and gastrointestinal infections which were mainly *C. difficile*. In all these infection types the key to protecting older people in healthcare settings is prevention.

Urinary catheter associated infection is best prevented by reviewing if the catheter needs to be put in at all. There is growing evidence of the unnecessary use of these devices

(Association for Practitioners in Infection Control 2008). International guidance on evidence based practice in all care settings indicates that if a catheter insertion is necessary during the patient journey in healthcare, ensuring a catheter is maintained in line with best practice to prevent infection, including removal as soon as possible, is important in preventing infection (Association for Practitioners in Infection Control 2008).

The best approach to preventing infected pressure ulcers is to prevent the pressure ulcer forming in the first place. Pressure area care is an essential nursing intervention in those at risk. Reviewing antimicrobial prescribing and ensuring prudent use of antimicrobials in older people is also an important nursing practice to protect health; when prescribing or administering antibiotics nurses should always consider whether the antibiotic is essential or could be avoided. A focus in these three practice areas – urinary catheterisation, pressure area care and antibiotic use – would be an important nursing contribution to protecting older people from HCAI.

To summarise so far, prevalence studies have shown that increased age alone puts older people at risk of HCAI. The most common infections in older people are related to indwelling urinary catheters, pressure sores and gastrointestinal infections with *C. difficile* following antibiotic prescription; nurses have a key role in preventing these infections.

Potential for nursing contribution

Applying a value base to infection prevention and management for older people

Protecting older people from HCAI cannot be separated from other fundamental aspects of care; awareness of and commitment to the core value base for nursing older people discussed in Chapter 1 applies equally to this issue as to the many other aspects of caring for, or working in partnership with, older people and their families. Infection control specialists are an invaluable resource for professional advice, although infection prevention and control should be viewed as the responsibility of every practitioner. Nurses who become expert in working with older people will draw on this specialised knowledge, integrating an understanding of microbiology and the pathophysiology of infection within the particular context of caring for older people.

A key concept discussed in Chapter 1 was adopting a value base for nursing care that centres on what older people want and believe is right for them. In the context of HCAI, older people and their families will have the same beliefs and expectations as any other member of the public, i.e. not to acquire an infection associated with their healthcare provision (Box 13.2).

Prevention of HCAI is important to patients. In a survey of patients in NHS Scotland, patients were asked to rank the top 10 most important aspects of healthcare and the top two were a clean environment and clean hands (Reeves & Bruster 2009).

However, there are specific clinical and ethical issues associated with the detection, prevention and management of HCAI which present particular challenges when caring for older people. The following section outlines the principles of infection control before returning to discuss specific challenges in applying these principles in caring for older people.

Box 13.2   Direct quote from older person

'I was in isolation. Now I was having to pull up doctors and nurses that was coming into my room with no gloves or no apron on and I didn't do it for to be smart, I done it because I didn't want somebody else to be going through what I was going through and passing the infection on to them and even Dr [consultant] one of the times, I pulled him up [laughter] I mean I did because he walked into the room with no apron, no gloves or nothing and I said, I just said to him "Excuse me Dr [name] but do you realise I'm MRSA" and he said "Oh I'm sorry, forgot all about it" but that's if I had been a patient that hadn't bothered and he'd come over and examined me, he could have passed that on to another patient and that was the only reason why I was doing it.'

Schofield *et al.* (2004)

Prevention is better than cure: principles of infection prevention and control

Infection control is a discipline that applies epidemiological principles to the prevention of infections. Effective infection control programmes have long been proven to reduce the rates of HCAI and to be cost-effective (Haley *et al.* 1985). The key components of successful infection prevention and control include intensive surveillance, feedback of data to clinicians, and ensuring clinicians are actively engaged in the infection control programme and control (with evidence based interventions). An important aspect of any infection control strategy is communicating risk to staff, visitors and patients themselves in order to promote compliance with infection prevention measures such as hand hygiene.

A useful way to help us understand how infection is spread is the *chain of infection* model, whereby each link in the chain represents a vital point at which appropriate action can be taken to break the chain of infection, thereby preventing transmission of organisms (Figure 13.1).

The previous section identified the range of infectious agents causing the most common infections in older people and highlighted the increased susceptibility to infection that advancing years brings. Understanding the nature of the other links in the chain of infection, depending on the infective agent, is crucial to ensure best practice is applied in preventing the transmission of organisms between individuals.

Interventions which will prevent and control HCAI require focus predominantly on extrinsic factors, i.e. healthcare interventions, in terms of patient care practices in hospital and community settings. Despite international differences in healthcare systems and in the strategies employed, the basic infection control and prevention interventions are universal and the evidence base has been developed internationally. However, the evidence base underpinning many infection control interventions is lacking or limited or of poor quality. This is because study design is usually observational and as such establishes

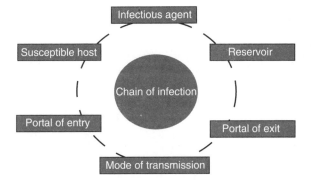

Figure 13.1 The chain of infection. (Adapted from NHS Education for Scotland *Cleanliness Champions*.)

association rather than cause and effect. The seminal work on epidemiology of HCAI was developed in this way during the 1970s and 1980s and this work set out the conceptual framework for future studies. Many studies in the infection control field examine multiple interventions at the same time and as such the role of individual interventions is not well established. There are some gaps in the evidence base, which might not ever be filled with robust evidence due to practical limitations and potential ethical dilemmas. An important note here is that absence of evidence is not absence of effect and as such best practice should be adopted at all times. There is little evidence that parachutes prevent death when freefalling from a plane, but very few of us would challenge the theory (Smith & Pell 2003).

The generic approaches to infection prevention and control can be broadly summarised as 'clean hands, clean environment, clean equipment, and clean techniques'. Standard infection control precautions (SICPs) have been widely adopted internationally as a policy and procedural framework for routine practice which minimises infection risk (Centers for Disease Control 2007; Health Protection Scotland 2009). The basic philosophy is that any patient (or staff member) could have an infection, and a minimum level of precaution is appropriate regardless of known or suspected infection risks. Some interventions apply to specific situations, for example *C. difficile* infections occurring in hospital settings require additional cleaning procedures (e.g. chlorine-based compounds), hand hygiene with soap rather than alcohol gel (which is less effective against spores) and prudent use of antibiotics in treatment of both *C. difficile* and other infections in older people. In older patient populations, where antimicrobial use is more prevalent, it is important that these prescriptions are monitored and reviewed regularly to protect patients against unintended consequences. It is also important that nurses are alert to the added risk that antibiotic prescription poses; whenever older patients who have had antibiotics experience diarrhoea, immediate screening for *C. difficile* should be initiated.

International experts agree that *the* most important activity to reduce the spread of infection is hand hygiene, using either soap or alcohol gels, before and between each and every patient contact (Allegranzi & Pittet 2008). The World Health Organization has captured this concept in its 'My 5 Moments for Hand Hygiene' campaign. Figure 13.2 illustrates the '5 moments' during which nurses, or any other healthcare professional,

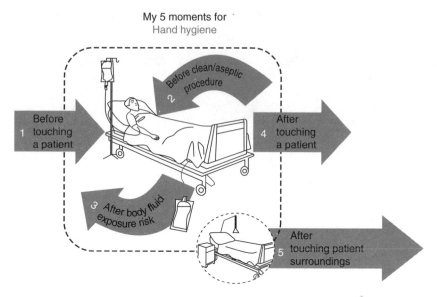

Figure 13.2   Five moments for hand hygiene.

should ensure that effective hand hygiene is carried out. The explanatory notes below provide the rationale for each action.

(1) *When?*   Clean your hands before touching a patient when approaching him or her.
　　Why?   To protect the patient against harmful germs carried on your hands.
(2) *When?*   Clean your hands immediately before performing a clean/aseptic procedure.
　　Why?   To protect the patient against harmful germs, including the patient's own, from entering his or her body.
(3) *When?*   Clean your hands immediately after an exposure risk to body fluids (and after glove removal).
　　Why?   To protect yourself and the healthcare environment from harmful patient germs.
(4) *When?*   Clean your hands after touching a patient and her or his immediate surroundings, when leaving the patient's side.
　　Why?   To protect yourself and the healthcare environment from harmful patient germs.
(5) *When?*   Clean your hands after touching any object or furniture in the patient's immediate surroundings when leaving, even if the patient has not been touched.
　　Why?   To protect yourself and the healthcare environment from harmful patient germs.

Whilst there is evidence from the World Health Organization that hand hygiene is the most important infection prevention activity in healthcare, there is no, nor will there ever be, randomised controlled trial evidence on hand hygiene: it would be unethical to withdraw hand hygiene as an intervention in healthcare to test this theory. In developed countries, there is an evidence base beginning to be established on hand hygiene compliance in healthcare (World Health Organization 2009). This evidence indicates marked variation in compliance between countries, some of which may be due to differing monitoring approaches. However, the challenge of ensuring staff, visitors and patients themselves comply with hand hygiene recommendations cannot be underestimated. The evidence suggests that multimodal implementation strategies using posters, and alcohol hand rub availability at the bedside can significantly increase hand hygiene compliance. However, at best, use of the correct hand-washing techniques at the right times can still only be expected to reach 65% compliance (World Health Organization 2009). Barriers to hand hygiene compliance in healthcare workers are not fully understood. Although it is acknowledged that these barriers can be physical ones (e.g. availability of sinks or hand gels), there is a clear behavioural component to this practice which requires further research.

Clean techniques and processes are also an important component of infection prevention and control. One of the most important areas of care in this regard is invasive device care. Device use is very prevalent in hospitals. Urinary catheters are used frequently in healthcare, although their use can lead to serious life-threatening complications. Care bundles as a mechanism for implementing evidence based practice have been promoted for the last few years as part of patient safety initiatives worldwide. With urinary catheter infection being a prevalent healthcare associated infection in older people, a bundle for this practice has been developed (Health Protection Scotland 2008; Institute of Healthcare Improvement 2008). Urinary catheters cause urinary tract infections and are the second leading cause of bloodstream infections. Complications arise directly from their use and in particular if the care is suboptimal. The risk of infectious complications increases the longer they are in use. The five elements of the care bundle proposed by Health Protection Scotland, after a systematic review of the literature, were as follows.

(1) Perform a daily review of the need for the urinary catheter.
(2) Check that the catheter has been continuously connected to the drainage system.
(3) Ensure patients are aware of their role in preventing urinary tract infection. (Alternative bundle criterion if the patient is unable to be made aware: Perform routine daily meatal hygiene).
(4) Regularly empty urinary drainage bags as separate procedures, each into a clean container.
(5) Perform hand hygiene and don gloves and apron prior to each catheter care procedure; on procedure completion, remove gloves and apron and perform hand hygiene again.

The care bundle approach suggests that if this is implemented with 95% reliability, then infections will be significantly reduced. There are some interesting data available in small-scale studies which suggest that this works (Institute of Healthcare Improvement 2009).

Additional infection control policies or procedures may be indicated. These are known as transmission based precautions, where airborne, droplet or contact spread is a recognised hazard of known cases of infection (Health Protection Scotland 2009). The evidence base for all these basic infection prevention and control practices is well described in international infection control guidance (Centers for Disease Control 2007; Health

Protection Scotland 2009). These guidelines note the lack of high-level evidence to support many of the practices. As a case in point, there is some evidence to support the use of isolation (Cooper *et al.* 2003) in reducing risk of cross-infection, but little or no evidence for the practice of cohorting patients. Cohorting, which is defined as separation of patients in an area where they are looked after by dedicated nurses, has a scant evidence base. Further, in reality it is frequently the same nurses looking after the patients in the cohort as the rest of the ward, a practice which causes challenges with bed management and for which there is no evidence base.

The evidence base for the contribution of environmental cleaning to infection control is thin, but the benefits of adequate cleaning of patient equipment and hand-touch surfaces near the patient are beginning to gather an evidence base (Dancer 2008). Some countries have formal technical guidance for environmental cleaning processes and procedures, but simple and objective measurement of 'cleanliness' remains problematic. Visual assessment is a poor indicator of bacterial or viral loading of surfaces (Dancer 2008).

Screening is a relatively new and emerging concept in prevention and control of HCAI. There is continuing debate in the literature over the place of screening at or before hospital admission for some specific infections such as MRSA. Modelling work (Ritchie *et al.* 2007) has suggested that screening all patients, isolating those colonised and decolonising those at high risk of infection, is both clinically and cost effective. However, the authors of this work called for more research in this field and for formal testing of the model, which is currently underway in NHS Scotland (Health Protection Scotland 2009). In addition, nurses have to be sensitive towards the potential for people to feel stigmatised if they are found to be harbouring an infectious organism.

Issues in protecting older people from HCAI

Nurses and other healthcare workers need to be sensitive to the particular needs of older people in terms of infection prevention and control issues. The challenge in ensuring that healthcare workers maintain compliance with hand hygiene recommendations is compounded when one considers the potential transmission hazard presented to, and by, older people with cognitive impairment who may suffer from agitation or confusion; ensuring patients wash their hands frequently and thoroughly and ensuring frequent cleaning of those surfaces that older people may use to support themselves when walking, such as locker or table tops, hand rails or other furniture, is crucial but not without difficulty. The imposition of isolation or barrier nursing of an older person, added to the physiological effects of infection, is well recognised as a trigger for acute delirium in people without a previous history of confusion (British Geriatrics Society 2006).

HCAI are clearly an international public health problem. Efforts to control infection focus on standard infection control precautions as well as organism or practice specific interventions, where required. The older person in hospital and care homes is uniquely susceptible to infections because of the physiological changes that occur with ageing, underlying chronic diseases and the institutional environment. In addition, infections may be more difficult to diagnose because of their subtle signs and symptoms in this patient population due to the presence of comorbidities. Delays in diagnosing and treating infections allow transmission to occur, and thus early detection of emerging threats to healthcare, ongoing measurement for management, and implementation of optimal patient care practices are the key to infection prevention and control. There are gaps in existing evidence, but practice should be based on best available evidence and it is important to note that absence of evidence is not absence of effect with regard to infection control practices. Further research is needed to continue to develop infection control practices in order that HCAI are prevented and to reach the irreducible minimum and achieve health protection.

Protecting older people by breaking the chain of infection relies firstly on an awareness of potential sources of infection in the specific care environment. However, applying SICPs when caring for frail older people, particularly when the person has cognitive impairment, requires the creative application of evidence based practice blended with nursing expertise; this is illustrated through discussion of the case study set out below.

Case study 13.1   Preventing infection

Making connections
Look carefully at the following case study scenario: think about the principles you have read about above and answer the questions at the end of the scenario.

Case study scenario
Mrs Smith is an 83-year-old care home resident with dementia, admitted to hospital with a respiratory tract infection and dehydration. On admission she was admitted to a medical ward for observation, and intravenous antibiotics. She had a cannula inserted for the intravenous therapy and a urinary catheter inserted to monitor her urinary output. She continued on her therapy and within a week was beginning to recover, her temperature had settled and she was hydrated. She was transferred back to the care home on oral antibiotics. Two days after returning to the care home, Mrs Smith developed diarrhoea. She had three episodes on the first day and by the third day was dehydrated and following review by her GP required readmission to hospital. On admission to hospital a diarrhoeal sample was taken and sent to the microbiology laboratory and she was put into isolation pending the results. She was again catheterised and had intravenous fluids administered and was closely monitored for fluid balance. She continued to have diarrhoea and was losing weight. Her Waterlow score was deteriorating and her pressure areas were red and excoriated with the continued diarrhoea. The sample came back from the laboratory as positive for *C. difficile* and therefore her antimicrobial treatment was reviewed and stopped. Mrs Smith's condition continued to deteriorate both physically and psychologically.

Key points for learning
- What key intrinsic and extrinsic factors put Mrs Smith at increased risk from infection?
- What types of infection should the nursing staff on the initial medical admission ward have been concerned about/screened for?
- What alternative nursing interventions might have prevented ongoing deterioration in Mrs Smith's condition?
- Write a scenario with an alternative ending that details the type of skilled nursing intervention at each stage of this patient's journey to provide holistic care, which could have tackled infection prevention issues whilst addressing the complex care needs of Mrs Smith.

Discussion of case study

This is a complex yet common scenario. Mrs Smith's cognitive impairment may have masked the early symptoms of respiratory tract infection, allowing the infection to gain ground beyond the point where simple oral antibiotics may have provided adequate treatment. Encouraging oral fluid intake in a scenario where the individual may have excess losses due to pyrexia, yet may be reluctant to drink, presents challenges for nursing staff. Providing small frequent amounts of whichever fluid Mrs Smith preferred may have averted the need for intravenous fluids. A key question here is whether more intensive observation and intervention at the very earliest stages of the infection could have averted the deterioration of the original condition, making hospital admission unnecessary. Intrinsic risk factors are, by their nature, unavoidable but the initial management of the infection could have been better, with early identification and management of the chest infection avoiding complications of severe infection and dehydration.

As the infection worsened, further questions relate to whether or not Mrs Smith required admission to an unfamiliar acute care environment. It is also important to consider which intravenous antibiotics were prescribed (taking account of antimicrobial prescribing guidelines that identify those antibiotics which place patients at greater risk of *C. difficile* infection) and whether the dehydration could have been treated without using an intravenous device. Furthermore, the insertion of a urinary catheter for fluid balance monitoring is questionable and adds to the challenge of continence management on return to the care home. After the resolution of the acute respiratory infection, care home staff should have been particularly alert for the potential of *C. difficile* infection, recognising the additional risk linked to advanced age and prior antibiotic treatment. The key point throughout this scenario is early identification to enable effective management.

Helping Mrs Smith to understand and carry out basic hygiene measures such as hand washing will require effective communication strategies that take account of her cognitive impairment. Professionals may be tempted in this scenario to avoid telling the patient and the family that the cause of the current infection is *C. difficile*, fearing the 'blame' associated with this infection. As discussed in Chapter 4, information sharing or not sharing is one way in which people can exert control over others; however, to prevent and manage infection, patients and their carers have to be viewed as partners in this process. Evidence from independent enquiries of outbreaks associated with *C. difficile* have highlighted concerns around the lack of communication, particularly with relatives, in relation to hygiene, for example laundry of patients' clothes. Effective management requires that patients and their families are told the truth about the circumstances surrounding cases of infection and understand the procedures used in their management.

Summary

There is a robust evidence base that HCAI are preventable. We understand the intrinsic risk factors associated with advancing age and are aware of the extrinsic risks that healthcare can bring to older people. Whilst there are still some gaps in the evidence base to support practices such as cohorting – and further research to explore the impact of isolation on older people would be valuable – much of the evidence to support infection prevention and control exists and has been presented in this chapter. The challenge for nurses working with older people is ensuring consistent implementation of best practice for every patient, every time. Applying key infection prevention and control interventions at each point in the patient pathway can minimise risk; however, applying these principles to the complex care needs of older people requires a skilled mix of technical knowledge and specialised gerontological caring principles.

Key messages

Key challenges in protecting older people from HCAI

- Creating a clinical environment in which everyone sees infection prevention as their responsibility: zero tolerance of HCAI.
- Reliable application of hand hygiene measures before and after every patient care practice. Support older patients and their visitors to maintain satisfactory hand hygiene.
- Early identification and management of the risk of infection.
- Addressing the gaps in the evidence base for practice, particularly in relation to the specific needs of frail older people or those with cognitive impairment.

Good practice points for protecting older people from HCAI

- Standard infection control precautions for all patients, all of the time.
- Early identification of risks and early intervention to manage those risks.
- Effective management of invasive devices such as urinary catheters to prevent primary infections and secondary bacteraemia in older people.
- Prevention of pressure ulcers to prevent HCAI.
- Prudent use of antimicrobials.

References

Allegranzi B, Pittet D (2008) Preventing infection acquired during healthcare delivery. *Lancet* **372**, 1719–1720.

Association for Practitioners in Infection Control (2008) *Guide to the Elimination of Catheter Associated Urinary Tract Infections*. Association for Practitioners in Infection Control, USA. Available at www.apic.org/Content/NavigationMenu/PracticeGuidance/APICEliminationGuides/CAUTI_Guide.pdf

British Geriatrics Society (2006) *Guidelines for the Prevention, Diagnosis and Management of Delirium in Older People in Hospital*. Royal College of Physicians, London.

Centers for Disease Control (2007) *Standard Precautions Infection Control Guidelines*. CDC, Atlanta. Available at www.cdc.gov/ncidod/dhqp/gl_isolation_standard.html

Chief Medical Officer (2004) *5 Top Tips for Visitors to Combat Healthcare Associated Infection in Hospital*. Available at www.scotland.gov.uk/Publications/2004/08/hai

Cooper BS, Stone SP, Kibbler CC *et al.* (2003) Systematic review of isolation policies in the hospital management of methicillin-resistant *Staphylococcus aureus*: a review of the literature with epidemiological and economic modelling. *Health Technology Assessment* **7**, 1–194.

Dancer S (2008) Importance of the environment in meticillin-resistant *Staphylococcus aureus* acquisition: the case for hospital cleaning. *Lancet Infectious Diseases* **8**, 101–13.

European Centre for Disease Prevention and Control (2008) *Annual Epidemiological Report on Communicable Diseases in Europe.* European Centre for Disease Prevention and Control, Stockholm.

Health Protection Scotland (2008) *Report on Review of* Clostridium difficile *Associated Disease Cases and Mortality in all Acute Hospitals in Scotland from December 2007–May 2008.* NSS, Scotland.

Health Protection Scotland (2009) *MRSA Screening: Interim Results from the NHS Scotland Pathfinder Project.* NSS, Scotland.

Health Protection Scotland (2009) *Model Policies for Infection Control.* NSS, Scotland. Available at www.documents.hps.scot.nhs.uk/hai/infection-control/sicp/handhygiene/mic-p-handhygiene-2009–09.pdf

Institute of Healthcare Improvement (2009) *Reducing Hospital-Acquired Infections in a Long-Term Acute Care Hospital.* Available at www.ihi.org/IHI/Topics/HealthcareAssociatedInfections/InfectionsGeneral/ImprovementStories/ReducingHAIinLongTermAcuteCareHospital.htm

National Audit Office (2004) *Improving Patient Care by Reducing the Risk of Hospital Acquired Infection: A Progress Report.* Report by the Controller and Auditor General, HC 876 Session 2003–2004.

NHS Education for Scotland (2010) *Cleanliness Champions Programme.* Available at www.nes.scot.nhs.uk/hai/champions/learning_units/ (accessed on 9 April 2010).

NHS Quality Improvement Scotland (2004) *Urinary Catheterisation and Catheter Care.* NHS Quality Improvement Scotland, Edinburgh.

Pittet D (2009) Hand hygiene promotion: 5 moments, 5 components, 5 steps. *International Journal of Infection Control* **5**(i1). Available at www.ijic.info/article/viewFile/3519/2875

Reeves R, Bruster S (2009) *Better Together: Scotland's Patient Experience Programme: Patient Priorities for Inpatient Care.* SGHD, Edinburgh. Available at www.scotland.gov.uk/Resource/Doc/278973/0083963.pdf

Reilly J, Stewart S, Allardice G *et al.* (2007) *NHS Scotland National HAI Prevalence Survey.* Final Report, Health Protection Scotland, Glasgow.

Ritchie K, Craig J, Eastgate J *et al.* (2007) *The clinical and cost effectiveness of screening for meticillin-resistant* Staphylococcus aureus *(MRSA).* NHS Quality Improvement Scotland, Edinburgh.

Schofield I, Tolson D, Knussen C, Flanagan U, Irwin A, Stewart C (2004) *An Exploration of Patient and Family Experiences and Care Preferences During the Treatment of Acute Uncomplicated COPD Exacerbations.* Department of Nursing and Community Health, Glasgow Caledonian University, Glasgow.

Smith G, Pell J (2003) Parachute use to prevent death and major trauma related to gravitational challenge: systematic review of randomised controlled trials. *British Medical Journal* **327**, 1459–1461.

Storr J (2009) Five moments for hand hygiene: a focused, targeted approach to patient safety. *International Journal of Infection Control* **5**(i2). Available at www.ijic.info/article/viewFile/3629/3200

World Health Organisation (2009) Online resources for hand hygiene available at www.who.int/gpsc/5may/tools/en/index.html
http://whqlibdoc.who.int/publications/2009/9789241597906_eng.pdf

Chapter 14

Pressure Ulcers

Janice Bianchi and John Timmons

Introduction

In this chapter we explore why older people are vulnerable to pressure ulceration, highlighting some of the underlying biological processes that affect skin integrity. Our key message is that most, but not all, pressure ulcers are preventable. Revision notes are included to remind readers of the multifactorial nature of the risks that contribute to pressure ulceration, drawing attention to a range of nursing interventions. We recognise that the evidence base can be confusing and that clinicians debate the value of assessment tools and therapeutic approaches, many of which have been developed from a relatively weak evidence base. In the final part of the chapter we present a case study of an older person with a sacral pressure ulcer. This complex case study illustrates the challenge for nursing when intervention needs to address the combined influences of the shared risks of several of the geriatric syndromes, namely loss of mobility, poor nutrition, depression and pain.

Definitions

International advisory groups (European Pressure Ulcer Advisory Panel and National Pressure Ulcer Advisory Panel 2009) have defined pressure ulcers as:

> *localised injury to the skin and/or underlying tissue usually over a bony prominence, as a result of pressure, or pressure in combination with shear. A number of contributing or confounding factors are also associated with pressure ulcers; the significance of these factors is yet to be elucidated.*

Pressure ulcers, also known as pressure sores, bed sores or decubitus ulcers, can occur at any age but older people, particularly over the age of 65 years, are considered to be at increased risk of developing these chronic wounds (Bergstrom *et al.* 1996). In Chapter 1, pressure ulcers were included in the list of geriatric syndromes (see Figure 1.2). Pressure

Evidence Informed Nursing with Older People, First Edition. Edited by Debbie Tolson, Joanne Booth and Irene Schofield.
© 2011 Blackwell Publishing Ltd. Published 2011 by Blackwell Publishing Ltd.

ulcers usually do not occur in isolation and are associated with a number of other conditions of older age, in particular reduced physical activity (Chapter 8), urinary incontinence (Chapter 7), under-nutrition (Chapter 11) and pain (Chapter 12).

Revision notes of the factors which may put an older person at risk of pressure ulcer development are summarised in Box 14.1. It is important to remember that most pressure ulcers develop because several intrinsic and extrinsic factors occur simultaneously and impact on skin integrity.

Box 14.1   Revision on the intrinsic and extrinsic factors which may contribute to pressure ulceration

Pressure (extrinsic factor)

The blood vessels in the skin supply oxygen and nutrients and are responsible for removing waste products. If high levels of pressure are applied, particularly to skin over bony prominences, the blood vessels can become compressed. If interruption to blood flow is sustained over a considerable period of time, the skin and underlying tissue can become damaged, leading to skin breakdown.

Shear (extrinsic factor)

In addition to unrelieved pressure, shearing forces can intensify the destructive effect on the skin. Shear is caused when the body slips down; the underlying structures move, but the skin stays in the same position. This may result in deeper layers tearing away from the top layer of the skin. An example of shear is when a person slides down the bed or chair; the skin stays stationary while the skeleton and surrounding tissues move.

Friction (extrinsic factor)

Skin damage can be caused by friction, produced by rubbing against sheets for instance. Pressure, shear and friction, in combination with moisture, can make an individual very susceptible to skin damage.

Moisture (intrinsic and extrinsic factor)

If an area of the skin is wet due to incontinence or even excessive sweating, it can become macerated. This may lead to alteration in the resilience of the epidermis to external force. This is known as excoriation. Further skin breakdown can occur if this condition is left untreated (Bours *et al.* 2003).

Health status (intrinsic factor)

People who suddenly become very unwell may be vulnerable to skin breakdown. Those who have had an illness for a longer period of time may also be vulnerable. This is especially the case for people with vascular/arterial disease, which causes reduced blood supply to the lower legs, and those with diabetes mellitus, who may have loss of sensation in their feet in addition to a reduced blood supply.

Mobility (intrinsic factor)

Immobility may be the greatest risk to skin integrity (Bours *et al.* 2003). A person's normal response to pressure is to move or reposition themselves. Ability to move may be affected by a number of factors.

Posture (intrinsic factor)

Proper posture when sitting is a key part of maintaining skin integrity. Anatomical changes in some people may mean the pelvis is tilted either forwards or backwards, which can cause unusual pressure distribution.

Sensory impairment (intrinsic factor)

Reduced awareness of pressure can lead to reduced spontaneous movement. People who have had strokes or a spinal cord injury are among those who may have sensory impairment.

Level of consciousness (intrinsic factor)

Post-surgical patients who have a reduced level of consciousness may not have the ability to reposition themselves. Others, such as people who have had a head injury, may also be at risk due to a reduced level of consciousness. Reduced spontaneous movement is similar to reduced mobility and can affect the skin's integrity.

Systemic signs of infection (intrinsic factor)

An elevation in body temperature, such as when a person has an infection, may affect tissue integrity. Although scientists do not fully understand the reasons for this, it is thought that it may be due to an increased need for oxygen to skin which already has a decreased supply of oxygen.

Nutritional status/body weight (intrinsic factor)

There is a link between poor nutritional status and the development of pressure ulcers (Clark *et al.* 2004). It is essential that we do not overlook the importance of a well-balanced diet. Additionally, vulnerable individuals may be at risk of pressure damage if they lose weight rapidly. Adequate nutrition for all individuals being treated within healthcare settings is seen as a priority by NHS Scotland, which has produced a guidance document called *Improving Nutritional Care*. This recommends that the Malnutrition Universal Screening Tool (MUST) be part of the admission procedure for anyone admitted to hospital and that a personal nutritional care plan related to the MUST score be developed. You can access the guidance document at www.nhshealthquality.org/nhsqis/files/Improving%20Nutritional%20Care%20June%2008.pdf and the MUST tool at www.bapen.org.uk/pdfs/must/must_full.pdf. Further details about preventing under-nutrition is available in Chapter 11.

Previous pressure damage (intrinsic factor)

Scar tissue from, for example, an old pressure ulcer is never as strong as undamaged tissue. It may have little or no blood supply, which makes it more vulnerable to breakdown.

Pain status (intrinsic factor)

People in severe pain may reduce the number of times they move or reposition. It is important to assess people's pain and if necessary make sure they have adequate analgesia to allow repositioning with comfort.

Psychological and social factors (intrinsic factor)

Very depressed people (acute depression) can have feelings of apathy and may become less active.

Medication (intrinsic factor)

Some medications, such as antihistamines or codeine-based analgesics, can make a person feel drowsy. The skin can become vulnerable if such medications are being used for long periods and the person is not able to move as freely as usual.

Cognitive status (intrinsic factor)

Cognitive status relates to thought processes. If thought processes are altered due to delirium or dementia, the person may be unable to recognise the risk of sitting or lying still for long periods without repositioning.

Blood flow (intrinsic factor)

It is essential for the skin to have a good blood supply to provide necessary oxygen and nutrients and remove waste products. Damage to skin integrity is more likely if the blood flow is reduced.

Extremes of age (intrinsic factor)

Very old people have more fragile skin. The skin gets thinner and can become dry with ageing.

Prevalence of pressure ulceration

A review of UK, US and Canadian prevalence and incidence studies indicate that pressure ulcer prevalence rates within the UK are lowest in the community setting, ranging from 2.5 to 6.8% and highest in palliative care at approximately 37% (Kaltenthaler *et al.* 2001). A recent study in Sweden (Gunningberg 2006) suggests a prevalence of 17.3% in surgical settings, 23.6% in medical settings and 50% in geriatric settings. Cost implications of managing patients with pressure ulcers are significant. Bennett *et al.* (2004) estimate that the NHS in the UK spends £1.4–2.1 billion annually on the treatment of pressure ulcers, with the cost per patient ranging between £1064 and £10 551. Additionally, for the individual and their families, the effects can be devastating. Pressure ulcers cause pain and distress and can lead to social isolation, and wound healing may be prolonged which could lead to economic hardship. They can also have serious complications that can lead to life-threatening infections. Redelings *et al.* (2005) carried out a descriptive study examining pressure ulcer associated mortality in the USA. Their data was obtained from national cause-coded death records. The researchers found that over an 11-year period (1989–2000) where pressure ulcers were reported as a cause of death, 39.7% had an associated septicaemia.

Skin changes in older people

Older people are at risk of pressure ulceration for a number of reasons. With ageing, body systems are affected and changes in the skin are often apparent. Intrinsic ageing of the skin occurs inevitably as a natural consequence of physiological changes over time. In a review of the literature on skin ageing, Farange *et al.* (2008) explored intrinsic ageing and identified changes in the skin and their consequences (Box 14.2).

Of course, the ageing process will affect more than the skin of the patient and changes can be noted in all the body's systems.

Box 14.2 Intrinsic skin ageing and its consequences

- Dermal thickness decreases: leads to skin thinning
- Decreased collagen: leads to loss of elasticity
- Dermal elastin reduced: leads to loss of elasticity
- Microcirculation decreased: reduced blood flow to tissue
- Reduced inflammatory response: wound healing may be delayed
- Reduction in sebum production: leads to compromised barrier function
- Dermoepidermal junction flattens: vulnerable to shear injury

---

Prevention

Most pressure ulcers are preventable and nurses play a major role in prevention in a variety of ways depending on the needs of the individual. This may involve health promotion, educating the older person and their carers in prevention techniques such as correct positioning, skin inspection, nutrition, or in frail people where nursing interventions are required ensuring that the care given is optimal to prevent pressure ulcers occurring. The level of intervention will be determined by the perceived risk of pressure ulcer development.

Risk assessment

A risk assessment policy should be in place in all healthcare settings. Over 40 pressure ulcer risk assessment tools have been developed to provide a structure and consistency to patient assessment. They raise awareness of risk factors, prompt risk assessment and provide a minimum standard for assessment and documentation. However, the majority were developed on the basis of expert opinion, literature review and/or adaptation of an existing scale, and therefore the evidence base for their use is weak. The most commonly used risk calculators include Braden, Norton and Waterlow. The Braden scale (Bergstrom *et al.* 1987) is the most widely tested across Europe and America in a variety of clinical settings. This scale has shown good reliability when used by qualified nurses (Bergstrom *et al.* 1987) and varying sensitivity (64–100%) (Nixon & McGough 2001). All risk assessment calculators have their limitations and thus should not replace clinical judgement, rather be an adjunct. Ongoing studies on modified scales are being conducted to increase sensitivity and usefulness of these calculators (Chan *et al.* 2008).

Where risk is considered to be present, depending on the care setting and equipment available, nurses will initiate measures to minimise risk. Positioning, equipment, patient education, skin care and nutritional care should all be considered.

Evidence based practice

There are many factors which may increase the likelihood of pressure ulcer development. Some of the evidence is based on expert opinion while other factors have been quantified by more rigorous research methods.

Recognising the importance of changes in the skin of older adults, and the additional impact incontinence may have on already vulnerable skin, Hodgkinson and Nay (2005) reviewed the best available evidence for the effectiveness and safety of topical skin care regimens for older people residing in long-term care facilities. Their extensive review indicated that results were variable depending on the skin condition outcome being assessed; the outcomes included rash, skin irritation, haematoma or tears. Patient satisfaction was also considered and the authors found reasonable evidence to support the use of disposable body-worn incontinence pads compared with non-disposable body-worn pads in the maintenance of skin integrity in older incontinent patients. Additionally, the use of non-rinse cleansers was more effective than soap and water in older incontinent patients. The use of the Bag Bath/Travel Bath no-rinse cleanser was also more effective in preventing overall dryness than soap and water in older people with dry skin.

In a single-centre open-label prospective study, a barrier film was compared with zinc oxide oil in the prevention of perianal/buttock skin breakdown in incontinent patients; total costs were also compared. Results indicated that both products resulted in improved skin condition after 14 days of treatment. However, the barrier film was more cost-effective as fewer applications were required, less time was spent in application and faster healing rates were achieved (Baatenburg de Jong & Admiraal 2004).

It is not uncommon for this patient group to have inadequate nutrition, and this, combined with poor living conditions and hygiene, adversely impacts on wound healing (Moffatt *et al.* 2004). Nutritional status and its importance in the development of pressure ulcers cannot be underestimated. A multicentre cross-sectional audit of nutritional status of a convenience sample of subjects was carried out as part of a large pressure ulcer audit in Queensland, Australia. This large audit included 2208 acute and 839 aged care subjects. The findings suggested that malnutrition was associated with at least twice the odds ratio of having a pressure ulcer. Moreover, the authors identified increased severity of pressure ulcers with increased severity of malnutrition (Banks *et al.* 2009).

Repositioning and frequency of repositioning has been debated by experts, although it was recognised that the evidence base is limited. As a result of this, Vanderwee *et al.* (2007) conducted a randomised controlled trial investigating turning regimes. The study was conducted in 16 Belgian care homes for older people. Subjects with non-blanchable erythema were recruited. Patients recruited to the experimental group were repositioned alternately 2 hours in a lateral position and 4 hours in a supine position. The control group were repositioned every 4 hours. In the experimental group 16.4% developed pressure ulcers, while 21.2% did so in the control group. The incidence was not statistically significant and therefore the authors concluded that repositioning more frequently than 4-hourly intervals cannot be considered more effective than repositioning every 4 hours. It should be noted that all the study patients were nursed on a foam viscoelastic overlay mattress, which is recommended for people with a higher risk of developing a pressure ulcer (McInnes *et al.* 2009). It is therefore reasonable to speculate that had this not been the case, the incidence of pressure ulcer development using these turning regimes and standard hospital mattresses may have been higher.

Despite what is known about prevention, pressure ulcers do occur. When avoidable or unavoidable ulceration occurs, the nurse's role is to prevent further damage and promote wound healing using the best-quality evidence based treatment available.

Pressure ulcer classification

As part of a guideline development process, the National Pressure Ulcer Advisory Panel and European Pressure Ulcer Advisory Panel developed a common international definition and classification system for pressure ulcers. The classification system (Box 14.3) was developed to aid comparison of inter-country data. Although there are some differences in the final grade (grade IV in Europe, unclassified/unstageable and deep tissue injury in the USA), there is agreement on four levels of injury.

Box 14.3   International definition and classification system for pressure ulcers (European Pressure Ulcer Advisory Panel and National Pressure Ulcer Advisory Panel 2009)

Category/stage I: non-blanchable erythema
Intact skin with non-blanchable redness of a localised area usually over a bony prominence. Darkly pigmented skin may not have visible blanching; its colour may differ from the surrounding area. The area may be painful, firm, soft, warmer or cooler as compared with adjacent tissue. Category I may be difficult to detect in individuals with dark skin tones. May indicate at-risk individual.

Category/stage II: partial thickness
Partial-thickness loss of dermis presenting as a shallow open ulcer with a red pink wound bed, without slough. May also present as an intact or open/ruptured serum-filled or serosanginous filled blister. Presents as a shiny or dry shallow ulcer without slough or bruising (bruising indicates deep tissue injury). This category should not be used to describe skin tears, tape burns, incontinence associated dermatitis, maceration or excoriation.

Category/stage III: full-thickness skin loss
Full-thickness tissue loss. Subcutaneous fat may be visible but bone, tendon or muscle are not exposed. Slough may be present but does not obscure the depth of tissue loss. May include undermining and tunnelling. The depth of a category/stage III pressure ulcer varies by anatomical location. The bridge of the nose, ear, occiput and malleolus do not have (adipose) subcutaneous tissue and category/stage III ulcer can be shallow. In contrast, areas of significant adiposity can develop extremely deep category/stage III pressure ulcers. Bone/tendon is not visible or directly palpable.

Category/stage IV: full-thickness tissue loss

Full-thickness tissue loss with exposed bone, tendon or muscle. Slough or eschar may be present. Often includes undermining and tunnelling. The depth of category/stage IV pressure ulcers varies by anatomical location. The bridge of the nose, ear, occiput and malleolus do not have (adipose) subcutaneous tissue and these ulcers can be shallow. Category/stage IV ulcers can extend to muscle and/or supporting structures (e.g. fascia, tendon or joint capsule) with potential for causing osteomyelitis or osteitis. Exposed bone/muscle is visible or directly palpable.

Additional categories/stages for the USA

Unstageable/unclassified: full-thickness skin or tissue loss, depth unknown

Full-thickness tissue loss in which actual depth of the ulcer is completely obscured by slough (yellow, tan, grey, green or brown) and/or eschar (tan, brown or black) in the wound bed. Until sufficient slough or eschar is removed to expose the base of the wound, the true depth cannot be determined; it will be either category/stage III or IV. Stable (dry, adherent, intact without erythema or fluctuance) eschar on the heels serves as the 'body's natural (biological) cover' and should not be removed.

Suspected deep tissue injury, depth unknown

Purple or maroon localised area of discoloration, intact skin or blood-filled blister due to damage of underlying soft tissue from pressure and/or shear. The area may be preceded by tissue that is painful, firm, mushy, boggy, warmer or cooler as compared with adjacent skin. Deep tissue injury may be difficult to detect in individuals with darker skin tones. Evolution may include a thin blister over a dark wound bed. The wound may further evolve and become covered by thin eschar. Evolution may be rapid, exposing additional layers of tissue with optimal treatment.

As previously discussed, the prevalence of pressure ulcers is higher in older people. Admission to long-term care facilities from a hospital may also be a marker for higher pressure ulcer risk. Baumgarten *et al.* (2003) carried out a prospective cohort study in America which recruited 2015 residents aged over 65 years who had been newly admitted to long-term care facilities. Of the 2015 residents studied, 208 (10.3%) had one or more pressure ulcers on admission to the facility. The authors did identify that residents admitted from hospital had more comorbidity and were more likely to be chair or bed bound and have faecal incontinence compared with residents admitted from other settings. This study demonstrates that high-risk individuals should be identified as early as possible to prevent pressure ulcer development or exacerbation of the problem and that admission from hospital may be a marker for higher pressure ulcer risk.

From the evidence reviewed here, whatever the setting, it is important to recognise risk of pressure ulcer development early and put appropriate actions into place. The following case study discusses an older person who found difficulties adjusting to life in a new environment and the subsequent deterioration in her health status. It also demonstrates the complexity of caring for someone with a pressure ulcer.

Complex case study of a patient with pressure ulcers

A 72-year-old woman was admitted to hospital from a care home with dehydration, a large sacral pressure ulcer and bilateral leg ulcers. Although she was overweight she was undernourished, as she had not eaten properly for a number of weeks.

The patient was a retired schoolteacher. Her obesity, combined with swollen legs and the presence of leg ulcers, had led to her admission to a care home. While the care home admitted residents with a wide range of medical and nursing needs, at that particular time the majority of residents were highly physically dependent or cognitively frail older people. On admission to hospital she was reported to have no known mental health issues. However, the lack of companionship and inability to form meaningful relationships with other residents within the care home had contributed initially to loneliness and insidious development of low mood leading to depression, over a period of 6 months. Subsequently, her emotional well-being was identified to be a major contributing factor to her current situation.

On admission to hospital, following an initial assessment by nursing staff, she was nursed on a pressure redistributing dynamic surface to reduce pressure on bony prominences. The large sacral pressure ulcer was the reason for admission and staff noticed that there were a number of small superficial ulcers present on her buttocks.

The patient had two leg ulcers one on either leg, and there was significant swelling in both legs. Swelling in the tissues can be the result of poor venous return and may be made worse by lack of mobility. Referral was made to the dermatology leg ulcer clinic for full assessment.

The wound at first review

At first review the patient had a large (6 × 7 cm) ulcer on her sacral area, which when probed ran to a depth of 8 cm towards the coccyx. There were numerous superficial ulcers on the buttocks, and as is often the case, these were more painful than the larger of the ulcers; this is due to the exposed nerve endings in the more superficial wounds.

The large ulcer had an area of necrosis, which can be seen in Figure 14.1. This tissue is devitalised and should be removed, as the wound will not heal properly while this tissue remains. The wound showed no signs of infection, there was no purulent drainage nor was there any sign of cellulitis around the wound margins, both of which indicate the presence of infection.

Additional health problems

Despite being overweight, the patient's albumin level indicated that she was undernourished. This is an important issue, as many of the staff wrongly assumed that she would benefit from a weight reduction diet. In fact this would be detrimental to a patient with a wound as it places extra demands on the immune system. In this situation, the individual requires an energy and protein rich diet to maximise healing (Lennard-Jones 1992). Poor nutritional state has also been linked to an increased risk of pressure ulcer development in patients living in nursing homes (Herbert & Hein 2007).

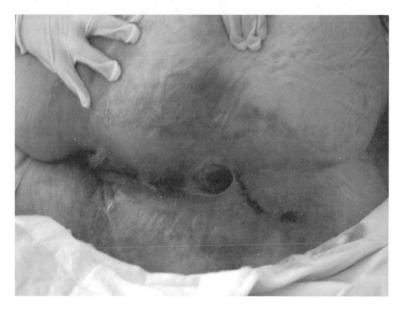

Figure 14.1 Wound on admission to ward.

The patient also had cardiac arrhythmias which the consultant attributed to her being dehydrated and lacking in essential electrolytes. An intravenous infusion was started to help address the dehydration and also to provide some energy in the form of glucose.

Treatment

Central to the wound treatment offered was the involvement of the multidisciplinary team. As well as nurses, there were medics, physiotherapists, dietitians and ECG technicians involved in caring for her. In addition, social services were involved in trying to find a more suitable 'home' environment for the patient where interaction with fellow residents was more likely.

Preventing further pressure damage was a primary aim and this was achieved by using a dynamic pressure redistributing mattress to minimise pressure on the patient's bony prominences. This also allowed her to be positioned in such a way that she was able to communicate with staff and relatives. This was important to the patient, in order for her to feel that she was involved in her care. Initially, she was catheterised in order to monitor urine output and renal function. This helped to reduce the risk of contamination of the wound bed from urine and the catheter was removed after 5 days.

Promoting wound healing

The wound consisted of a large deep pressure ulcer, an area of necrosis and some small superficial areas of skin damage. The superficial wounds were treated with thin hydrocolloid dressings, which maintain a moist wound healing environment, protect the wounds from external pathogens and contribute to wound healing by providing an optimum pH for healing.

The large wound was treated with Intrasite Gel (Smith and Nephew, Hull). This hydrogel was used to support granulation in the cavity and also to encourage gentle debridement of the necrotic tissue that was covering part of the wound. A shaped sacral dressing was applied to cover the whole area. Using large shaped dressings can be helpful as they are designed to contour to the patient's shape, and they provide a larger surface area than would be afforded by a square dressing. There is also a larger adhesive border on these dressings which allows better adherence and the dressing is therefore less likely to be accidentally removed when repositioning in bed or when mobilising. The foam dressing is able to trap exudate from the wound within the cells of the dressing and results in less fluid being trapped next to the skin, which can cause maceration and skin damage.

The patient's leg ulcers were assessed by the leg ulcer clinic nurses, who carried out a full vascular assessment including Doppler Ankle–Brachial Pressure Index (ABPI) in accordance with guidelines (Royal College of Nursing 2006). This assessment aids in identifying whether arterial disease is present. If the patient has significantly reduced blood supply, then compression bandaging may be unsafe; however, if the blood supply is adequate to both limbs, then compression bandaging can be applied.

As the patient had good arterial blood supply to both legs, compression bandaging was applied. Compression therapy works by helping to move fluid which is trapped in the legs towards the heart and into more efficient veins which are responsible for carrying waste products and metabolites away from the limbs.

Progress

Within 3 days of admission to the ward, the patient's overall condition had improved. Her intravenous infusion was discontinued and she was eating and drinking normally. The nurse specialist in tissue viability and the dietitian had also requested for the patient to have protein supplement drinks to help healing and build up her strength.

Figure 14.2 shows the initial impact of the hydrogel dressings after 1 week of treatment. The necrotic tissue has been debrided from the wound, exposing a large area of granulation tissue. Initial impression of this tissue was not reported as good, as the tissue colour is darker than would be normal for a healthy wound and this could have indicated infection. However, the first stage of treatment had been successful and the patient showed no signs of systemic infection. Both leg ulcers were healing, and there was a significant decrease in the size of both limbs, indicating that excess fluid was being moved back into the circulation.

Because of the improvement in the patient's condition, it was decided to change the bed to a mattress replacement system that would allow the patient to get in and out easily for physiotherapy and exercise. After 2 weeks of treatment with the hydrogel and foam dressings the wound was healing well, with good healthy granulation tissue present in the wound bed and the smaller wounds were showing signs of epithelialisation (Figure 14.3).

The patient was mobilising with assistance and she was eating and drinking well. Both legs remained in compression and continued to improve. Her mood was also gradually improving and this was one of the most notable and encouraging changes. Given these improvements, her requirement to live within a facility providing 24-hour nursing care had reduced and moving into an environment suited to her renewed independence became a reality. It was anticipated that treatment for her sacral and leg wounds could be provided from community nurses once suitable accommodation was located.

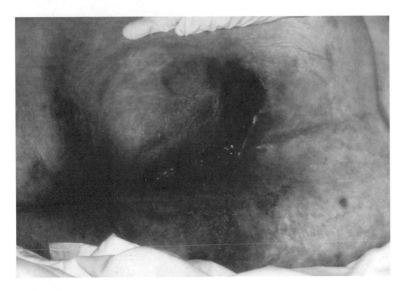

Figure 14.2 Wound after 1 week of treatment.

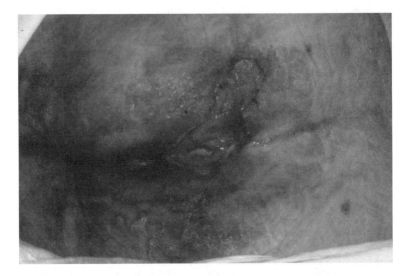

Figure 14.3 The wound showing healthy granulation.

This patient's story helps to illustrate the value of a multidisciplinary approach to the care and treatment of people with complex and enduring health problems. In addition it highlights the interdependence of health and social care needs and the benefits of taking an integrated approach. The patient's wounds were likely to have been caused by her immobility, with depression, possibly due to her change in circumstances and sense of hopelessness, as a contributing factor. By providing a care package which addressed a combination of needs the team was able to change this patient's physical condition and improve her outlook from a psychosocial perspective by offering alternative living arrangements.

Summary

Pressure ulcers can have devastating effects on older people. It is important that nurses are aware of the risk factors of pressure ulceration and that they know how to minimise risk. Nurses are also educators and as such need to make sure that patients are aware of risk and prevention. Key messages arising from the chapter are summarised below.

Key messages

- Pressure ulcers are prevalent in older people and can have a significant effect on an individual's well-being.
- There is much than nurses can do to prevent pressure ulcers developing both through interventions and education.

References

Baatenburg de Jong H, Admiraal H (2004) Comparing cost per use of 3M Cavilon No Sting Barrier with zinc oxide oil in incontinent patients. *Journal of Wound Care* **13**, 398–400.

Banks M, Bauder J, Graves N, Ash S (2010) Malnutrition and pressure ulcer risk in adults in Australian health care facilities. *Nutrition* 26, 896–901.

Baumgarten M, Margolis D, Gruber-Baldini AL *et al.* (2003) Pressure ulcer and the transition to long term care. *Advanced Skin and Wound Care* **16**, 299–304.

Bennett G, Dealy C, Posnett J (2004) The cost of pressure ulcers in the UK. *Age and Ageing* **33**, 230–235.

Bergstrom N, Braden BJ, Laguzza A, Holman V (1987) The Braden Scale for predicting pressure sore risk. *Nursing Research* **36**, 205–210.

Bergstrom N, Braden B, Kemp M, Champagne M, Ruby E (1996) Multi-site study of incidence of pressure ulcers and the relationship between risk level, demographic characteristics, diagnosis and the prescription of preventative measures. *Journal of the American Geriatrics Society* **44**, 22–30.

Bours GJ, Halfens RJ, Huijer Abu-Saad, Grol RT (2003) Development of a model for case-mix adjustment of pressure ulcer prevalence rates. *Medical Care* **41**, 45–55.

Chan WS, Pang SMC, Kwong EWY (2008) Assessing predictive validity of the Modified Braden Scale for prediction of pressure ulcer risk of orthopaedic patients in an acute care setting. *Journal of Clinical Nursing* **18**, 1565–1573.

Clark M, Schols JM, Bennati G *et al.* (2004) Pressure ulcers and nutrition: a new European guideline. *Journal of Wound Care* **13**, 267–274.

European Pressure Ulcer Advisory Panel and National Pressure Ulcer Advisory Panel (2009) *Prevention and Treatment of Pressure Ulcers: A Quick Reference Guide.* National Pressure Ulcer Advisory Panel, Washington, DC.

Farange MA, Miller KW, Elsner P, Maibach HI (2008) Intrinsic and extrinsic factors in skin ageing: a review. *International Journal of Cosmetic Science* **30**, 87–95.

Gunningberg L (2006) EPUAP pressure ulcer prevalence survey in Sweden: a two year follow-up of quality indicators. *Journal of Wound, Ostomy and Continence Nursing* **33**, 258–266.

Herbert GR, Hein T (2007) The pressure ulcer prevention diet. *Long Term Care Management* **10**, 40.

Hodgkinson B, Nay R (2005) Effectiveness of topical skin care provided in aged care facilities. *International Journal of Evidence Based Healthcare* **3**, 65–101.

Kaltenthaler E, Whitfield MD, Walters SD, Akenhurst RL, Paisley S (2001) UK, USA and Canada: how do their pressure ulcer prevalence and incidence compare? *Journal of Wound Care* **10**, 530–535.

Lennard-Jones JE (1992) *A Positive Approach to Nutrition as Treatment. Report of a Working Party on the Role of Enteral and Parenteral Feeding in Hospital And home*. King's Fund, London.

McInnes E, Cullum NA, Bell Syer SEM, Dumville JC, Jammali Blasi A (2009) Support surfaces for pressure ulcer prevention. *Cochrane Database of Systematic Reviews* (4), CD001735.

Moffatt CJ, Franks PJ, Doherty DC *et al.* (2004) Prevalence of leg ulcers in a London population. *Quarterly Journal of Medicine* **97**, 431–437.

Nixon J, McGough A (2001) Principles of patient assessment: screening for pressure ulcers and potential risk. In: Morrison M (ed.) *The Prevention and Treatment of Pressure Ulcers*. Mosby, Edinburgh, pp. 55–74.

Redelings MD, Lee NE, Sorvillo F (2005) Pressure ulcers: more lethal than we thought. *Advances in Skin and Wound Care* **18**, 367–372.

Royal College of Nursing (2006) *The Nursing Management of Patients with Venous Leg Ulcers*. RCN, London.

Vanderwee K, Grypdonck MHF, De Bacquer D, Defloor T (2007) Effectiveness of turning with unequal time intervals on the incidence of pressure ulcer lesions. *Journal of Advanced Nursing* **57**, 59–68.

Chapter 15

Achieving Evidence Informed Nursing with Older People

Debbie Tolson, Joanne Booth and Irene Schofield

Introduction

We began our exploration of evidence informed nursing with an assumption that nurses make a major contribution to the health and social care of older people. Our basic premise, set out in Chapters 1 and 2, is that the nursing contribution is optimised when practice is informed by evidence and delivered in accordance with agreed gerontological practice principles. Furthermore, we recognised that practice should have a sound theoretical basis and be delivered with sensitivity to the local context. Acknowledging the broad scope of gerontological nursing, we proposed that it is important to delineate and advance the specific contributions of nursing within later life healthcare.

We believe that positive clinical outcomes for older people are achieved through advancing knowledge and practice in the management and supported self-management of later life syndromes and conditions. Accordingly, the content of this book is framed around selected prevalent conditions of old age where nurses can make a difference to patient care. These include incontinence, loss of mobility, pain, sensory impairments, pressure ulcers, malnutrition, healthcare associated infections and delirium, all commonly termed 'geriatric syndromes' (Tinetti *et al.* 1995; Inouye *et al.* 2007).

We have examined the evidence base related to these later life conditions, and uncovered their complexity and interconnectedness. We have also described the challenges for nurses in developing their knowledge and skills to deliver safe and dignified care to older people experiencing these later life conditions. Opportunities to enhance practice by evidence application in the context of principle-led gerontological nursing are illustrated throughout Chapters 5–14. In shaping the practice improvement agenda it is also important that we embrace partnership working and relational care. This will enable standards to be raised and promote perceptions of quality among individuals and their family carers. Key components influencing perceptions of the care experience relate to reciprocity, trust and truth-telling in relationships between nurses, older people and family members. We have explored these conceptual issues and ethical dilemmas in Chapters 3 and 4.

This final chapter offers a synthesis of the key messages from the book in relation to evidence, theory and practice values. We propose that to progress the unique contribution

Evidence Informed Nursing with Older People, First Edition. Edited by Debbie Tolson, Joanne Booth and Irene Schofield.

that nurses can offer to older people's care, we need to build on our professional heritage and demonstrably strengthen our clinical contribution. An important element of this involves preventing the development of conditions of later life, which contribute to developing frailty and dependence and which, if ignored, can lead to the patient's death. This notion of 'failure to rescue' is coming under increasing scrutiny in terms of care processes and outcomes (National Confidential Enquiry into Patient Outcome and Death 2009). Early recognition of opportunities to delay onset or reverse deterioration in health manifested as one or more of these conditions is a sentinel indicator of quality in nursing older people. Evidence informed practice in support of such quality nursing is presented throughout the book but particularly the case study Chapters 5–14.

This final chapter will conclude with a brief consideration of global challenges for nurses working with older people and the professional opportunities afforded to them through evidence informed nursing with older people.

Essential connections for practice

In our introductory chapter (see Figure 1.1), five inextricably connected components of gerontological nursing were identified:

(1) theory
(2) evidence base
(3) caring values
(4) relational care
(5) later life conditions.

The first four chapters focused on exploring theoretical and philosophical dimensions of these. In the opening chapter, Tolson *et al.* discussed and described the principles of gerontological practice. In Chapter 2, Booth *et al.* explored evidence use in day-to-day practice and highlighted the merits of forming communities of practice to accelerate evidence application. In Chapter 3, Brown *et al.* focused attention on the enrichment of the care environment through relationship-centred approaches, and in Chapter 4 Tuckett and Tolson highlighted the role of truth-telling practices in defining the integrity of work and relationships with older people. The key messages from the four introductory chapters are summarised in Table 15.1.

One of our early contentions, stated in the first chapter, was our belief that nurses are uniquely positioned to provide care and influence care outcomes and perceptions of quality in older people with later life conditions. Mindful of earlier debates about the nature and status of nursing older people, we recognise the importance of distinguishing the contribution and expertise of nurses equipped with gerontological practice knowledge and skills from the generic skills of other nurses. However, we stress that it is important for all adult nurses to be familiar with and committed to the underlying principles of gerontological practice. Moreover, practice that is aligned with the principles presented in Chapter 1 (see Box 1.3) is more likely to display compassion and a positive attitude towards older people than practice which is not informed by an explicit and shared value base. The contemporary value base for nursing older people in many countries is rooted

Table 15.1 Key messages from the introductory chapters 1–4.

Chapter	Message
1 Principles of gerontological nursing	The interconnectedness of theory, evidence, values, relational care and knowledge of age-related changes, challenges and conditions equips nurses to deliver safe and effective care with older people
2 Applying evidence to practice	Evidence informed decision-making that reflects agreed practice values is best practice The Caledonian Improvement Model, centred on a community of practice framework, enables nurses to achieve best practice
3 Understanding dynamics of relationships within care	Relational care recognises partnerships within care and interdependency, as core values and its achievement in practice is demonstrably enriching
4 Truth-telling	Truth-telling is central to the development of trust between nurses and older people, without which relationship-centred care is undermined

in internationally agreed rights (United Nations 1991) and often expressed in terms of the underlying principles for practice. Focusing on a unique example of a nationally agreed value base grounded in the views of nurses, older people and family carers described in Chapter 1 (Kelly *et al.* 2005), we went on to illustrate in Chapter 2 how such shared values can be used as a lens through which to shape the presentation of evidence based care guidance (Booth *et al.* 2007). A remaining challenge is to find ways of combining caring values with evidence based review criteria in processes that are used to judge the quality of nursing care and outcomes for older people and their family carers.

In most countries nursing older people occurs within a multi-professional and multi-agency context, and the shared values of the collective team will ultimately determine the predominant culture of care. Caring attributes and displays of compassion and relational care, while key to perceptions of care quality, are insufficient ingredients on their own to influence the outcomes and effectiveness of care. For this reason we argued it was timely that nursing re-focuses and invests in research and the development of practice related to common later life conditions, comorbidity and multiple age-related changes. As acknowledged by Inouye *et al.* (2007), geriatric syndromes are multifactorial and challenge traditional ways of viewing clinical care and research. Approaches to nursing older people need to be responsive to both specific pathological conditions and the often non-specific changes in health status associated with the different geriatric syndromes.

In Chapter 2 the discussion of the processes by which evidence can be converted into practice know-how and skills, developed through the Scottish Gerontological Nursing Demonstration Project, highlighted the importance of ensuring care guidance is in tune with practitioner values (Booth *et al.* 2007). This is important for the credibility, relevance, acceptability and ultimate ownership of the guidance. It is achieved where values are explored, reconciled and applied as the 'lens' to focus the wider evidence base in order to ensure clarity and definition. It also confirms that the evidence is fit for practice through context and cultural sensitivity.

The challenges facing practitioners accessing appropriate evidence have been frequently rehearsed since the inception of the evidence based practice movement and have resulted in a range of evidence based guidelines being developed and made available across the globe. However, as suggested by Rycroft-Malone *et al.* (2009):

> *The successful implementation and judicious use of tools such as protocols and guide-lines will likely be dependent on approaches that facilitate the development of nurses' decision making processes, in parallel to paying attention to the influence of context.*

Working with older people, as all of our contributors testify, requires a collaborative approach between practitioners from different disciplines working with the older person and, where appropriate, their family and friends. There are many situations in which nurses can lead and design strategies to enable partnerships in practice, although as Ross and Redfern (2006, p. 738) admit there are probably more examples in the UK where nurses play a reactive provider role rather than leading and innovating from the front. Health and social care policy is replete with calls for partnership approaches, and inter-professional working. On the ground there is more evidence of dyadic partnerships between different professionals than there are examples of triadic approaches which con-nect the person with the family and the professionals. Brown *et al.* in Chapter 3 explore relationship-centred care, arguing that it is time to move beyond person-centred frame-works. Their arguments and research base are persuasive of the need to advance practice in this area and in line with calls for future developments towards quality healthcare for older people (Potter 2009). They describe a conceptual framework and outline toolkits which are under development to assist in the enrichment of the practice environment through the promotion of the Senses Framework.

Caring is indisputably a core value within nursing and the concept of the caring conver-sation, espoused by Fredriksson and Eriksson (2003), is arguably key to the formation of relationships with therapeutic potential for older people and family carers. In considering the caring conversation we must engage with another important dimension, that of truth-telling within care. As Tuckett and Tolson argue in Chapter 4, there is more evidence to suggest that truth-telling contributes to physical and psychological well-being than there is evidence to support the myth that it is harmful. However, it is important, as they cau-tion, to temper this with the realisation that the capacity of an individual to cope with the truth varies and nurses should ask older people how much information they want rather than make assumptions.

Evidence informed practice

A consistent assertion within this book is that evidence informed practice is the fusion between the scientific and the know-how of practice. Rycroft-Malone's (2006) discus-sion of the politics of evidence based practice highlights how it has become the policy mantra in many countries and that the public expect nurses to be informed about, and use, the latest evidence. In Chapter 2 of this book we explored the connections between the evidence and the decisions which nurses make daily within their work with older people. We have acknowledged that in practice there are many influences on decision-making processes, including what is known from research, clinical experience, the immediate situation confronting the practitioner and the preferences of older people. As increasingly noted, what is not clear is how these influences are weighted and to what extent they impact on patient outcomes (Rycroft-Malone *et al.* 2009; Hajjaj *et al.* 2010). Promoting a culture of evidence generation, synthesis and application is the contemporary and accepted way forward. Given the investment in what is often described as the evidence based practice movement, it is somewhat ironic that this has not been matched with investment in the development of evidence based implementation methods. Achterberg *et al.* (2008) are critical of this situation, arguing for the prioritisation of nursing implementation science. We believe that the Caledonian Improvement Model, which has featured in several of our chapters, makes a promising contribution (Tolson *et al.* 2008). This theoretically informed community of practice model is grounded in user experience. Its unique genesis involved social participatory research methods inclusive of nurses and other professionals, older people and family carers. Its components include equal attention to values and different forms of evidence, including the tacit knowledge of practice.

Later life conditions: synthesis of practice messages

We have dedicated two-thirds of this book to a consideration of the evidence and evidence implementation in practice related to selected later life conditions. This emphasis is justified by the large number of older people who are affected by abrupt-onset conditions such as delirium (acute confusion) and healthcare associated infection or more enduring conditions. The latter includes chronic pain and conditions with an insidious onset that may go unnoticed, such as often happens with the development of age related hearing loss. Although many of the chapters cite imprecise prevalence figures, it is possible to estimate the scale of risk and potential impact of the conditions on the health and well-being of older people. Nursing intervention is therefore warranted in terms of the numbers of older people affected, the detrimental consequences to the individual and economic costs to society. The prevalence of some of the conditions escalates with advancing years, while for others the presence of multiple later life conditions, general decline and frailty are more important determinants for nursing care than age alone.

Delirium is a case in point. In Chapter 5, Schofield and Hasemann report estimates of delirium in adults ranging from 7 to 61%, highlighting the greater vulnerability of people with dementia. That older people with dementia are at increased risk of developing delirium is not always addressed in reports and studies on patients with dementia in the acute hospital. As the ongoing intervention study in Switzerland illustrates, nurses have much to contribute to the prevention and management of this condition, which should be viewed as a medical emergency.

In Chapter 7, a recently completed survey of community-living older people revealed that lower urinary tract symptoms were more common than actual urinary incontinence, which was reported by 42%. Nocturia, for example, affected 85% of the respondents, frequency 68% and urgency 53% (Booth *et al.* 2010).

Prevalence data on hearing impairment, discussed by Tolson *et al.* in Chapter 9, estimated that functional hearing problems affect 60% of people aged 71–80 years, escalating to 93% in people aged over 81 years.

Levels of depression and low mood noted by Lowndes *et al.* in Chapter 10 are generally believed to be gross underestimations, but available figures in the UK suggest that between 10–15% of older people experience depressive symptoms rising to 30–40% in the institutionalised group.

Jackson and Polding-Clyde (Chapter 11) revealed unacceptably high levels of malnutrition in frail older people, with estimates from the UK for example indicating that one in four older people in long-term residential care is malnourished (Clinical Research and Audit Group 2000). The situation in care homes will not improve while food intakes remain below estimated requirements (Leslie *et al.* 2006).

The complexity of pain management and assessment was elaborated by Jones and Schofield in Chapter 12. Evidence was presented that justified the call by pain experts to consider pain as the fifth vital sign. For many older people chronic pain is a feature of their lives and is a source of prolonged distress. Given the distress associated with pain, the reluctance among some older people to admit to pain or accept adequate analgesics is difficult to understand and justifies continuing efforts to understand pain from both physiological and psychosocial perspectives. Nurses must be alert to the likelihood of chronic pain and its impact on an individual's life and the part that pain plays in illness recovery and the maintenance of independence.

In Chapter 13 Currie and Reilly highlight the vulnerability of older people to healthcare associated infections. It is particularly worrying that 80% of the cases of *Clostridium difficile* affect older people receiving healthcare and the case fatality rate has been estimated to be around 10% in the UK (Health Protection Scotland 2008).

In Chapter 14, Bianchi and Timmons reported pressure ulcer prevalence rates within acute European hospitals of approximately 23% (European Pressure Ulcer Advisory Panel 2002). Studies from the UK, Canada and the USA consistently reveal higher rates of around 37% within palliative care settings.

Parker and Froggatt commenced their consideration of palliative care in Chapter 6 by exploring the leading causes of death among older people. In Australia, ischaemic heart disease is the leading cause of death in older people, closely followed by cerebrovascular disease then lung cancer. In the UK the three main causes of death are circulatory disease, cancer and respiratory disease. The authors went on to reveal that in Australia only 5.5% of older people die in a hospice; in the UK the figure is 4%. Most older people die in hospitals (approximately 49% in Australia, 56% in the UK) or care homes (16% in Australia, 20% in the UK). Management of many of the later life conditions discussed in this book is integral to palliative care. Moreover, given the high percentage of deaths within hospitals and care homes, nurses will need to understand how to ameliorate the negative impact of these conditions, often in the presence of disease or trauma, if they are to provide quality support to older people in the final stages of life.

A striking feature about the later life conditions is their cumulative impact and shared risks as described in our first chapter. If we take a closer look at the conditions in turn, for example falls, we can see that it has been linked with urinary incontinence, delirium, visual and hearing problems, and depression; tissue damage sustained on falling may trigger ulceration. A pressure ulcer is less likely to heal in someone who is malnourished. Furthermore, it is painful and an open sore increases the risk of a healthcare associated infection. The interdependency of the conditions and shared risks explains why a fall can have a devastating effect on the life of an older person. Moreover, it can trigger what at first may seem a disproportionate level of decline and loss of independence. Recognising the role and interplay of multiple syndromes and adverse outcomes has prompted calls for more unifying approaches to practice and research (Tinetti *et al.* 1995). There is growing interest among researchers to explore the relationship between geriatric syndromes such as urinary incontinence and the disablement process (Coll-Planus *et al.* 2008). Understanding the role of specific syndromes in the disablement process is complex and there remain many research gaps and challenges. However, for nursing practice it is important that we appreciate the growing consensus that geriatric syndromes are linked to functional decline and increase the person's predisposition to frailty and loss of independence. Any prevalent factor which diminishes health and undermines the quality of life for older people justifies a proactive commitment from nursing to develop effective interventions.

In focusing on the later life conditions it is important that we keep in perspective the fact that there are many fit and active older people, whose exposure to the conditions discussed in this book may be limited to accepted deterioration in their hearing and eyesight. Nonetheless, it is important that individuals who currently enjoy good health know how to reduce their risk of developing such conditions as falls, malnutrition, incontinence and depression and this remains a goal of health promotion with this population.

Global challenges

As we write this final chapter, we are aware of the prediction that globally health and social care services will come under pressure as a result of the crisis in many international financial institutions. This is happening at a time when demand for healthcare is increasing, as a result of technological innovation, new drugs and increasing numbers of very old people with complex conditions. One of the consequences of financial pressure on services is likely to be the requirement that nurses achieve and demonstrate care which leads to predetermined, measurable outcomes.

This calls for nurses who work with older people to be able to demonstrate both quality in the experience of care and in clinical outcomes. Establishing nursing sensitive indicators to measure outcomes is not without its challenge. Griffith *et al.* (2008) identified possible evidence based indicators to measure outcomes delivered by nurses and patient experiences within acute care to be:

(1) patient safety indicators (failure to rescue associated with preventable deaths, healthcare associated infections, falls, pressure ulcers);
(2) patient experiences of compassionate care (an important outcome in its own right);
(3) staffing and skill mix indicators linked to patient outcomes;
(4) process indicators.

Use of these nursing metrics is advocated as the route to demonstrate the impact of nursing within acute care, albeit mindful that this occurs within a multi-professional context. The taskforce suggest that these metrics may be applicable beyond acute care. The anticipated arrival of robust metrics, from ongoing work, signals the beginning of a new era where the nursing contribution can be measured in ways that bring together measures of safety, effectiveness and compassion. It is thus timely and no coincidence that throughout this book we have focused on these three dimensions to demonstrate the impact of nursing older people. Firstly, our call to engage with later life conditions and syndromes is related to rescue and prevention, and hence the safety of the older person. Secondly, we have highlighted the benefits of equipping adult care nurses with appropriate expertise that includes knowledge of both ageing and common later life changes, conditions and challenges in order to provide effective nursing interventions. We have also argued for nurses with specialist gerontological knowledge and skills to provide expert practice leadership. Thirdly, we believe that delivering care mindful of the principles of gerontological nursing emphasises relational care concerns, improves the quality of care experience and promotes compassion.

Many countries are facing nursing workforce shortages and this reality must be recognised in future developments. A key policy consideration for all countries must be the goal of national self-sufficiency and sustainability of the nursing workforce (International Centre for Human Resources in Nursing 2007). As older people are major users of health and social care services, it is reasonable to assume that demands for nursing will increase as numbers of older people around the world increase. A major concern for nursing is to ensure that older people have access to expert gerontological nursing and that practice is informed by an age appropriate evidence base.

Population ageing makes it imperative to prioritise preventative strategies and self-care to limit the known shared risks from the geriatric syndromes that lead to health loss and poor outcomes. Nursing is uniquely positioned to make a major contribution to working with older people to support them to adapt and adjust to these changes and to develop effective interventions. Internationally, healthcare policy is replete with calls to shift the balance of care and maintain older people in their own homes, reduce hospital admissions and avoid unnecessary use of health and social care resources. We believe that focusing attention on developing the evidence base, particularly for non-pharmacological solutions, will strengthen the nursing contribution in relation to geriatric condition management, and preventative activities will help in the realisation of this imperative.

Conclusion

Responding to the needs of older people and promoting health in older age is one of the biggest challenges facing nursing internationally. There is no doubt that the rising numbers of older people will place increasing demands on health and social services and that this in turn will call for the deployment of nursing knowledge and skills. Historically many countries have under-invested in services for older people and undervalued the nursing contribution. We recommend to nurses that they take up the resources contained in this book as a means of achieving relational care and improving care experiences and care outcomes for older people. To achieve what will be a major shift for many countries we need high-level strategic commitment and effective leadership. Demonstrating the worth of expert nursing with older people has been overshadowed by many historical twists and turns.

Over the past two decades the nursing focus has moved away from clinical to more conceptual dimensions of caring such as quality of life and compassionate elements of care. Whilst we acknowledge their importance, it is possible that they have shifted attention from the common age related changes that undermine health and well-being, including the geriatric syndromes. We have argued in this book that it is time for nurses working with older people to re-focus on these conditions, whilst retaining their commitment to compassionate approaches. A failure to recognise and manage later life malnutrition, falls, incontinence, depression and healthcare associated infections imposes high costs on society. In addition we would argue that there is a moral imperative to lessen the negative impact and personal misery associated with these conditions. Such complex conditions require skilled nursing to enable older people to achieve effective self-care, or to successfully manage the person's health. It involves combining evidence informed knowledge of geriatric conditions with compassionate approaches to caring: the essence of gerontological nursing.

References

Achterberg T van, Schoonhoven L, Grol R (2008) Nursing implementation science: how evidence-based nursing requires evidence based implementation. *Journal of Nursing Scholarship* **40**, 302–310.

Booth J, Tolson D, Hotchkiss R, Schofield I (2007) Using action research to construct national evidence-based nursing care guidance for gerontological nursing. *Journal of Clinical Nursing* **16**, 945–953.

Booth J, O'Neil K, Lawrence M, McMillan L, Munro A, Godwin J (2010) The prevalence and impact of nocturia in community living older people. Oral presentation at Scottish School of Primary Care Conference, April 2010.

Clinical Research and Audit Group (2000) *National Nutritional Audit of Elderly Individuals in Long Term Care, Scotland*. Clinical Research and Audit Group, Scotland.

Coll-Planus L, Denkinger M, Niklaus T (2008) Relationship of urinary incontinence and late-life disability: implications for clinical work and research in geriatrics. *Zeitschrift fur Gerontologie und Geriatrie* **41**, 283–290.

European Pressure Ulcer Advisory Panel (2002) Summary report on the prevalence of pressure ulcers. EPUAP Prevalence Working Group. Available at www.epuap.org/review4_2/page8.html

Fredriksson L, Eriksson K (2003) The ethics of the caring conversation. *Nursing Ethics* **10**, 138–148.

Griffith P, Jones S, Maben J, Murrells T (2008) *State of the art metrics for nursing: a rapid appraisal*. National Nursing Research Unit, London.

Hajjaj FM, Salek M, Basra M, Finlay A (2010) Non-clinical influences on clinical decision-making: a major challenge to evidence based practice. *Journal of the Royal Society of Medicine* **103**, 178–187.

Health Protection Scotland (2008) *Report on Review of* Clostridium difficile *Associated Disease Cases and Mortality in all Acute Hospitals in Scotland from December 2007 to May 2008*. NSS, Scotland.

Inouye S, Studenski S, Tinetti M, Kuchel G (2007) Geriatric syndromes: clinical, research, and policy implications of a core geriatric concept. *Journal of the American Geriatrics Society* **55**, 780–791.

International Centre for Human Resources in Nursing (2007) *Nursing Self Sufficiency/Sustainability in the Global Context*. Report developed for the International Centre on Nurse Migration and the International Centre for Human Resources in Nursing. Available at www.ichrn.com/publications/policyresearch/SelfSufficiency.pdf

Kelly T, Tolson D, Schofield I, Booth J (2005) Describing gerontological nursing; an academic exercise or prerequisite for progress? *International Journal of Nursing Older People* **14**, 1–11.

Leslie WS, Lean M, Woodward M, Wallace F, Hankey C (2006) Unidentified under-nutrition: dietary intake and anthropometric indices in a residential care home population. *Journal of Human Nutrition and Dietetics* **19**, 343–347.

National Confidential Enquiry into Patient Outcome and Death (2009) *Caring to the End? A Review of the Care of Patients who Died in Hospital Within Four Days of Admission*. NCEPOD, London.

Potter C (2009) What quality healthcare means to older people: exploring and meeting their needs. *Nursing Times* **105**, 49–54.

Ross F, Redfern S (2006) *Nursing Older People*, 4th edn. Churchill Livingstone, London.

Rycroft-Malone J (2006) The politics of the evidence based practice movements: legacies and current challenges. *Journal of Research in Nursing* **11**, 95–108.

Rycroft-Malone J, Fontenla M, Seers K, Bick D (2009) Protocol-based care: the standardisation of decision-making? *Journal of Clinical Nursing* **18**, 1490–1500.

Tinetti ME, Inouye SK, Gill TM, Doucette JT (1995) Shared risk factors for falls, incontinence and functional dependence. *Journal of the American Medical Association* **273**, 1348–1353.

Tolson D, Booth J, Lowndes A (2008) Achieving evidence-based nursing practice: impact of the Caledonian Model. *Journal of Nursing Management* **16**, 682–691.

United Nations (1991) General Assembly resolution 46/91 of 16 December 1991. Implementation of the International Plan of Action on Ageing and related activities, annex. Available at www.un.org/documents/ga/res/46/a46r091.htm (accessed 19 April 2010).

Index

Evidence Informed Nursing with Older People, First Edition. Edited by Debbie Tolson, Joanne Booth
and Irene Schofield.
© 2011 Blackwell Publishing Ltd. Published 2011 by Blackwell Publishing Ltd.